Barefoot Doctors and Western Medicine in China

Rochester Studies in Medical History

Senior Editor: Theodore M. Brown
Professor of History and Preventive Medicine
University of Rochester

ISSN 1526-2715

Barefoot Doctors and Western Medicine in China

Xiaoping Fang

UNIVERSITY OF ROCHESTER PRESS

First published 2012
Reprinted in paperback 2015

University of Rochester Press
668 Mt. Hope Avenue, Rochester, NY 14620, USA
www.urpress.com
and Boydell & Brewer Limited
PO Box 9, Woodbridge, Suffolk IP12 3DF, UK
www.boydellandbrewer.com

ISSN: 1526-2715
hardcover ISBN: 978-1-58046-433-8
paperback ISBN: 978-1-58046-521-2

Library of Congress Cataloging-in-Publication Data

Fang, Xiaoping.
    Barefoot doctors and western medicine in China / Xiaoping Fang.
        p. cm. — (Rochester studies in medical history, ISSN 1526-2715 ; v. 23)
    Includes bibliographical references and index.
    ISBN 978-1-58046-433-8 (hardcover : alk. paper) 1. Medicine, Chinese—China—
History. 2. Medicine—China—Cross-cultural studies. I. Title.
    R601.F29 2012
    610.951—dc23

                                                                        2012030654

A catalogue record for this title is available from the British Library.

This publication is printed on acid-free paper.
Printed in the United States of America

Contents

Illustrations

Acknowledgments

My earliest memory of barefoot doctors dates back to the late 1970s when I was a little boy growing up in a small village high in the mountains of Zhejiang Province in Eastern China. Whenever I became ill, my father would go to the barefoot doctor of our village to ask for a few medicinal tablets. Because a tablet was too big for me to swallow, my father would crush it into powder and mix the powder with water. But when he asked me to drink it, I always refused since it tasted awful. My father was left with no other option than to take me in his arms and hold my mouth open with one hand while pouring the medicine in with the other. My mother held my legs tightly to keep me from kicking. I screamed loudly, while my aunty stood by and laughed. Needless to say, I have not forgotten these experiences, even after all these years. At that time, I could never have imagined that one day I would write a book on the barefoot doctors who gave those tablets to my father.

I sincerely thank all the former barefoot doctors, their fellow villagers, former commune clinic doctors, and other informants who allowed me to interview them from 2003 to 2011. By sharing their life stories, they provided me with vivid oral historical accounts that became essential material for this book. I am especially grateful to Chen Hongting, Chen Zhicheng, Yan Shengyu, Zhou Yonggan, Luo Zhengfu, Shen Qingyang, Hong Jinglin, Xu Peichun, and Fang Shunxi, to name just a few. My conversations with these doctors and villagers gave me a great deal of inspiration. I do hope that this book accurately represents their experiences and that they will be pleased to know that people all over the world will now be able to read about them. I am also very grateful to Wu Yuegen, Lin Jun, Jiang Lihong, and Lu Qun for accompanying me during my fieldwork in their home villages.

My archival materials came from many sites, including the Fuyang City Archives, the Chun'an County Archives, the Yuhang District Archives and the Xiaoshan District Archives of Hangzhou Prefecture, the Hangzhou Prefecture Archives, the Sandun Township Integrated Chinese and Western Medicine Hospital, the Lin'an City Archives, the Jiande City Archives, the Shaoxing Prefecture Archives, the Zhejiang Province Archives, the Shanghai Municipality Archives, the Pudong New District Archives of Shanghai Municipality, the Jiangsu Provincial Archives, the Nanjing Prefectural Archives, the Changyang County Archives of Hubei Province, the National Archives in London, and the Rockefeller Archival Center in New York. This study could not have been completed without the generosity of these archives in providing me access to their collections. All the local gazetteers of Zhejiang Province used in this book were found in the Local Documents Department of Zhejiang Province Library. I am especially grateful to Liu Hang, who generously provided me with various and valuable assistance since the very beginning. The provincial gazetteers used in this book were from the Universities Service Center of the Chinese University of Hong Kong, where thanks go to Jean Hung for her assistance.

I started working on this book in the Department of History of the National University of Singapore (NUS). I am deeply indebted to Gregory Clancey for his unwavering patience and advice in guiding me through developing analytical perspectives, discussing the drafts with me chapter by chapter at different stages, and revising the text for final publication. Huang Jianli recommended that I read two books related to this topic on the first day I met him. His kindness and help in my research and life at the NUS were broad and enormous. Thomas Dubois deeply impressed me with his devotion to and methodology of his study of China's rural religion. In the Department of History, I also owe a debt to Ng Chin Keong and Tan Tai Yong for their intellectual stimulation and moral support. At the Needham Research Institute at the University of Cambridge, I benefited greatly from the rich library collection and my proximity to Christopher Cullen, Geoffrey Lloyd, and John Moffett. I thank Tatjana Buklijas and her colleagues for allowing me to audit courses in the Department of History and Philosophy of Science for a year. At the University of Technology, Sydney, I would like to acknowledge the China Research Centre's intellectual and funding supports, which allowed me to concentrate on the manuscript revision. I am very grateful to Maurizio Marinelli, Lesley Farrell, Yingjie Guo, Andrew Jakubowicz, and other colleagues for their generous assistance and valuable advice for the revision.

Without the generous funding of many institutions, this book would have been impossible. I would like to thank the NUS Faculty of Arts & Social Sciences and the Asia Research Institute (ARI) in Singapore for granting me a scholarship to study at NUS and for travel grants for my fieldwork in China. At the University of Technology, Sydney, I am very grateful to the Faculty of Arts and Social Sciences for offering me a research development grant to conduct three fieldwork trips in China to revise the manuscript and a dissemination fund to cover the editing costs. The faculty and the Social and Political Change Group also funded my attendance at many conferences, where I benefited from valuable comments from colleagues in the field of medical history. My thanks also go to the Rockefeller Archival Center for offering me a travel grant to visit its archives for my research concerning rural reproduction and granny midwives and to the New York Li Foundation Fellowship for funding my study at Cambridge.

Over the years of the writing process, numerous people have helped me in so many different ways. Andrew Wear of University College London, Liew Kai Khiun of Nanyang Technological University, Bruce Lockhart of NUS, and Geoffrey Wade of Nalanda-Sriwijaya Centre at the Institute of Southeast Asian Studies, Singapore, Yongming Zhou of the University of Wisconsin–Madison, and Nathan Sivin of the University of Pennsylvania read the draft and offered me constructive suggestions relating to the framework and arguments. I have been benefited from many scholars' assistance and advice during my studies and fieldwork, including Zhu Baoqin, Zhang Xianwen, Gao Hua, and Chen Hongmin of Nanjing University, Luo Weidong and Lang Youxing of Zhejiang University, Anthony Reid of Australian National University, Lin Wenbiao of Shaoxing College of Arts and Science, Liu Hong and Lee Lai To of Nanyang Technological University, Yu Keping of China Central Compilation and Translation Bureau, Ma Boying of the Federation of Traditional Chinese Medicine in the UK, Bridie Andrews of Bentley University, Mary Bullock of the China Medical Board, and Mobo Gao of Adelaide University. Erik Holmberg of NUS and Xiaorong Han of Butler University gave me unfaltering help over the past decade. Francesca Bray of the University of Edinburgh never hesitated to give me her timely and invaluable suggestions through all the stages of my revision process. Louise Edwards of the University of Hong Kong supported me in too many ways to list. I offer all of you my sincere thanks.

At the University of Rochester Press, I am very grateful to the series editor Theodore Brown and editorial director Suzanne Guiod for accepting this book for publication in the Rochester Studies in Medical History series; to Ryan Peterson, Carrie Watterson, Julia Cook, and Tracey Engel for their invaluable work in improving the manuscript as it underwent the editing process. I am also very grateful to two anonymous readers' constructive and incisive comments and suggestions for the final revisions of the manuscript. Thanks also go to Victoria Patience, who provided meticulous and serious proofreading of the final manuscript; to Fang Jianxin, for preparing three maps; and to the Fuyang City Archives, the *Zhejiang Daily*, the *Hangzhou Daily* and Chen Aikang for generously granting me permission to reproduce their figures in this book. Earlier versions of parts of chapter 1 appeared in an article entitled "From Union Clinics to Barefoot Doctors: Healers, Medical Pluralism, and State Medicine in Chinese Villages, 1950–1970," published in the *Journal of Modern Chinese History* 2, no. 2 (2008). Revised versions of these materials are reprinted in this book by permission of Taylor & Francis Ltd.

No words can fully express my gratitude for the support of my family. My parents grew up and spent their lives in an isolated mountain village. Although they did not even have the chance to finish their primary school education like their fellow villagers of that era, they are kind and diligent, and I hope I have already inherited these qualities from them. I am also very grateful to my wife, Huajuan He, who quit her job in China so that she could join me during my years abroad in Singapore, Britain, and Australia. We have shared much happiness and endured many hardships together. Without her sacrifices, I could not have finished this book. I dedicate this book to our daughter, Xinlin Fang.

Sydney, Australia

Maps

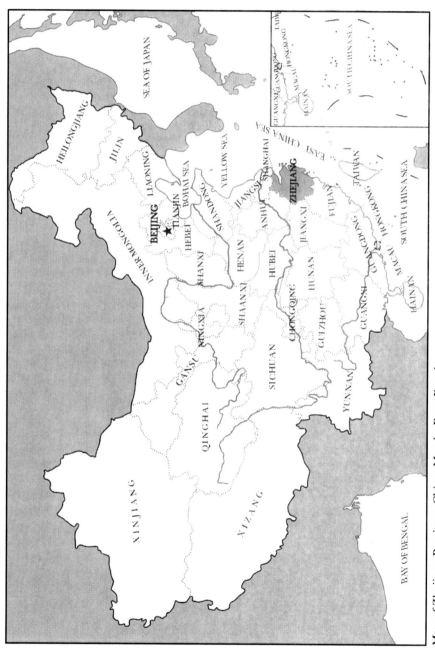

Map of Zhejiang Province, China. Map by Fang Jianxin.

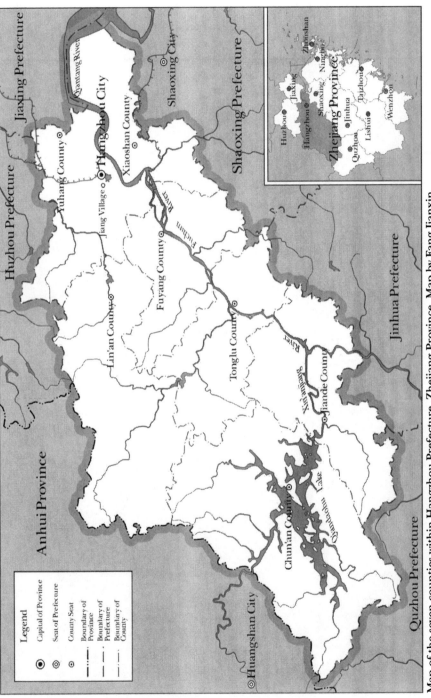

Map of the seven counties within Hangzhou Prefecture, Zhejiang Province. Map by Fang Jianxin.

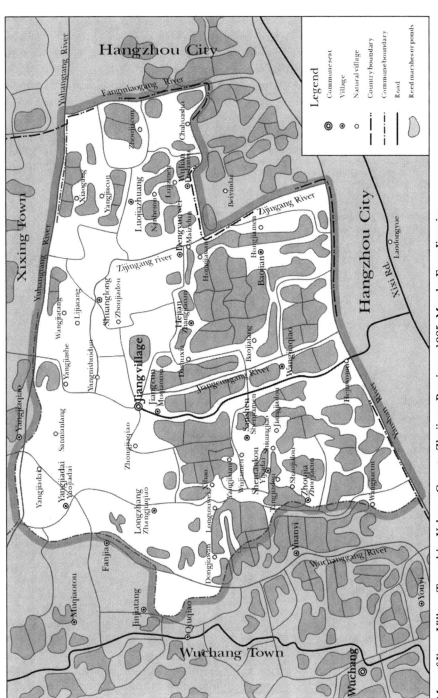

Map of Jiang Village Township, Yuhang County, Zhejiang Province, 1985. Map by Fang Jianxin.

Introduction

The year 1968 saw the publication of Ralph Croizier's *Traditional Medicine in Modern China: Science, Nationalism, and the Tensions of Cultural Change*, which would become one of the most cited books on twentieth-century Chinese medical history. It focused on one "central paradox and main theme": why twentieth-century intellectuals, committed in so many ways to science and modernity, insisted on upholding China's ancient "prescientific" medical tradition.[1] From the perspective of cultural nationalism, Croizier argued that these intellectuals were influenced by "the interaction of two of the dominant themes in modern Chinese thinking—the drive for national strength through modern science, and the concern that modernization not imply betrayal of national identity."[2] However, 1968 also marked the inauguration of a massive public health initiative in China that would have far-reaching consequences for the medical development of the world's most populous country: a rural medical program inspired by the principles of revolutionary socialism and promoted nationwide. This new medical program pitted Chinese and Western medicine against one another and, more importantly, eventually determined the future of the two types of medicine in Chinese villages. This social transformation has been largely overlooked by scholars of Chinese medical history. The centerpiece of the program was the introduction of "barefoot doctors" (*chijiao yisheng*) into Chinese villages at the height of the Cultural Revolution (1966–76).

The barefoot doctors were members of commune production brigades who were given basic medical training so they could provide treatment and perform public health work in their home villages. They formed the lowest level of a three-tiered state medical system comprised of county, commune, and brigade levels. The concept of barefoot doctors was introduced to the public through newspaper pieces, particularly "Fostering a revolution in medical education through the growth of the barefoot doctors," an investigative report published on September 14, 1968, in the *People's Daily*, an organ of the Central Committee of the Chinese Communist Party. It described the work of barefoot doctors in Jiangzhen Commune, Chuansha County, Shanghai Municipality.[3] On December 5, 1968, the same newspaper carried a report with the headline "Cooperative medical service warmly welcomed by poor and lower-middle peasants." This article introduced the new cooperative medical service of Leyuan Commune, Changyang County, Hubei Province.[4] As one of the "newly emerged things" (*xinsheng shiwu*) that reflected the political ideologies and rural development strategies of the Cultural Revolution, the barefoot doctors were rapidly popularized, and cooperative medical stations were set up in villages nationwide with revolutionary zeal. Villagers paid fees to form local "cooperative medical services" (*hezuo yiliao*) to cover the costs of establishing these medical service stations presided over by barefoot doctors. When villagers sought treatment at these stations, they were administered certain services and medicines free of charge. With the implementation of rural-reform policies and the dismantling of the people's commune system after 1978, the barefoot doctor program began to gradually disintegrate. Barefoot doctors who passed medical examinations and continued practicing medicine in villages were renamed "village doctors" (*xiangcun yisheng*). By 1983, cooperative medical services had basically ceased to function in most Chinese villages.

From their first appearance, the barefoot doctors attracted the attention of scholars and social commentators. The barefoot doctor program was regarded, both inside and outside China, as "a low-cost solution built around easily available indigenous medicines."[5] They presented a suitably revolutionary image: young people wading undaunted through the mud of rice paddies to provide medical services in answer to Mao's call to "stress rural areas in medical and health work."[6] Their basic equipment was popularly described as "one silver needle and a bunch of herbs" (*yigen yinzhen, yiba caoyao*), a reference to acupuncture and Chinese herbal medicine, but they combined Chinese and Western medicine in practice.

Together with the three-tiered rural medical system, barefoot doctors and cooperative medical services are associated with improvements in basic health indicators under socialism after the founding of the People's Republic of China (PRC) in 1949.[7] In the late 1970s, the World Health Organization (WHO) promoted the Chinese system as a model of health care for developing countries.[8] It is widely argued that the rural medical system collapsed as a result of the reforms initiated in 1978 and that the commercialization and marketization of medical provision have reduced the accessibility, affordability, and equity of public health care in rural China.[9] Meanwhile, in recent decades, both academic studies and public opinion have contrasted the current state of crisis in China's medical sector with the supposedly halcyon days of the barefoot doctor program.[10]

This book reaches beyond a nostalgic view of barefoot doctors and calls into question the orthodox interpretations that dominate present scholarship on public health in China. It retrieves Western medicine in rural China from potential historical oblivion through the perspective of the social history of medicine. It contextualizes barefoot doctors in the history of debates about the challenge posed by Western medicine to the legitimacy of Chinese medicine since the early twentieth century. As a village-centered and fieldwork-based ethnographical study, this book draws evidence from local archives of the Cultural Revolution period and personal interviews with villagers and doctors, and it places this data into a broad history of medicine in revolutionary and postreform China. It demonstrates that a key impact of the barefoot doctor program was facilitating the entry of Western medicine into villages hitherto dominated by Chinese medicine through scientificization, institutionalization, and professionalization, which led to a marginalization of Chinese medicine.

First, this book challenges the government propaganda, which presents barefoot doctors as a revolutionary vanguard consolidating Chinese medical knowledge and treatments on par with biomedicine. In contrast, it shows how a shifting constellation of factors (among them, knowledge transmission, pharmaceutical prices and supply chains, and healing styles and medical beliefs) indicates that the barefoot doctors effectively converted rural populations to a preference for Western medical treatments. Second, this book discards the standard interpretation of the roles of barefoot doctors in the three-tier medical system. It argues that the establishment of the rural medical system through barefoot doctors implanted medical institutionalization in Chinese villages through the construction of a hierarchical medical system, the formalization of medical encounters, and the codification of the medical community. It proposes a dumbbell-shaped structure to the evolution of the medical system and the origin of the current crisis in rural medicine, which the system has been undergoing since 1978. Third, this book argues that the development of barefoot doctors was a process of medical professionalization initiated by a political campaign developed in an enclosed village society and strengthened by the barefoot doctors' survival of profound social changes. In contrast to the negative assessments of rural medicine and health care since the early 1980s, this book argues that the reforms consolidated the position of barefoot doctors as a result of their further professionalization as "village doctors." The reforms also guaranteed a remarkable continuity in medical and public health provision, even though rural Chinese still face serious challenges in accessing health-care services.

Healers and Patients in Chinese Medical History

Henry Sigerist describes medicine as nothing more than the manifold relations between physicians and patients. Because of this, medical history should be seen as social history.[11] Regarding healers and patients in Chinese medical history, Nathan Sivin points out that

> classical medicine deserves the adjective 'scientific' no less (but no more) than its counterparts in Western culture until recent times. It provided health care for a small portion of the Chinese populace. The majority of its patients and

its more eminent practitioners belonged to the upper crust of society. Most of the afflicted among the Chinese population over the course of history had no access to the fully qualified physicians. They depended on a great variety of less educated healers, ranging from herbalists to priests.[12]

However, research on Chinese medical history based on written documents tends to deal with healers throughout the social and medical hierarchy in inverse proportion to their total numbers—that is, a great deal of attention has been given to a relatively small number of elite practitioners, while relatively little has been paid to the far greater number of practitioners who treated the masses. In Chinese history, medical records have long focused on elite medical traditions or, more exactly, on so-called Confucian and hereditary physicians.

Low-status healers are generally dismissed as incompetents or quacks. Furthermore, as Francesca Bray suggests, since they were neither scholars nor philosophers nor gentlemen, they did not have the kinds of disciples or clients who could transmit and publicize their medical knowledge and writings.[13] Thus, though elite physicians constituted only a tiny percentage of all healers,[14] they have long been the protagonists of studies of Chinese medical history. Nonelite healers, including ordinary Chinese medicine doctors, are absent from historical records and thus remain nameless to us.[15] On the rare occasions they do appear in the historical records, it is generally because a patient consulted them unsuccessfully before eventually deciding to see a "proper" physician, who then administered an effective treatment.[16] These healers were presented as the despised competitors of elite physicians, particularly in the case of women medical practitioners like the socially marginalized granny healers known as *chanpo* or *jieshengpo*.[17]

Available written texts present certain stereotypes among elite (and urban) physicians and their patients, who are said to have resorted to multiple doctors and to have changed physicians frequently.[18] For example, more than two-thirds of the patients of the mid-Ming physician Wang Ji had consulted at least one other healing practitioner, and many had availed themselves of the services of several practitioners.[19] By the 1930s, this practice was criticized as a bad habit, and patients and their families were called upon to become modern patients, which meant being loyal to one modern, scientifically trained physician.[20] These historical texts also describe patients and their relatives as being well versed in judging the prescriptions made by various physicians—to the extent that they were prepared to negotiate the nature and treatment of their illnesses with them.[21] Furthermore, the patients and their families documented in these encounters were well enough off to be able to afford the various medicines suggested by their physicians.[22] In contrast, the health services available to ordinary Chinese people, if any, remain less well documented. As late as the 1930s, one-third of the citizens in the Nationalist government capital Nanjing died without any medical care at all.[23] If residents in such a key urban area did not obtain quality medical treatment, it would have been almost impossible for rural Chinese villagers to do so.

During recent decades, the study of Chinese medical history has turned from the "great physicians" and "great inventions" perspective to the social history of medicine, which was first proposed by Henry Sigerist in 1947. Nonetheless, the field's main focus has still been elite healers and patients.[24] Scholars therefore need to take the further step of studying rural Chinese medicine healers in a broad sense, including ordinary clinic medical practitioners, itinerant doctors, shamans, acupuncturists, and granny midwives, all of whom are quite absent from the present elite-centered Chinese medicine studies. Such research should also include villagers, who have been largely ignored in medical history studies. Despite this academic emphasis, the reality of the social history of medicine in China was actually dominated by rural healers and patients who constituted the bulk of China's practitioners and consumers.

Chinese and Western Medicine in the Countryside

Ironically, the large-scale emergence of rural Chinese medicine as a topic in academic research and media was associated with Western medicine as a result of the barefoot doctor program: the integration of Chinese and Western medicine has emerged as a fashionable, widely promoted trademark of barefoot doctors in studies from both developed and developing countries.[25] The simultaneous emergence of Chinese medicine and Western medicine in Chinese villages is of great significance in the history of the legitimacy controversy posed to Chinese medicine by Western medicine in modern China. Before interpreting the history of the legitimacy debates, a few key concepts should be defined. Medical anthropologist Arthur Kleinman defines "medicine" as a cultural system. He points out that in every culture illness, the responses to it, the individuals experiencing it and treating it, and the social institutions relating to it are all systematically interconnected. The totality of these interrelationships is the health-care system.[26] This system includes the beliefs and behaviors that constitute the activities influenced by particular social institutions (e.g., clinics, hospitals, professional associations, and health bureaucracies), social roles (e.g., patients and healers), interpersonal relationships (e.g., doctor-patient, patient-family, and social network), and the settings of interactions (such as homes and doctors' offices).[27]

The term "Chinese medicine" has only been used since the arrival of Western medicine in China.[28] Prior to the nineteenth century, the term "medicine" (yi) could refer to any form of medicine from different medical schools and social strata in China. After Western medicine arrived in China, the terms "Chinese medicine" (*zhongyi*), "old medicine" (*jiuyi*), and "national medicine" (*guoyi*) appeared. The latter two were coined in the Republic of China,[29] but all references to "national medicine" were dropped after 1949 because it had too strong an association with Nationalist rhetoric. The term "old medicine" then died out because it seemed derogatory and was inconsistent with the Communist Party policy of promoting the benefits of Chinese medicine.[30] The term "Traditional Chinese Medicine" (TCM) first appeared in 1955,[31] but as Volker Scheid points out, it is found only in Western-language literature. No equivalent term is applied in China, where "Chinese medicine" (*zhongyi*) remains the more proper term.[32] Regardless of terminology, according to Paul Unschuld, Chinese medicine encompassed a wide range of practices, including oracular therapy, demonic medicine, religious healing, pragmatic drug therapy, Buddhist medicine, and the medicine of systematic correspondence in a broad sense.[33] Its key features included the home-based medical encounter mode and the doctor-patient relationship, which were embedded in the culture and customs of Chinese village society prior to the institutionalization and professionalization of Chinese medicine.

Western medicine, expressed in Chinese as *xiyi xiyao* or "modern medicine," mainly refers to modern biomedicine (with its related theories), vaccines, and the associated medical instruments in theory and practice. The hospital-based encounter is one of the key components of medical institutionalization, as is medical professionalization. Western medicine was introduced into China in the mid-nineteenth century, mainly through Christian missionaries. There Western medicine encountered its Chinese counterpart, which had existed for thousands of years and on which it made a great impact. The advent of Western medicine in China gave rise to new ideas about "the presence, nature, and causation of disease; over appropriate therapies; over the legitimacy of native, foreign, and foreign-trained healers; over the imposition of policing measures in the name of public health; over the need for a particular institutional infrastructure; over the intellectual presuppositions themselves of Western medicine."[34] More significantly, Western medicine started to challenge the legitimacy of Chinese medicine from the early twentieth century onward. In 1929, the proposal for "abolishing old-style medicine in order to clear away the obstacles to medicine and public health" was passed by the first National Public Health Conference of the Nationalist government. It became the hallmark event of the legitimacy crisis in the first half of the twentieth century.

Though Chinese medicine doctors were not deprived of their status and their legal right to practice medicine, the state was reluctant to give them legitimacy, and their precarious position was continually challenged throughout the Republican period.[35] The situation did not change much until the mid-1950s, in the early years of the new Communist regime.[36]

Chinese medicine was given, and is still given, very little administrative power within the higher echelons of the party structure.[37] However, Chinese medicine finally acquired legitimacy under the new regime, when it was transformed from the marginal, sidelined medical practice it had been in the early twentieth century to an essential and high-profile aspect of the national health-care system. The institutionalization and standardization of Chinese medicine in Communist China was completed by 1963, by which time it had begun to be admitted into the primary health care system.[38] During the 1960s, Chinese medicine was practiced in hospitals and clinics and taught in schools. Its knowledge was systematically recorded in textbooks, and it was divided into categories that parallel those of Western medicine.[39] By the 1980s, C. C. Chen—who led a rural medical experiment in Ding County, Hebei Province, under the leadership of James Yen in the 1930s and was opposed to Chinese medicine—reluctantly admitted that "each system has its own representation in the central government, as well as its own nationally or provincially administered urban clinics, hospitals, and medical schools . . . as of 1987, organizational conflict had almost entirely disappeared."[40]

More significantly, since the mid-1950s the integration of Chinese and Western medicine has been promoted as a key feature of the Chinese medical system, one in which barefoot doctors were said to play a pivotal role during the 1970s. Medical anthropologists and sociologists have suggested various interpretations for this integration. Sydney White proposed a theory of "syncretism from above" as the state-formulated policy and "syncretism from below" as local practice. According to this theory, integrated medicine within rural China scientificized TCM practices while giving Western medicine more flavor by adding TCM to it.[41] Stella Quah and Li Jingwei proposed the concept of a "marriage of convenience,"[42] and Quah put forward the concept of "pragmatic acculturation" to explain the dual use of traditional and modern health services in third-world societies with more than one medical system.[43] The advantage of the integration of medicines, WHO points out, is that "it offers reciprocal benefit[s] to each system."[44]

However, these overly simplified, stereotypical views have cast the relationship between Chinese and Western medicine during the Cultural Revolution as superficial, static, and unchanging, rather than complex, dynamic, and flexible. These arguments fail to account for Chinese medicine's continued domination of the rural medical world at least up to the mid-1960s. However, by the time the barefoot doctor program disintegrated in the early 1980s, Western medicine predominated Chinese villages in terms of medical knowledge and practice, the institutionalization of medical encounters, and the professionalization of medical practice. Certain historical questions that may influence how we think about social issues relating to rural medicine under socialism remain unanswered: Under what circumstances was Western medicine introduced into Chinese villages? How did Western medicine challenge Chinese medicine in these aspects, and how did Chinese medicine respond to this challenge? How did the introduction of Western medicine shape the social transformation of rural medicine in China under socialism and postsocialism?

The Dynamics of Plural Medical Systems

Paul Unschuld argues that the medical system of a culture is made up of a spectrum of resources that meet the demand for health-care services as well as the distribution and control over these resources.[45] The government obviously plays an important role in resource distribution, and in Chinese medical history the extent of this role has fluctuated over time.[46] Generally speaking, the imperial government did not show any real awareness of a modern state's medical responsibilities until the very end of the Qing Dynasty.[47] The state's role in medicine changed in response to the rise of modern public health systems in nineteenth-century Europe. The mass health problems created by large-scale urbanization and industrialization there prompted the notion that the state had an obligation to intervene directly to safeguard public health.[48] When this concept took root in China during the late Qing and early years of the Republic, it was associated with modernization and nation building. In other words, the government's promotion of Western-style public health activities had as much to do with national sovereignty as with the health of the people or with industrial efficiency.[49] The founding and development of the state medical system was clearly the main theme of medical modernization in twentieth-century China under both the Nationalist and Communist governments.

As China had a largely rural population, the establishment of the state medical system in rural areas was highly significant. The rural medical system was proposed and implemented experimentally in the 1930s by the Nanjing-based Nationalist government and the Rural Construction Movement, which was represented by C. C. Chen in Ding County, north China. In both the governmental and nongovernmental blueprints and practices, village health workers were at the lowest level of the organization. These lay people were selected from general village organizations and given brief training in the reporting of births and deaths, the administration of smallpox vaccinations, and simple sanitation, including methods of applying ordinary antiseptics.[50] After the founding of the People's Republic of China in 1949, a new rural medical system was gradually established from the top down. By 1970, the three-tier medical system (comprising the county, commune, and brigade levels) had been fully implemented throughout rural China with the popularization of the barefoot doctors and the implementation of cooperative medical services nationwide.

An Elissa Lucas thoroughly analyzed the policy continuities in Chinese state medicine through the chaotic thirty-year period from the beginning of the Sino-Japanese War in 1937 through the founding of the People's Republic of China, to the start of the Cultural Revolution in 1966. Lucas argues that, despite the many changes in political leadership during this period, the forms and functions of Chinese medical organizations and policies continued to follow the blueprints first drawn up for Chinese state medical modernization in the 1930s by League of Nations health reformers for the Nationalist government in Nanjing.[51] Lucas demonstrates that the Chinese system after 1968 was a replica of the Yugoslav state medical system between the wars. More specifically, China's village medical stations—run by the barefoot doctors—were based on the model health center in Mraclin, in what is now Croatia.[52] Lucas also points out that the larger lesson learned from the failure of medical modernization under the Nationalists is that effective national political leadership and social mobilization are prerequisites to rapid medical modernization in a highly populated country like China.[53] The Communist government had certain advantages over its Nationalist predecessor in the field of rural health in terms of ideology and experience in political mobilization and ideological manipulation, as demonstrated by the organization of mass public health movements like the Patriotic Hygiene campaign.[54] Therefore, the rural medical system was founded in the villages only after the advent of the Communist regime, though the "politics of medicine" among the top leadership were complex with regard to stressing rural areas or urban areas, as David Lampton thoroughly analyzed.[55] His scholarly work presents the historical contexts and institutional frameworks for understanding the state medical system in rural China after 1949 and barefoot doctors between 1968 and 1983. However, several outstanding issues still need to be addressed: How did the Communist government respond to the shortage of medical personnel described above? How exactly were the medical units of the new top-down state medical system implemented in Chinese villages? In what medical context did the barefoot doctors emerge, and what was their relationship with other village healers?

The conceptual tools needed to answer these questions might be found in the theory of "plural medical systems" or "medical pluralism," first theorized by Arthur Kleinman in his study of Taiwan Chinese society during the 1970s. In it, Kleinman categorizes all healers into professional, folk, and popular medical systems.[56] In China the professional sector of the health-care system, or the organized healing profession, includes doctors of both Chinese and Western medicine.[57] Folk medicine is classified into sacred and secular sectors, but in practice this division is often blurred, and the two sectors usually overlap in such areas as herbalism, traditional surgical and manipulative treatments, special systems of exercise, and symbolic nonsacred healing.[58] The popular health care system contains several levels, including individual, family, social network, and community beliefs and activities. According to Kleinman, this last sphere—the nonprofessional, nonspecialist arena of popular culture—is where illness is first defined and health-care activities are initiated.[59] This theory suggests that the study of Chinese medical history should also pay attention to folk healers and the popular health-care system.

Chinese medical anthropologists and historians have applied Kleinman's theory of plural medical systems to the social history of Chinese medicine.[60] Christopher Cullen used it to analyze how members of the Ximen family interacted with healers in the classical Chinese novel *Golden Lotus* (*Jinpingmei*).[61] Elisabeth Hsu's study of medical pluralism in contemporary Yunnan included temple monks, fortune tellers, herbalists, *Qigong* healers, and doctors of both Chinese and Western medicine.[62] Sydney White explored the narrative of modernity in the Lijiang Basin, Yunnan, by examining the Naxi people's acquisition of Chinese and Western medicine from the Republican era to post-Mao China. White argues that "medical pluralism is, in essence, the politics of therapeutic practices—that is, how relationships of power and meaning are played out between diverse therapeutic practices in a given context and how they shift over time. As such, medical pluralism is integrally linked to the politics of cultural identities."[63] These works offer insights into the state medical system's establishment in rural areas after 1949 through the dynamic differentiation of professional and folk healers according to both political ideology and practical needs, by including them in or excluding them from the state medical system during the continuous political campaigns of the new socialist regime. This process started when private Chinese medical practitioners established union clinics (*lianhe zhensuo*) after 1952 and continued to the outbreak of the Cultural Revolution, which completely reshuffled the plural medical systems. Barefoot doctors emerged in the reconstructed village medical world as a national health program after 1968.

Contesting Forms of Medical Knowledge and Practice

Traditional Chinese medicine has always been a dynamic discipline that has constantly redefined itself.[64] Chinese medical doctrines changed regularly, perhaps even more so than their premodern European counterparts in imperial China.[65] When missionaries introduced Western medicine into China in the early nineteenth century, it was not highly regarded among the Chinese,[66] because its technological and clinical skills were not superior to those already available in China and its therapeutic advantages at the time were limited to a few areas, such as quinine therapy for malaria, analgesia and anesthesia, and a certain number of medicinal plants not employed by Chinese doctors.[67] Although some Western surgical procedures, especially eye surgery, seem to have gained quick acceptance because they solved problems beyond the skill of native medical practitioners,[68] Western medicine offered no "modern" technology-intensive clinical medicines or relatively safe surgical procedures.[69] As a result, when missions first began to offer medical services, the patients who sought them were usually poor people attracted by the fact that these services were free or very cheap. Officials or the gentry took longer to seek Western medicine, and they regarded it as a "minor art" or last resort.[70]

Many of the Western physicians practicing in Western hospitals in China during this period admitted the effectiveness of certain Chinese medicines.[71] However, Western medical science made great achievements in the second half of the nineteenth century that enabled doctors to diagnose humankind's most important disease conditions, for the first time in history, on a scientific footing.[72] These medical advances include Robert Koch's discovery of the bacillus that caused tuberculosis in 1882 as well as the establishment of the therapeutic effectiveness of the rabies vaccine by Louis Pasteur in 1885 and of the diphtheria antitoxin by Emil von Behring in 1890. As Charles Rosenberg argues, "the image of medicine itself had changed radically in the last third of the nineteenth century."[73]

After these scientific achievements, Western medicine in China was no longer limited to destitute Chinese patients but instead became the treatment of choice for urban elites and gradually extended to less affluent city-dwellers.[74] Technological developments—including the microscope (from the 1840s), the medical thermometer (from the 1880s), and the X-ray machine (in 1896)—were applied as aids for diagnosis, treatment, and monitoring when medical missionaries were able to raise the necessary funds to acquire them.[75] However, a gap always existed between the scientific technology of medicine and its practical application. In 1920 a study by the China Medical Missionary Association, which encompassed 80 percent of urban and rural missionary hospitals, revealed that 73 percent of the hospitals had no means of sterilizing bedding or mattresses and 87 percent of the hospitals had no X-ray machines.[76] Even when the legitimacy of Chinese medicine was being challenged by Western medicine in the late 1920s and early 1930s, the former was still popularly perceived as more therapeutically effective than the latter. As C. C. Chen recalled, "at that time, it was commonplace to hear someone assert that missionary physicians and Western medicine were competent in surgical cases, but that one should still rely on indigenous medicine for treatment of disease."[77]

From the 1940s Western medicine expanded dramatically in terms of theory, practice, and pharmaceuticals, particularly regarding the development of antibiotics and sulfanilamide to treat common diseases and vaccines for the worst epidemic diseases.[78] Yet access was still quite difficult for ordinary Chinese, so it is easy to understand why Western medical knowledge, pharmaceuticals, and practices were of no real significance to most villagers for until the 1950s. All the same, the knowledge, pharmaceuticals, and healing styles of Western medicine eventually entered into Chinese medicine-dominated villages, albeit at a snail's pace. The process picked up speed with the gradual establishment of the state medical system in the 1950s, which promoted Western medicine as "modern." The significance of this shift lay not only in the contents of Western medical knowledge but also in the changed ways that knowledge was transmitted, notably the introduction of school-based training. These changes led to an increased number of doctors, which in turn further disseminated Western medicine through the villages. Western pharmaceuticals—mainly antibiotics and vaccines—also started to enter the countryside and even reached border areas.[79]

As Western medicine advanced into the countryside, Chinese medicine also underwent a revival in villages due to its legitimization by the socialist medical system through the Chinese herbal medicine campaign (*zhongcaoyao yundong*). This campaign is often claimed to have been launched nationwide when cooperative medical services were implemented during the 1970s. As discussed above, acupuncture and herbal medicine were at the heart of this campaign, as reflected by the saying mentioned above, "one silver needle and a bunch of herbs." In the other campaign slogan, "the three folks and the four selves" (*santu sizi*), the term *santu* refers to folk medicines, doctors, and prescriptions, while the second term *sizi* encourages people to collect, plant, make, and administer herbal remedies themselves.[80]

The advent of new knowledge and pharmaceuticals and the encounter of Chinese and Western medicine in these programs naturally brought about new healing styles. The popularization of barefoot doctors in Chinese villages nationwide after 1968 comprehensively accelerated this trend. While it may seem that state directives led to an integration of modern and indigenous medical knowledge in Chinese villages during the 1970s, the encounter of Chinese and Western medicine in these programs actually led the two to contest one another in ways obscured by the political rhetoric of the Cultural Revolution. The advent of the barefoot doctors meant that Western medicine effectively won this battle, while Chinese medicine was steadily marginalized, even though it is still consumed and appreciated today. In other words, the supposed integration of Chinese and Western medicine was actually a dynamic, unbalanced process rather than a static, symmetrical juxtaposition.

The Evolution of a Medical Community

The introduction of Western medical knowledge, pharmaceuticals, and healing into rural China also implanted medical institutionalization. As the institution that unites clinical treatment, medical research, and training, the modern hospital is the lynchpin of medical institutionalization, especially as it replaced the home as the site of medical encounters.[81] In modern European history, hospitals developed from hostels for pilgrims, travelers, and foreigners, and from poor houses for the destitute, the infirm, and the aged.[82] These hospitals provided of food, bedding, and nursing care (during both the day and night) as well as physicians to minister to patients suffering from illnesses and injuries.[83] In Chinese medical history, a germ of the hospital idea may have existed in earlier times in institutions like the Peace and Happiness Hospital (*anle bingfang*) in the Song Dynasty. However, it is not known how widely these hospitals were implemented.[84] Furthermore, according to K. C. Wong and Wu Lien-Teh, the development of such establishments cannot be compared with those of Europe and America, which were organized on an elaborate and extended scale.[85]

The introduction of the modern hospital into China, as a concept and as a reality, coincided with a revolution in the theory and practice of Western medicine.[86] Western medicine hospitals were the most conspicuous institution brought by medical missionaries to China,[87] where they emerged sporadically from the mid-nineteenth century onward.[88] Meanwhile, Chinese medicine also attempted to adopt Western models of hospital organization in metropolitan areas such as Shanghai, where Chinese medicine hospitals were established to offer both in-patient and out-patient treatment.[89] At the start of the People's Republic of China in 1949, many public county hospitals had already been established by the Nationalist government since the 1930s. Private clinics also existed in rural areas, mainly in county seats. Though these hospitals were poor in terms of both medical staff and instruments, they displayed the basic features of modern Western medical institutions: bureaucratic management, the division of medical expertise, and clinic-based medical encounters. However, most villagers lived too far from such hospitals or were too unfamiliar with their treatment style for the majority to adopt hospitals as their medical reality. Instead, the home-based medical encounters that were still the key feature of Chinese medicine predominated.

After 1949, the world of village medicine was transformed through the gradual establishment of the three-tier medical system. This top-down process took over the Nationalist government's public county hospitals and renamed them county people's hospitals, formed union clinics in district and township seats after 1952, and established the medical stations over which barefoot doctors presided after 1968. Scholars have proposed a few interpretative concepts for this three-tier medical system. According to Ray Elling, the ideal structure of any medical system includes the concepts of "medical regionalization" and "concertion." A regionalized system is a graded hierarchy of interdependent services with a two-way flow of patients, information, supplies and the like between the periphery and the center of the system. Concertion is a tight interweaving of political will in the creation of policy, such that political authority is empowered to coordinate and implement the structure and possesses the necessary funding to do so or the ability to appropriate and control resources.[90]

After their visits to Guangdong in 1978, Li Peiliang and Xu Huiying developed Elling's notions of "medical regionalization" and suggest "a hierarchical structure of medical networks" (*yiliao wangluo chaxu geju*) to explain the three-tier system. According to this concept, the whole country was divided into several regions for the provision of comprehensive and cheap medical services. A hierarchy of proficiency was established among the different medical units, and cooperation could be implemented for the treatment and prevention of diseases as well as for research and education. Other countries that attempted to implement this model met with difficulties due to administrative regionalization and issues of power and cooperation. In China, two factors contributed to its successful implementation. The first was the existence of clear borders at the county, commune, and brigade levels, which helped the formation of a hierarchical network. The second was the integrated political and medical authority structure.[91] Similarly, Pi-Chao Chen proposed the concept of a "cellular pattern of health organization." In his opinion, China wove its rural medical services into the existing social and economic fabric at the grassroots level, rather than setting up a new bureaucracy.[92] It has been widely argued that this system was very effective in providing medical services, particularly in combating epidemic and pandemic diseases through Maoist mass mobilization tactics and political campaigns.[93] This argument was repeated in the critiques of the postsocialist health system that followed the SARS (severe acute respiratory syndrome) pandemic in early 2003.[94]

These concepts have provided a macrostructural interpretation of the three-tier medical system, particularly in terms of public health campaigns. However, it is still not clear how villagers and private medical practitioners coming from "old society" experienced the changes brought by the establishment of hospitals, clinics, and the new medical system in general. These new top-down institutions and the system itself need to be understood from a bottom-up perspective. In traditional Chinese village society, as in other premodern societies, medical encounters were usually based in the patients' homes because of the individualized nature of medical service delivery. A medical community could not be said to exist in theory or practice because of the absence of hierarchical proficiency and cooperation. This lack of community was the feature setting Chinese medicine apart from Western medicine in terms of medical institutionalization. After 1952, following the principle of "one clinic per township," union clinics were established to function as minihospitals beneath county hospitals—in other words, the second tier of the three-tier medical system. As a result, a medical community emerged in rural China based on the townships (or the communes after 1962). This brought changes for both villagers, whose medical encounters started to move from their homes into clinics, and for rural medical practitioners, who began to form part of a hierarchical system that stratified medical proficiency and coordinated the treatment.

The arrival of the barefoot doctors in 1968 further accelerated this trend. As the medical staff at the lowest level of the three-tier medical system, the barefoot doctors and their counterparts at the commune and county levels finally accomplished and enhanced the technical stratification and cooperation of the medical system through the patient referral system. As a result of their presence, villagers' encounters with doctors increased, and they began to receive treatment outside their home villages and communes at county hospitals, sometimes even prefectural and provincial hospitals above the county level. More significantly, the advent of the barefoot doctors caused the three-tier system to evolve into the dumbbell-shaped structure that this book proposes: the barefoot doctors' medical stations and the county hospitals grew in importance, while commune clinics—the middle level of the three-tier system—experienced a dramatic decline. Barefoot doctors were thus at the heart of the radical changes that implanted medical institutionalization in Chinese villages.

Starting a Medical Profession from Scratch

Professionalization is the third key feature of the modernizing influence of Western medicine on Chinese medicine. Eliot Freidson argues that the formation of a medical profession depends on several basic elements, which include educational requirements, medical knowledge, the establishment of criteria for acceptance and dismissal from a society of professionals, and the struggle for reputation and social recognition. This process unfolds distinctively at different times and in various locations around the world.[95] However, some scholars suggest that the sociological approach to analyzing the professionalization process is of little help to medical historians, especially non-Western ones, because the idea of a medical profession outside the West is at best vague.[96] There have been many debates about how the notion should be defined and applied, including some heated arguments— in the context of late imperial China—about whether it is even proper to apply it. Nathan Sivin argues that it is inappropriate to see classical medicine in China as a "profession" prior to the twentieth century and the arrival of Western medicine.[97] Sivin's key argument is that elite doctors in premodern China made no organized attempt to prevent people unlike them from practicing medicine.[98] According to Francesca Bray, the key features of a medical profession are self-regulation and self-certification. She argues that "the nearest to professional physicians were those who took the medical examinations instituted by the state at various periods from the ninth century, and who then served as state medical officers; but even they did not constitute a self-regulating body."[99] As these factors were absent, Bray suggests that a physician in late imperial China was not a professional in the modern sense. Furthermore, their medical language was not as impenetrable to nonspecialists as it is in the West today.[100]

Notwithstanding, Yüan-ling Chao asks in her study of Suzhou physicians in late imperial China "whether the concept of professionalization can transcend cultural boundaries. Can there be a universal concept of professionalization?" Chao argues that, despite the absence of licensing laws, formal medical instructions, and the growth of the political and social power of physicians in traditional China, elites' increasing participation in medical practice in the late imperial era contributed to demarcating boundaries for inclusion and exclusion. In her opinion, Confucian physicians created a dominant ideal of medicine by emphasizing ethics and classical knowledge, as well as by forming a consciousness of identity.[101] Meanwhile, social and literary networks as well as the writing and publication of medical texts facilitated the development of group consciousness and a sense of community and identity among medical practitioners.[102] The state was absent from this process, which was led principally by elite physicians. In the meantime, medical practice regulations were applied during different dynasties to imperial court physicians.[103] Outside the court, the Song dynasty government briefly attempted to set unified standards and to examine physicians,[104] but Sivin argues that these initiatives did not have any lasting effect and were not revived by subsequent governments.[105]

The state began to facilitate the development of a modern medical profession only with the spread of Western medicine at the start of the twentieth century. As a byproduct of government involvement in public health, epidemic prevention, and medical education, both Western-style physicians and Chinese medical practitioners organized themselves into separate medical associations.[106] Within this process, the gradual professional association of Chinese medicine physicians was more significant than that of the Western medicine physicians because the former had operated independently and were geographically scattered and unregulated.[107] At the time, Chinese medicine doctors were facing a major crisis. According to Angela Ki Che Leung, the reasons for this were twofold. Firstly, the government's initiative to abolish Chinese medicine in 1929 called the legitimacy of Chinese medical knowledge into question. Secondly, and more seriously, Chinese medicine doctors had to contend with an increase in the professional management of medicine instigated by the government to promote modern (i.e., Western) medicine.[108] However, the medical legitimacy crisis did have some positive outcomes in terms of professional development, as it awakened Chinese medicine doctors' consciousness of modern medical professionalization.[109] This gave rise to the formation of professional associations that—with the active or passive concurrence of the state—set the rules for licensure, certified specialized expertise, and disciplined deviant members of the profession.[110]

After 1949, the socialist state demonstrated remarkable power in the professionalization of medicine, driven largely by the scarcity of medical resources.[111] Judith Farquhar recounts how the governments organized the previously diverse and scattered practitioners of traditional medicine into a rapidly growing national hierarchy of clinical and academic institutions. Traditional Chinese medical practitioners suddenly acquired a clear-cut professional identity.[112] In this sense, the process of the Chinese medicine practitioners joining the union clinics in the early 1950s can be understood to some extent as the formation of a professional identity in rural China. The state disciplined and regulated the relationships of these rural medical practitioners from the "old society" with their counterparts and their patients by impressing professional codes and socialist ideologies on them.

The emergence of the barefoot doctors after 1968 occurred in a context of the concurrent penetration of state power and Western medicine into Chinese villages. New kinds of village healers, the barefoot doctors, were inserted into the reshuffled and reorganized medical world of the Chinese villages as one of the "newly emerged things" of the Cultural Revolution. They undertook medical and health work in the specific social environment of the people's commune system, which the implementation of the household registration system dividing urban and rural areas organized into an enclosed village society. Introducing the basic concepts of medical professionalization into the analysis of the barefoot doctors' rise will reveal the very particular development path of a medical profession starting from scratch. It will help us understand the state's role in this process in terms of the formation of a group identity among the barefoot doctors, the power relationships that emerged, and the claims to medical legitimacy, which involved competitors, counterparts, patients, and the state respectively. More importantly, it will shed light on why rural reform and medical examinations—which led to the so-called disintegration of the barefoot doctor group—actually further enhanced their group identity, power, and legitimacy as a medical profession. As such, the barefoot doctors can be said to have continued playing positive roles in rural medicine and health, despite facing serious challenges in the postsocialist era.

Methodology and Structure of This Book

This book is a study of seven counties in Hangzhou Prefecture, Zhejiang Province, in eastern China and is based on oral interviews and archival documents. The main thread of discussion is the development of medicine and health since 1949 in Jiang Village, Yuhang County, which is now a suburban area under the jurisdiction of Hangzhou, the provincial capital city of Zhejiang. From 1912 to 1961, Jiang Village was under the jurisdiction of Hang County, the most important county in Zhejiang Province, as the location of the provincial capital. In 1961, Hang County was made part of Yuhang County, which was under the jurisdiction of Hangzhou Prefecture.[113] Jiang Village People's Commune was established in the same year and was renamed Jiang Village Township in January 1984. Jiang Village was made up of thirteen administrative villages and seventy-nine villager teams, which were scattered throughout 146 natural villages containing a total of 3,574 households and 14,762 people. In 1996, Jiang Village Township was allocated to Xihu District of Hangzhou City and became a suburban area.[114]

I chose to center my study on Hangzhou Prefecture for simple but practical reasons. First, the vastness of China would make it impossible to analyze in detail the experiences of barefoot doctors in each corner of the country. I thus felt it best to concentrate my research on a single prefecture, albeit a large one, which I could then explore in depth. Second, Hangzhou was one of many "ordinary" prefectures in which the barefoot doctor program was implemented during the 1970s—in other words, it lacked the showpiece model villages that attracted national attention, such as those in Changyang County of Hubei Province and Chuansha County of the Shanghai Municipality.[115] A systematic analysis of an ordinary prefecture (while also paying attention to the general situation throughout the country) should reflect the trends and features of the barefoot doctor program nationwide. Third, as the son of an ordinary peasant from the Hangzhou area, I speak the local dialect and have access to the necessary social network to make fieldwork possible, particularly in procuring interviews with barefoot doctors and ordinary villagers and gathering information relating to the Cultural Revolution from local archives.

My decision to focus specifically on Jiang Village was based on similar reasons. Moreover, as Jiang Village is a wetland, before the 1950s it was seriously affected by a key infectious disease, schistosomiasis. Jiang Village has undergone all the new regime's medical and health campaigns, including the schistosomiasis eradication campaign. More importantly, my interviewees from Jiang Village—including preliberation Chinese medicine doctors, union clinic staff, former barefoot doctors, commune clinic doctors, and ordinary villagers—were happy to share their life histories with me and offer me assistance, even though I am not a native of their village. China's vastness and diversity calls into question the representativeness of any particular case study. But, without detailed research of specific locations, we are left with broad generalizations that are of limited utility in deepening our knowledge of rural China. This book seeks to balance the specific and the general and in so doing provides evidence of how the actual experiences of health practitioners and patients challenge existing preconceptions of health-care programs in rural China.

Chapter 1 provides historical background by analyzing the dynamic differentiation and reorganization of village healers under the plural medical systems. It charts this process from the birth of the union clinics in the early 1950s to the advent of the barefoot doctors in 1968 when the rural medical world experienced a major reconstruction in which barefoot doctors were positioned as new and revolutionary healers.

Chapters 2, 3, and 4 focus on the contestation between Chinese and Western medicine—in terms of knowledge, pharmaceuticals, healing styles, and medical beliefs—which the advent of the barefoot doctors brought to a head. Chapter 2 explores how the selection criteria for the barefoot doctors changed traditional ways of knowledge transmission in the villages in the context of a gradual confluence of Chinese and Western medicine and examines the evolution of a Western-influenced medical knowledge structure for the barefoot doctors themselves and their villages. Chapter 3 opens with a discussion of the social epidemiology of rural Hangzhou before the barefoot doctor program. It goes on to address how the establishment of medical stations and the presence of medical kits from 1969 to 1970 extended the pharmaceutical network into the villages, effectively opening the door for Western medicine into the villages, where it met—and came into conflict—with Chinese medicine and government-promoted practices. Chapter 4 discusses how the barefoot doctors developed healing styles that were more oriented toward Western medicine and how villagers, as patients, formed comparative ideas about Chinese and Western medicines. It also examines the fundamental changes barefoot doctors brought to the structure of medical consumption in Chinese villages, which have endured since then.

Chapter 5 explores how the advent of the barefoot doctors extended and stratified medical encounters across the villages, contributing to the shift in their location from home bedsides to hospital wards, which depended on the formation of a medical coordinating scheme. This chapter also addresses how the work of barefoot doctors changed the three-tier medical system into a dumbbell-shaped structure.

Chapter 6 analyzes how the barefoot doctors created a medical profession from scratch within an enclosed village society. It explores how the state, together with the aggressiveness of Western medicine, contributed to their formation of group identity and their ascendance in power relationships. It analyzes how changes in the definition of medical legitimacy under rural reform had a positive impact on barefoot doctors and rural medicine as a whole.

The concluding chapter first briefly describes barefoot doctors and the plural medical world in the postsocialist era. It then explores the significance of rural medicine's transformation by the barefoot doctors in the context of the continuity of medical changes in twentieth-century China and the interrelationships between barefoot doctors, the socialist state, and villagers.

Chapter One

Village Healers, Medical Pluralism, and State Medicine

One chilly morning in the early spring of 1952, former Nationalist Party member Chen Hongting and his father Chen Changfu got up early and began their day as usual. The Chen family lived in Jiang Village, Hang County, in the eastern Chinese province of Zhejiang, in a house dating back to the Tongzhi reign of the Qing dynasty. There they carried on the sixty-year-old medical practice started by Hongting's grandfather. Yet, on that day in 1952, this tradition was about to be transformed. For the past two years, new songs had echoed through the village:

> The sky of the liberation area is bright.
> The masses in liberation areas love it very much;
> the democratic government loves the masses;
> the kindness of the Communists is too enormous to be described.

On that fateful morning, the Chens once again welcomed several special guests into their clinic: a group of doctors from the neighboring villages. After continuing the discussion they had begun a few days earlier, the group finally agreed to use the Chens' existing facility as a base for the new clinic, which would be known as the Jiang Village Union Clinic. Two rooms of the ground floor were set aside for treatment and the dispensary, while the top floor would serve as living quarters for the medical staff. The Chen's family-operated private practice was thus transformed into a union clinic—that is, a public health station officially sanctioned by the new Communist government. The village celebrated the official opening of the Jiang Village Union Clinic with firecrackers.[1]

The Plural Medical World on the Eve of the New Regime

Prior to the Communist victory in 1949, the medical world of rural China was largely plural and unregulated. Most professional doctors were individual practitioners of Chinese medicine who worked from "clinics" that were their own homes, although most consultations actually took place in their patients' homes. Usually each doctor worked alone, specializing in a particular kind of medicine.[2] Patients then went to Chinese medical halls to obtain the medicine their doctor had prescribed. Alternatively, some Chinese medicine doctors worked within such medicine halls and were known as *zuo-tangyi* (literally, "doctors who sit in the pharmacy"). They carried out their diagnoses over the counter and prescribed medicine that patients collected directly from the same pharmacy. These doctors were not paid directly by the pharmacy; rather, they simply used the pharmacy premises as consulting rooms in which to earn their own livelihood.[3] Pharmacy owners were often also doctors. In addition to these doctors who practiced from fixed venues were itinerant doctors called *guolu langzhong* (literally, "street-side healers"), some of whom used large, white umbrellas with red borders to signal their presence in a market street.[4] In the eyes of villagers, these itinerant healers were less prestigious than the type of doctors who made house calls, and this hierarchy is reflected in the use of the title "Doctor" or "Mister" for the latter, an honor that was not afforded to itinerant healers.[5] Chen Hongting and his father belonged to the more prestigious category, so the Jiang villagers usually called Chen Hongting "Mr. Ah Bao" (*Ah Bao xiansheng*).

By the late 1940s, the majority of professional medical practitioners were loosely regulated by Nationalist government departments and guilds through various forms of licensing and certification.[6] From 1946, registered medical practitioners joined the County Doctor Association,[7] a guild-oriented network that depended on the County Social Department and was organized by town. In May 1947, the 254 Chinese medicine doctors of Hang County were grouped into fifteen guild branches. Jiang Village—and thus the Chens—belonged to the sixth of these branches.[8] However, according to Chen Hongting, he and his father "owned a business, made a living by ourselves, and didn't care about the state before the liberation."[9] Nonetheless, like other guild members, the Chens did provide some patients with free prescriptions from time to time, particularly in the summer, the peak season for disease. Their philanthropic actions often earned them official acknowledgment at the end of the year, when the county magistrate presented them with ritual calligraphic memorials extolling their excellent medical proficiency (*miaoshou huichun*).[10]

As in other societies in which traditional medicine predominates, folk healers always supplemented the medical services provided by doctors like the Chens. In rural Hangzhou, folk healers were very popular among villagers and included herbalists, bonesetters, and snake doctors, as well as fellow villagers known for successfully using folk methods to treat common illnesses, such as tumefaction, heat stroke, bone fractures, and bloating due to overeating. In Shentankou, in the southwest corner of Jiang Village, lived a famous folk healer of this sort named Shen Fengxiang, who had learned medicine from Buddhist and Daoist monks and started practicing in 1903.

His main areas of expertise were treating heat stroke, bone setting, and bloodletting, at which he was particularly good.[11] He was assisted by his teenage grandson Shen Jinrong, who carried his medical kit.

Religious and supernatural healers were also very popular in rural areas. Indeed, for most Chinese people, the rituals such healers practiced were the first therapies to which they would turn. Temples and nunneries were therefore medical centers as well as places of religious worship. Religion played a stronger role in medicine in Jiang Village than elsewhere because temples and nunneries had flourished there since the twelfth century, when Hangzhou was made the capital of the southern Song dynasty. Peasant pilgrimages to the area were popular for centuries.[12] Many wives, concubines, and young ladies also built personal temples to regain the favor of their husbands or lovers.[13] By the late Republican era, there were still sixty-eight nunneries, fifteen temples, and fourteen ancestral halls in Jiang Village—an area of only about twenty square kilometers.[14] Villagers and pilgrims worshipped Buddha with incense to treat illnesses and begged him to protect their family members' health. In rare cases, monks and nuns even had special medical skills, much like secular professional practitioners. For example, the monks at the Bamboo Temple (zhulinsi) in Xiaoshan County, near Jiang Village, were famous for their gynecological expertise, which was unusual, given that religious and social norms generally forbade Chinese monks from touching women.[15] Villagers also sought health advice from the blind or disabled fortune-tellers outside temples. One such man in Jiang Village had no legs and was famed for treating patients through fortune telling and sorcery, so his fellow villagers called him a living Buddha (huopusa).[16]

The Birth of the Union Clinics

The plural village medical world gradually began to change with the advent of the Communist regime in 1949. With the establishment of the new government came an initial improvement in the number of doctors practicing medicine in rural areas. This increase was partly due to military doctors from both the Nationalist Army and the People's Liberation Army returning home after the war. Likewise, people who had studied medicine but never practiced now started to do so. Medicine became a popular way of making a living among the elites who would come to be known as "landlords" and "members of the bourgeoisie" after the land reform period.[17] From the end of 1949, the Communist government began to investigate medical practitioners and register medical agencies in each county, though the process was almost the same as that conducted by the Nationalist government two years earlier.[18] There were a total of 349 registered, government-approved social medical practitioners (shehui kaiyeyi), who were categorized into Chinese medicine doctors, dentists, druggists, nurses, midwives, and so on.[19] Of these, 285 were so-called old-style doctors (*jiuyi*), or Chinese medical practitioners, while 64 were new-style doctors (*xinyi*), or Western medical practitioners.[20] In January 1951, the Hang County Medical Practitioners and Workers Association was founded. All the doctors from the county were enrolled in the association except those who were excluded either on political grounds (those regarded as counterrevolutionaries, landlords, and rich peasants) or professional grounds (such as itinerant doctors). Chen Hongting was among the 228 old-style doctors who joined the association, but another 57 old-style doctors were not included for one of the two reasons above or simply because they had no interest in joining. The county association was then divided into nine district subassociations corresponding to rural administration districts in Hang County.[21] Although the form of the new association was the same as that of the former guild-oriented association, its main tasks were changed to "uniting Chinese and Western medicine . . . , guiding and promoting medical practitioners' political studies . . . , leading cooperation within the medical profession . . . , [and] helping the government implement social health care and epidemic prevention."[22] In the meantime, the founding of a state medical system—which had been proposed as early as the 1930s but never undertaken—was part of this broad political agenda.

Within this process, county hospitals were generally established by taking over existing county clinics, which had mainly been run by the Nationalist government, though their staff and facilities were quite poor.[23] To form medical units below the county level, the county medical units dispatched groups of one to three medical staff members to provide mobile medical service but also organized private medical practitioners into establishing mobile medical stations in villages. These groups also made medical services available at fixed locations on regular schedules.[24] Gradually, the various social medical and health workers (*shehui yiwu gongzuozhe*), such as Chinese medicine doctors, Western medicine doctors, heatstroke acupuncturists, and even itinerant healers, were—in the government's words—"mobilized" and encouraged to "walk the collective road." As Chen Hongting recalled, "after Chairman Mao came, all peasants believed in the Communists. Peasants were organized into mutual aid teams that strongly influenced us."[25] Another union clinic doctor said that when the union clinic was first established, medical personnel were told that they would receive no payment for their work. However, they were glad to be accepted as members, since they believed that they could survive only by joining the organization.[26]

As described in the opening of this chapter, Chen Hongting and his father were among the medical practitioners who formed a union clinic in Jiang Village in 1952. There were five doctors in total at this clinic: Chen Hongting, his father Chen Changfu, Shen Ahmei from Sanshen Village, Zheng Buying from Laodongyue Village, and Sun Juzhuang from Wangjiaqiao Village.[27] By May

1954, a total of twenty union clinics and eight clinic branches had been set up by similar means in towns all over Hang County. These clinics and branches fell into two basic categories: Chinese medicine union clinics and Chinese-Western medicine union clinics.[28] Thus, a two-tier state medical system was formed in the countryside, consisting of county hospitals and numerous township-level union clinics.[29] In this sense, union clinics partially established a state medical system in rural areas, as had first been proposed by the Nationalist government and the Rural Construction Movement in the 1930s.

The Chens' new clinic was completely different from the one they had run before. According to the *Regulations for Organizing Union Clinics* issued by the Ministry of Health in 1956, a union clinic was a socialist health and welfare entity under the ownership of a doctors' collective (*yisheng jiti suoyou-zhi*) and established voluntarily by doctors under the leadership of the party and the government. The union clinics' personnel, finance, distribution, and management were all run by the medical collective, which established fees for services, undertook individual accounting, managed the facility democratically, and distributed salaries according to the contributions of each member.[30] Each clinic was responsible for its own profits and losses, and, in this sense, the union clinics were self-supporting and self-managing entities.[31] Chen Hongting recalled the situation in 1952:

> Take a look, just two rooms. Anyway, there were no things at all in the clinic. Each doctor came here to form the clinic bringing only himself. There were benches and tables already here. If you had some money, you could contribute some of it [to the clinic]. Those higher up didn't care and invested nothing at all. We [Chen and his colleagues] had worked here for a long time. The clinic paid me one yuan for each room per month as rent for the house. . . . The state didn't care about us. We had to make a living by ourselves and feed ourselves."[32]

Clinics set aside a certain percentage of profits for future investment in the clinic, including building work and supplies, a pension fund for the families of doctors who died, and other welfare payments. The remainder was used to pay members' salaries, which were defined using an evaluation method. Each member was given a certain number of points according to his or her medical proficiency, medical licenses, reputation among the masses, and family financial burdens. These were called fixed points, and they were relatively stable from year to year. A fixed point's financial value each month was the ratio of the profits to the total of all members' points. Each member's monthly salary was calculated by multiplying his or her fixed points by the fixed point value for that month, which obviously varied according to profit levels. This system was known as "fixed points and flexible values" (*sifen huozhi*).[33] In 1955, Chen was paid an average monthly salary of RMB 55, which was very high in the 1950s, according to his brother-in-law Zhu Shouhua.[34]

Although the union clinics did not receive state funding, the state nevertheless assigned public health work as their members' compulsory daily duty. They were responsible for treating the masses, protecting mass health, and serving agricultural production by guaranteeing villagers' health. At the same time, union clinic medical personnel were required to be actively responsible for preventive medicine, maternal and child health care, public health instruction, and health worker and midwife training, all while carrying on their regular medical practice.[35] According to statistical data from 1957, union clinics undertook 90 percent of treatment and epidemic prevention in the rural areas of Zhejiang Province.[36]

Differentiation, Reorganization, and Extension

Union clinics established the basic form of the state medical system in China's villages from the early 1950s onward. Their creation also sparked a general differentiation and reorganization of the various healers in the villages. The registration process and enrollment in the county medical practitioners and health workers association brought most professional doctors under state management. While the union clinics made some professional medical practitioners undertake public health work in villages under the leadership of the health departments, other medical practitioners continued their private practices and did not join the union clinics. Of the total 349 registered medical practitioners in the Hang County association in 1950, 157 did not participate in union clinics but instead continued to make their living through private practice up to 1954.[37] They were officially recognized by the Ministry of Health, which announced that "private medical practitioners will exist for a long time to come, and their earnings should be respected."[38] However, demand for their services began to decline as union clinics were further consolidated when the medical collectives that owned the clinics signed health-care contracts with agricultural cooperatives. The number of private medical practitioners therefore decreased, and more and more joined union clinics.

The implementation of the people's commune system in the Great Leap Forward campaign in 1958 incorporated some township union clinics and other district health facilities into the health clinics of people's communes (which were based on original district health clinics) or health clinics of management districts (which were based on a former township union clinic or the combination of a few township union clinics).[39] As a result of these changes, Chen Hongting left the Jiang Village Union Clinic when it was annexed by Liuxia Management District Health Clinic, where he was appointed deputy director.[40] From 1958 to 1960, a veteran of the People's Liberation Army was in charge of Jiang Village Clinic, as it was now known, and clinic staff still worked there. The clinic's income was submitted to Liuxia Health Clinic, which paid the staff's salaries.[41] More importantly, private medical practitioners were no longer allowed to practice medicine from their own practices, so many were incorporated into clinics during this period.

However, these changes proved temporary. With the beginning of economic retrenchment in 1961, the people's commune or management district health clinics were dismantled and health-care provision reverted to district health clinics and commune union clinics, respectively, under the new and downsized people's commune system.[42] These commune union clinics were under the double leadership of the communes and the county health department and were responsible for their own profits and losses.[43] At this time, Chen Hongting left his position as deputy director in Liuxia to follow a cadre-training course held by the Zhejiang Provincial Health Department. One year later, he returned to Jiang Village Commune Clinic to resume his work.[44] The situation also changed for private medical practitioners: according to an official document, "they are individual intelligent workers and complement socialist health. A few private medical practitioners should be allowed to exist."[45] In 1962, private medical practitioners received approval after registration and review if they were over twenty years of age, had certain types of medical knowledge, and had practiced for more than three years.[46] As a result of these changes, many of those who had joined management district clinics during the Great Leap Forward campaign resumed their private medical practice, as this allowed them greater freedom and the opportunity to earn more money than their counterparts at the union clinics.[47] Nonetheless, despite these movements, the general trend was toward a decrease in the number of individual practitioners because of increasingly strict administration and decreasing space for their daily medical practice. Furthermore, private medical practitioners were encouraged to "walk the socialist road" during the Socialist Education campaign from 1964 to 1965.[48]

When professional medical practitioners were absorbed into the state medical system, the lives and practices of other healers in the villages, such as bonesetters and heat-stroke acupuncturists, were largely unaffected. The bloodletting healer Sheng Fengxiang and his grandson continued to wander the area treating their fellow villagers. In contrast, healers from religious sects were affected to some degree by the social and political changes taking place. Beginning in 1949, nunneries, Buddhist temples, and ancestral temples were gradually destroyed, and their buildings were used to house pigs or commune canteens and schools. Others survived successive political campaigns until the outbreak of the Cultural Revolution and provided shelter for monks and nuns whose establishments had already been destroyed.[49] These temples and nunneries had their own land, which the monks and nuns had inherited from their predecessors in the Republican era. The people's commune and production brigades lay outside the sphere of these establishments, but the secular and sacred worlds coexisted peacefully. Chen Zhicheng, who joined the clinic as a Chinese medicine apprentice in 1959, still remembers accompanying his master Zheng Buying to treat old nuns in the early 1960s. In his words, "the conditions [in the nunnery] were excellent, and the environment was very good." They were treated to a lunch of ten delicious vegetarian dishes.[50]

The birth of the union clinics also represented a significant downward extension of the state medical system. With the beginning of agricultural collectivization, villagers were selected to become health workers within mutual aid teams and cooperatives as part of the program of enhancing agricultural productivity.[51] The selection criteria for these initiatives were the possession of both basic primary educational qualifications and the right political credentials. Selected candidates were required to follow an informal training program entailing the "Four Principles of Health Work," which pertained to basic first aid and preventive medical treatment.[52] Usually the candidates also labored in the paddy fields like other commune members, hanging their medical kits on nearby trees. Jiang Jingting (who was known as Mr. Cat-Dog) was selected as one of the health workers in 1958. He recalled that Jiang Village health workers followed the union clinic doctors in disseminating preventive medicines, collecting blood samples, and helping to instruct villagers on how to provide stool samples to be analyzed for schistosomiasis.[53] Though it was not yet institutionalized, the basic structure of the state medical system based on the union clinic model had already taken shape in Chinese villages by the early 1960s.

Through the establishment of union clinics, villagers' health was brought under the state's supervision and control. Sun Kuijin, who was seventy-seven in 2004 and the last surviving schistosomiasis patient in Gao Village of neighboring Fuyang County, recalled this moment:

> When the People's Liberation Army came to our village, they were scared. They said, "There are no normal [uninfected] men in your villages." The army men taught us to put the pigs into the pigsty and not let them run in the villages . . . Later, no one came to the village from the higher levels in the years following liberation. Chairman Mao just became an emperor at that time. He was busy at that time and had no time to pay attention to schistosomiasis.[54]

In 1956, a campaign named "Exterminating Pests and Eliminating Diseases" was proposed as the way to increase agricultural production. In the same year, sanitation and epidemic prevention stations were set up in each county, and the system for infectious disease prevention and local disease treatment was basically established. According to *The Study of Schistosomiasis* by Chen Fangzhi of the Central Health Experimental Institute in 1934, Jiang Village was once listed as an area seriously affected by schistosomiasis.[55] From the mid-1950s onward, stool samples were tested in order to identify patients with schistosomiasis: villagers were asked to wrap their feces in paper or leaves on which their names were written, then leave these packages outside their doors for union clinic doctors and health workers to collect for testing. Villagers complained of the inconvenience, and some even called the union clinic doctors "feces doctors" and cursed that "the Communists managed so many things that they even managed feces."[56] When recalling the experience of collecting feces in the 1950s and 1960s, Chen Hongting sighed.

> Usually, we had to go to door to door to persuade [commune members] to provide stool samples. In the beginning, they would run away immediately when they saw us. During the time of "eating in the big canteen" [*chi dashitang*, the Great Leap Forward campaign of 1958–60], we found a way of getting commune members to submit their stool samples: If members didn't submit the samples, they were not allowed to have dinner in the canteen. The situation improved a great deal.[57]

Union Clinics and the Politics of Rural Medicine in the Mid-1960s

In the mid-1960s, union clinics were still the core of the state medical system in Chinese villages. However, the clinics' isolation from the modern urban medical systems at the county level and above meant that the union clinic model was formed by constantly absorbing the internal medical resources of Chinese villages. There were still a number of serious problems with the system. Though the union clinics were theoretically organs of the state charged with public health duties, they remained autonomous and did not receive substantial funding from the government. As such, they had to earn their own revenues through their medical services. When Chen Hongting recalled his work experiences before the mid-1960s, he always sighed.

> At that time, there were a lot of epidemic prevention tasks assigned by the higher-ups. You know, there were the four diseases (*sibing*): schistosomiasis, hookworm, filariasis, and malaria. We worked on epidemic prevention all day and all night, but we still had to treat patients and support ourselves. The state didn't take care of us. One year, I went to the county seat to attend a meeting held at the County Health Bureau. The bureau director criticized us for not working hard enough to meet the requirements for epidemic prevention. I was so angry that I beat the table and shouted at him. Alas, I was young at that time and had a bad temper.[58]

Chen Hongting's words were confirmed by the Hangzhou Prefectural Health Bureau: "Union clinic medical staff members are the sole force in medical and health care. They undertake the tough tasks of pest and disease control. As they must make a living from giving treatment, they emphasize treatment and neglect preventive health work." In 1965, the poor and lower-middle peasant representative by the surname of Zhou from Jiang Village Commune complained at the Hangzhou Health Work Meeting that Chen Hongting's union clinic served only those who had money. In Zhou's village, when the family of a seriously ill fifteen-year-old girl was unable to pay for medical services, the Jiang Village Union Clinic told them, "No money, no treatment!" The young girl died two days after she returned home.[59] In addition, medical facilities and conditions were generally poor in the union clinics, as medical personnel, instruments, and medicine were all in short supply. In 1965, the Hangzhou Prefectural Committee admitted that "only a third of the commune union clinics' medicine demands can be met."[60]

This state of affairs at union clinics was entangled with the unequal distribution of health-care resources in both rural and urban areas, which came under serious criticism in the political context of the mid-1960s. Like the Nationalists, the new Communist authorities faced the challenge of serving a burgeoning population with scarce medical resources. While the Nationalists had claimed to offer "state medicine" for all, the Communists claimed "to serve workers, peasants, and soldiers."[61] However, the new regime made institutional arrangements for certain sections of the population to be given priority in receiving the scarce medical resources available. In 1952, the State Council began granting free medical services (*gongfei yiliao*) to civil servants at each government level, as well as to party and association members and disabled revolutionary veterans.[62] In the same year, labor insurance medical services (*laobao yiliao*) were granted to workers in state-owned enterprises.[63] However, the peasants who comprised the majority of the Chinese population had no public medical provision, except for infectious disease inoculation, local disease treatment, and sporadic free clinical services. With the establishment of the household registration system (*hujizhi*), this "inequality of treatment based on social distinction"[64] continued until the late 1990s.[65] More seriously, the free medical services described above took up a huge percentage of total public health expenditures because of extravagance and abuse. For example, in Fuyang County, free medical services represented between 32.5 percent and 73.2 percent of the total expenditure on health care from 1955 to 1965, with a yearly average of 48.8 percent. However, only 2 percent of the total county population enjoyed these subsidized services, which cost RMB 32 per capita each year, while the overall county health expenditure was RMB 0.37 per capita.[66] As for state investment in health infrastructure, this was registered as nil in rural areas at the county level after economic adjustment in 1963. In Hangzhou Prefecture, 97 percent of the state infrastructure investments went to the county level and above, leaving only 3 percent for the countryside.[67]

Starting in 1965, the Socialist Education campaign targeted this inequality in the distribution of health-care resources, along with inequality in rural politics and other social issues, including education. In January 1965, plans were put forward to organize mobile medical service teams for rural areas and to train rural health workers in order to improve the rural medical situation.[68] Each production brigade was required to have two "half-peasant, half-doctors" (*bannong banyi*), one of whom was to be a woman, who would be in charge of delivering babies.[69] Youths with primary- and middle-school educations and "good" family origins, "correct" political thoughts, and "love for the countryside" were selected after being nominated by the masses, recommended by the association of poor peasants, approved by a party branch or commune, and interviewed by a training unit. After receiving training, they returned to their own brigades (*duilai duiqu*), where they were required to diagnose and treat a number of common diseases using their basic pharmaceutical knowledge as well as conduct the Patriotic Hygiene campaigns.[70] Training half-peasant, half-doctors was the main work of the urban mobile medical teams, while union clinics also undertook training work. In Jiang Village, Chen Hongting's union clinic began training health workers, who studied under him and other doctors in the clinic.[71]

The aim of these efforts was to introduce the medical personnel and facilities of the urban medical system into the rural system and to train the half-peasant, half-doctors to be extensions of the union clinics. Subsequent criticism from Mao soon drew attention to the situation, effectively promoting these measures:

> The Ministry of Health is only able to serve 15 percent of the total population, and this 15 percent is made up mostly of the privileged. The broad ranks of the peasants cannot obtain medical treatment and also do not receive medicine. The Ministry of Health is not a people's ministry. It should be called the Urban Health Ministry, the Ministry of Health for the Lords, or even the Urban Ministry of Health for the Lords. . . . Stress rural areas in medical and health work!

Mao's statement, made on June 25, 1965, later became known as the "June 26 Directive."[72] However, the measures adopted in 1965 both before and after Mao's statement did not fundamentally change the union clinic model and the structure of the village medical world, in which plural medical systems still predominated, despite the presence of the state medical system. It was only after the outbreak of the Cultural Revolution that the union clinic model changed completely.

Barefoot Doctors: From "Old Things" to "Newly Emerged Things"

When Wang Guizhen started out as a health worker, she could never have imagined that she would become an overnight celebrity and eventually be appointed vice minister of the Ministry of Health in Beijing in spite of her humble educational and social background. Similarly, as an ordinary doctor in a union clinic high in the mountains, Qin Xiangguan could never have foreseen that he would meet Chairman Mao several times in Tiananmen Square and be promoted to vice director of the International Chinese Health Delegation in 1974.[73] Not only did the Cultural Revolution bring these two figures unimaginable fame and status, it changed the medical world of rural China, including Jiang Village.

These extensive changes came about largely because of broader educational reforms, one aspect of which was the reform of medical education. In the mid-1960s, in keeping with his criticism of the health sector, Mao criticized the urban-oriented education system for its failure to bridge urban-rural inequalities.[74] The discussion of education was interrupted by the chaotic stage of the Cultural Revolution but resumed when this ended. On July 22, 1968, the *People's Daily* published an investigative report which explained how the Shanghai tool plant trained technicians using methods different from those used before the Cultural Revolution. In his comments on the report, Mao said, "Students should be selected from among workers and peasants with practical experience, and they should return to production after a few years' study." Mao's comment was called the "July 22 Directive," and it "pointed out the direction for the revolution in education."[75]

Against this background, a revolution in medical education became a topic of discussion in the press. On September 14, 1968, the *People's Daily* published an investigative report entitled "Fostering a revolution in medical education through the growth of the barefoot doctors." It introduced readers to barefoot doctors in Jiangzhen Commune, Chuansha County, Shanghai Municipality. Wang Guizhen was one of the barefoot doctors praised in the report. The barefoot doctors were young commune members who were selected to receive basic medical training and then returned to their brigades to serve their villages. The term "barefoot doctor" was thought to come from the fact that villagers called for help from these health workers who labored barefoot in the rice paddy fields but were ready to do medical and health work as needed.[76] However, a former barefoot doctor by the surname of Fang has a different interpretation of the origin and meaning of this term. He argued that the character *chi* in *chijiao* did not mean "bare" but rather "red," rendering the whole as "red-footed doctor." Because red is the symbolic color of Mao Zedong Thought, the term "red-footed doctor" is very revolutionary and ideologically loaded. Later, some barefoot doctor training classes were also called "red doctor classes."[77] No matter how the term *chijiao* is interpreted, the people to whom it was applied in the report in the *People's Daily* were the same health workers or "half-peasant, half-doctors" who had been selected to help the union clinics in villages from the 1950s to the mid-1960s.[78] In this sense, they were one of the "old things" (*jiushiwu*). However, the idea of barefoot doctors was consistent with Mao's ideological positions on "the direction of the Education Revolution" while also answering his call for medical work to focus on rural areas. Soon the barefoot doctors were described in charismatic terms by the press, which called them "newly emerged things."[79]

Although health workers experienced no intrinsic changes to their role as they went from being "old things" to "newly emerged things," the new contexts in which they worked within the cooperative medical service became institutionalized, a shift that also evolved out of the discussion on education in 1968.[80] From the mid-1950s, a hybrid education system was implemented to expand rural education: known as "walking on two legs"(*liangtiaotui zoulu*), it consisted of state-run schools and collective-run schools.[81] The latter, known as "people-run schools," had been expanded during the Great Leap Forward campaign, but their numbers declined when the campaign subsided. A discussion about rural education was also initiated in late 1968. On November 18, the *People's Daily* published a letter suggesting that "all state-run primary schools in the countryside should be run by the production brigades."[82] The letter argued that the intrinsic feature of collective-run schools (that is, the fact that they were run by the people) should also be applied to other aspects of life in rural areas, and the barefoot doctor initiative reflected this. In other words, there was a definite search for a medical model which would reflect the people-run aspect of Mao's ideology.[83]

On December 5, 1968, the *People's Daily* published an investigative report entitled "Cooperative medical service warmly welcomed by poor and lower-middle peasants."[84] It introduced the cooperative medical service of Leyuan Commune, Hubei Province, which was set up in December 1966.[85] The report described how the doctor Qin Xiangguan returned from the commune union clinic to his home brigade, where he set up the cooperative medical service. To finance the program, each commune member personally submitted one *jiao* (RMB 0.10) to the cooperative medical service fund, which production teams matched, totaling two *jiao* for each person. A management committee was established, consisting of commune cadres, representatives of the poor and lower-middle peasants, and commune union clinic doctors, who were sent down to work on the production brigades. When commune members sought treatment, they only had to pay five *fen* (RMB 0.05) as a registration fee, after which their medicine was free.[86] Therefore, the Leyuan program was in essence the health care equivalent of a "people-run school." The *People's Daily* held the Leyuan program up as a model for the whole nation, even after it suffered a serious financial crisis that nearly led to its dismantlement just two months after it was established.

Thus, barefoot doctors and cooperative medical services addressed the needs for medical personnel and funding for health care in rural areas, respectively, in a way that accorded with Mao's ideology and the strategy of the Cultural Revolution. Potential barefoot doctors were usually selected from commune members in the villages. After receiving basic medical training, they returned to their home villages to preside over the cooperative medical service stations, which were supported by the medical fund. As such, these cooperative medical service stations became fixed venues from which barefoot doctors operated, using medical kits purchased by production brigades (i.e., villages). In this way, the structure of the state medical system underwent a massive downward extension to the village level, as compared with the union clinic model. As official propaganda claimed, barefoot doctors and cooperative medical services were "great inventions made by poor and lower-middle peasants to combat diseases by depending on collective forces." Moreover, they "solved the problems of poor and lower-middle peasants seeking doctors, medicines, and health care."[87]

Under these circumstances, the government initiated a nationwide campaign to promote these "newly emerged things," notably through wide-scale media propaganda.[88] At the same time, various party and revolutionary committee documents instigated the establishment of barefoot doctors and cooperative medical services all over China.[89] Learning from model villages (those that implemented policies exceptionally well) was another key method of promoting these "newly emerged things." So great was the fervor that the report on Leyuan's medical program inspired that, only a few days after it was published, Qin Xiangguan and his fellow villagers in the snow-covered mountains were surprised to find that a delegation from Hebei Province had arrived in their village on horseback, headed by the vice governor, to learn from Leyuan's experience.[90] Wang Guizhen, now the representative of Jiangzhen Commune, made a speech about how barefoot doctors served peasants in front of thousands of people at a public rally in Shanghai.[91] Though the pace at which the barefoot doctor program spread through China varied, it was generally quite rapid. For example, by 1970 there were 11,152 barefoot doctors and 3,681 cooperative medical stations in Hangzhou Prefecture serving 83.6 percent of the total production brigades.[92]

Reconstructing the New Medical World of Socialist Villages

Like his family prior to the liberation, Chen Hongting was very influential in Jiang Village under the new regime. The commune party secretary Weng was a close friend of his, and they often had dinner and drank together at Chen's home. Party committee member Shen even borrowed money from Chen Hongting, whose high salary enabled him to lend. Sometimes the commune party committee conference and commune cadre meeting convened at Chen's clinic, and Chen himself was once selected to be the Township Committee member for Jiang Village.[93] However, Chen could not hide from the successive waves of political campaigns. In 1962, the commune committee confiscated radios belonging to Chen Hongting and Shen Ahmei, another founding member of the Jiang Village clinic, because they had been listening to enemy radio broadcasts from Taiwan. The commune returned the radios after the two doctors wrote self-criticisms.[94] By the outbreak of the Cultural Revolution in 1966, the Jiang Village Union Clinic was still located in Chen Hongting's house, and Chen himself was still in charge of daily operations. But in contrast to previous campaigns, the Cultural Revolution would soon cause the clinic and its staff to experience tremendous revolutionary upheaval.

These events were witnessed by Shen Xianbing, who was the clinic's accountant from 1962 to 1996. Jiang Village Commune was greatly influenced by the factional fighting in nearby urban Hangzhou. Villagers were brought fully into the revolutionary turmoil. According to Shen Xianbing, the villagers debated which faction they should support, Red Storm (*hongbao*) or United Headquarters (*lianzong*)—discussions so heated that they carried on from dinner into bed.[95] In Jiang Village Clinic, a large slogan was painted in yellow characters on a red background on the wall which read "Holding up the great flag of Mao Zedong Thought and striding bravely." As Shen recalled, "Our clinic did not have the money to buy red paint. We used pig blood and red powder to write on the walls and gate of our clinic. At that time, there were so many red flags in the street of Jiang Village that it was an ocean of red. The district health clinic distributed *Quotations from Chairman Mao* to each clinic staff member. We were not allowed to say 'buy.' We had to say 'invite.'"[96]

In 1966, a rebellion took place at the clinic. It was led by Chen Zhicheng, a young Chinese medicine doctor who was apprentice to Zheng Buying and the nephew of Chen Hongting.[97] This internal rebellion, which was supported by Red Guards from Hangzhou urban areas and local villages, overthrew Chen Hongting as clinic manager. He was criticized as being "the district director of the Nationalist Party," a "member of the Three People's Principles Youth League," and "a power holder," because he was in charge of the union clinic.[98] After being stripped of his position, Chen was forcibly paraded through the streets wearing a dunce cap, and his monthly salary was cut from RMB 80 to RMB 40.[99] Zheng Buying was accused of having served as a "Nationalist district secretary" and criticized for a year. In 1967, he died as a result of "criticism" and "struggle" (*pidou*).[100] Shen Ahmei, an acupuncturist specializing in heat stroke and one of the five founding members of the clinic, was accused of having both a "bad political origin" and for allegedly listening to Taiwanese radio broadcasts. He was escorted to parade barefoot through the village.[101] Another clinic member, Chen Naixing, was accused of supporting reactionary speeches and for being eager to do private medical practice. All the accused men's houses were also searched. In Chen Hongting's house, a land inventory, land contracts, and high-quality clothes were discovered, while in Shen Ahmei's house, cotton, liquid medicine, and gauze from the hospital were found, along with RMB 100 in cash. The search of Chen Naixing's house revealed mercury and medicines, some of them extremely poisonous.[102] Chen Naixing and Shen Ahmei were sent down to production brigades to serve as barefoot doctors.[103] During this period, Xu Aher, the first newly trained midwife of Jiang Village Union Clinic and its only Communist member, was appointed to take charge of the clinic's daily operations. However, she was dismissed with the beginning of the Cleansing Class Enemies campaign in 1968, when it was disclosed that her husband had been a secretary of the Nationalist district committee.[104] She was ordered to go to a production brigade to raise chickens.[105] In October 1968, a Revolutionary Leadership Team was set up in Jiang Village Union Clinic, of which rebel leader Chen Zhicheng became the director, a position he held until the end of the Cultural Revolution in 1976.

In the days that followed the rebellion, Chen Hongting "treated patients in the daytime and wrote self-criticisms by night in preparation for criticism meetings held by the clinic." He ended up as an ordinary medical staff member at the clinic until his retirement in 1979.[106] His nephew Chen Zhicheng, the new revolutionary leader, "treated patients in the morning and cleansed class enemies in the afternoon."[107] The remaining clinic members congregated to read *Quotations from Chairman Mao* before they began work each morning and read newspapers and reported their thoughts to the clinic in the evening. In early 1969, Chen Zhicheng began preparations to establish the cooperative medical service. Later that year, the Jiang Village Commune held a Chinese Communist Party member representative meeting, which was attended by five to six hundred party members and production team leaders. At the meeting the commune called on the masses to launch the cooperative medical service, in which the cadres mobilized villagers to participate once they had returned to their home brigades.[108] The cooperative medical service started formally in Jiang Village in 1971, after a year of preparation.[109]

While such internal changes were taking place in the union clinics, the Cultural Revolution also completely changed the union clinic model itself. First, the union clinics were renamed commune clinics, and Communist Party branches were systematically set up within them.[110] Second, the financial system was changed from one in which each clinic had sole responsibility for its profits and losses to a system that was subsidized by local commune finances, at which point the state began to supply medical equipment.[111] It was subsequently pointed out that "enforcing commune clinic construction was an important measure in implementing Chairman Mao's June 26 Directive."[112]

Meanwhile, the identities of the union clinic doctors also changed. Because union clinics were collective entities with no state funding or subsidies, some union clinic doctors were also commune members in the villages. As a result, they all had rural household identities and could not enjoy a number of welfare benefits that were provided to workers and staff of state-owned enterprises and agencies, who had urban household identities. However, the government decided that all official medical workers in commune clinics would attain urban household status and enjoy state benefits, except those with serious historical and political faults.[113] The changes to clinic names, the establishment of Communist Party organizations, financial investment, and the granting of "urban household" status to union clinic doctors, comprehensively incorporated the union clinics into the state medical systems. As the second-tier medical units above the barefoot doctors in the villages, union clinics were strengthened, while barefoot doctors replaced the clinics model as the front line in medical and health work.

The Cultural Revolution had a tremendous impact on the plural medical systems of rural China. No matter how healers were reorganized or recategorized after 1949, private medical practitioners not associated with union clinics continued to exist. However, with the outbreak of the Cultural Revolution, private medical practitioners were criticized as being the "wind of individual work"(dan'ganfeng) and the "tails of capitalism"(zibenzhuyi weiba). They were then either incorporated into the state medical system or forbidden from practicing medicine. During the Cultural Revolution, there were no longer any private medical practitioners in any of the other six counties of Hangzhou Prefecture. In Yuhang County, however, fifty-nine private medical practitioners still remained, but they were subjected to close surveillance.[114]

Like professional medical practitioners, folk healers also experienced great changes. As mentioned earlier, before the mid-1960s, herbalists, bonesetters, snake doctors, and heat-stroke acupuncturists were important medical providers for villagers because of medical traditions and customs. After the Cultural Revolution broke out, the official instructions pointed out that "in order to consolidate and develop the cooperative medical service and enlarge the medical group, the folk healers in the rural areas should be organized."[115] Folk healer Shen Fengxiang's grandson, Shen Jinrong, who learned medical skills by following his grandfather from the age of 14, later participated in rural medical and health work and attended many training classes to improve his medical proficiency during the Great Leap Forward campaign. Like his grandfather, his expertise included treating heatstroke and joint problems, and bonesetting. In 1969, he was selected as the barefoot doctor for Shentankou Village.[116] The incorporation of folk healers into the barefoot doctor program consequently legitimized folk medicine. In theory, they became the barefoot doctors' instructors in folk (or indigenous) medical knowledge, while the barefoot doctors became agents for continuing folk medicine in the villages.

Meanwhile, the local government smashed temples and statues and denounced so-called feudal and superstitious behaviors, prohibited healers from supernatural and religious sects, and eradicated their practices for being "superstitious." In Jiang Village, the man known as the "living Buddha" was one of those who were severely criticized during the Cultural Revolution. Commune cadres put him at the prow of a boat they rowed along a canal near the commune's fields while they beat drums to attract the attention of commune members who were laboring there, to his humiliation.[117] Similarly, the Yuanjue Temple, which was located near the center of Jiang Village, was completely destroyed, while the Temple of Lord Jiang was dismantled and reconstructed as a commune machinery factory.[118] The nuns and monks were forced to return to secular life (*huansu*), and the land that had been allocated to them was confiscated. Chen Zhicheng, the rebellion leader and new director of the commune clinic, could no longer enjoy the delicious vegetarian food cooked by the old nuns.

Accompanying the internal changes within the rural medical world, the outbreak of the Cultural Revolution brought external changes that came to affect the village medical world. The medical systems of rural and urban China in the 1950s and 1960s were still fundamentally different, in that they conformed to traditional and modern practices, respectively. The governments made efforts at one point to introduce urban medical personnel and facilities into rural areas by sporadically sending out mobile medical services, but the results of these initiatives were quite limited. Prior to the Cultural Revolution, far fewer than half of China's county seats, let alone their outlying rural villages, were served by urban medical teams.[119] Furthermore, until the mid-1960s, few medical graduates from urban areas were assigned to rural medical and health agencies.

After the Cultural Revolution commenced, these outreach measures were resumed and emphasized, in keeping with the new political ideology. Urban medical graduates were assigned to rural areas, and urban doctors were "sent down" (*xiafang*) to rural areas (either temporarily or permanently) following Mao's instructions for "educated youth to go to rural areas to be reeducated by the poor and lower-middle peasants" and "stress rural areas in medical and health work." According to Mao's instructions, the Zhejiang Revolutionary Committee decided in 1968 that "medical graduates should be assigned to the people's commune clinics to serve the rural medical and health-care agencies in mountainous and remote areas. In general, they should not be assigned to medical and health agencies at the county level or above."[120] A former official of the Hangzhou Prefectural Health Bureau by the surname of Wu, who graduated from Zhejiang Medical University in Hangzhou in 1967, recalled that no graduates were assigned jobs in urban areas that year. A total of 320 students from 10 graduate classes were sent down to rural areas; he himself was sent down to Shaanxi in northwestern

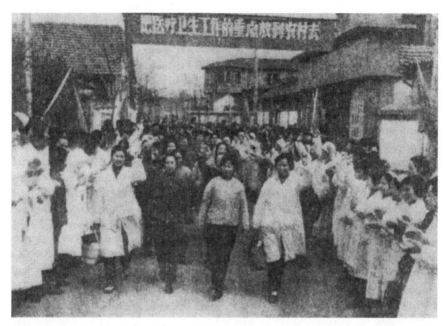

Figure 1.1. Hangzhou urban medical personnel leaving for rural areas to implement the revolution. *HZRB*, March 18, 1972. Reproduced with permission.

China.[121] As part of this sending-down policy, in 1971 the Hangzhou Prefecture government planned to mobilize 50 percent of the medical personnel in urban areas to go to work in the countryside, either permanently or on two-year rotations.[122]

However, the real history and practice of sending down is more complicated than official discourse suggests. Urban medical personnel were not willing to be sent to rural areas because it meant the loss of status, financial security, access to the benefits of urban life, as well as separation from family and the knowledge that their painful new rural resident status would be inherited by their children.[123] When the Hangzhou City No. 4 Hospital discussed who should be sent down to the countryside, some staff complained that "it is alright to discuss this topic during meetings of Communist Party members and cadres, but it is really very difficult to discuss this openly." When hospital colleagues recommended that one doctor go to the countryside, he became very angry and shouted,"Why are you happy about my suffering?"[124] More importantly, the selection of candidates to be sent down was closely entangled with the political power struggle inside the medical units. Wu said that when one faction captured political power in a medical unit, the faction it had overcome was asked to go to work in a rural area. These prospective sent-down medical staff could not protest because Mao had specifically instructed emphasizing medical and health work in rural areas.[125] Eight sent-down doctors wrote complaint letters to Hangzhou revolutionary committees that confirmed Wu's description. They complained that the leader of some medical units used implementing Mao's June 26 Directive as an excuse to exile new and rebellious cadres to rural areas. For these reasons, the sending-down plan changed repeatedly. After these periods of persuasion and mobilization, a total of 230 medical personnel were sent to rural areas in March 1972, the first and only batch of medical personnel from urban Hangzhou sent down during the Cultural Revolution.[126]

The incomplete statistical data of 1965–74 reveals the complexities inherent in the sending-down process (see table 1.1), which current scholarship does not describe in detail.[127] In terms of destinations, the majority of the roughly 360 sent-down urban medical personnel from Hangzhou's prefectural medical units were sent to Hangzhou's suburban counties, including

Table 1.1. Statistical data of sent-down medical staff of hospitals at county level and above working in rural commune clinics in seven counties within Hangzhou Prefecture, 1965–74 (unit: clinic and person)

County	Commune clinics		District clinics		County hospitals
	Clinic numbers	Number sent down	Clinic numbers	Number sent down	Number sent down
Xiaoshan	56	73	5	74	
Yuhang	49	0	9	43	
Fuyang	38	0	4	70	Fewer than 100
Lin'an	45	0	1	8	51
Tonglu	30	1	8	14	
Jiande	37	22	6	0	
Chun'an	53	0	6	0	39
Total	308	96	39	209	
Average		0.31		5.6	

Sources: Hangzhoushi weishengju [Hangzhou Prefecture Health Bureau], "Hangzhou diqu nongcun shengchan dadui shengchandui weisheng zuzhi qingkuang" [Survey of health organizations in production brigades and production teams in Hangzhou Prefecture], 1974, HZA, vol. 87-3-298; Yu, *Chun'anxian weishengzhi*, 20; Xu, *Fuyangxian weishengzhi*, 17–18; Lin'anxian weishengzhi bianzhuan weiyuanhui, *Lin'anxian weishengzhi*, 26–27.

Xiaoshan, Yuhang, Fuyang, and Lin'an. The mountainous counties far from Hangzhou's urban areas, including Chun'an, Jiande, and Tonglu Counties, received only about 130 sent-down doctors. Furthermore, the distribution of urban medical personnel was uneven: medical staff members were basically sent to district clinics and county hospitals. Commune clinics had few medical staff members—indeed, there was only one sent-down urban doctor in the commune clinics of five counties. In terms of the gender balance, more women urban medical personnel with lower designations were sent down than men. Of these, nurses ranked the highest, comprising 32 percent of the total sent-down medical personnel.[128] The urban doctors who moved to district clinics and county hospitals did not remain there for very long, either. According to local gazetteers, thirty-nine and one hundred medical personnel from urban Hangzhou were sent down to Chun'an and Fuyang counties, respectively, in 1972.[129] Three years later, twenty-seven and seventy of them had left the two counties and returned to Hangzhou's urban area.[130] There was only one sent-down urban doctor in the Jiang Village Commune Clinic during the entire Cultural Revolution period.[131]

Compared with sending down urban doctors, dispatching mobile medical teams to rural areas was much easier. Such deployments were regularly conducted by health bureaus at different levels, particularly during the summer harvesting and planting time in late July and early August. Deploying medical teams and sending down urban medical personnel to rural areas began to connect China's rural and urban medical systems. Urban medical personnel became major sources of Western medical knowledge in the villages, which the barefoot doctors then disseminated further.

The barefoot doctor program and cooperative medical services fulfilled the designs for state medicine that had been proposed by the Nationalist government and the Rural Construction Movement in the early 1930s. The difference between the policies of the Chinese Communist Party and the Nationalist government lay in their attitudes toward plural medical systems. For the Nationalists and the Rural Construction Movement, the goal was to establish a new modern medical system in the villages without utilizing existing plural medical systems. This policy was based on Nationalist ideologies and strategies as well as its capacity to impose reforms in the countryside. Likewise, followers of the Rural Construction Movement intentionally aimed to avoid conflicts with the existing system in order to sustain the operations of their social experiment.

In contrast, the Chinese Communist Party constantly reorganized the existing plural medical systems in order to build the state medical system. The pace and nature of these changes depended on variations in state coercive forces and the impacts of various political campaigns. From the birth of the union clinics in the early 1950s to the advent of the barefoot doctors in 1969 and 1970, the gradual establishment of the state medical system was based on the constant reorganization of healers under the plural medical systems. The union clinics, which were formed by registered professional medical practitioners, were the first centers of this dynamic process. The Cultural Revolution finally propelled the incorporation of the entire plural medical systems into a state medical system. Former peasant health workers were reevaluated according to revolutionary ideology and strategy, given the new title of "barefoot doctors," and accorded advantageous positions within the reconstructed rural medical world.

The health implications of the advent of the barefoot doctors were three-fold. First, barefoot doctors became agents for the introduction of modern medicine into China's villages while continuing to provide villagers with access to traditional medicine. This situation forced the two types of medicine to confront each other and interact. Second, the barefoot doctor program signified the implantation of an institutionalized and hierarchical medical network in the villages. This process correspondingly transformed a previously isolated medical world and the medical encounters and medical community structure of which it was composed. Third, barefoot doctors were situated in the social and medical context of a political campaign and developed a new medical profession while forming a new medical identity from scratch in the villages. Taken together, these developments enabled the barefoot doctors to fulfill the social transformation of rural medicine through the introduction of Western medicine and the marginalization of traditional medicine in Chinese villages across the spheres of knowledge, pharmaceuticals, healing, institutionalization, and professionalization.

Chapter Two

Revolutionizing Knowledge Transmission Structures

The healers who made up the plural Chinese medical world prior to 1949 followed long-standing traditions of knowledge transmission. These traditions were mainly either family based (parent-to-child transmission) or apprenticeship based (master-to-disciple transmission), and in both cases were confined to the local community. The personal nature of these transmission methods limited both the breadth of the dissemination of medical knowledge and the number of recipients of that knowledge. The People's Republic of China's newly established state medical system constantly reorganized existing plural medical systems, and the state sought to replace these traditional ways of acquiring medical knowledge to meet the demands of a modern, integrated national health program with more numerous medical personnel. The changes in the ways knowledge was transmitted were accompanied by the introduction of Western medicine into villages where Chinese herbal medicine had hitherto dominated, initially through Chinese medical practitioners and later through the barefoot doctors. This chapter contextualizes barefoot doctors at the confluence of Chinese and Western medicine and the new ways of transmitting medical knowledge, and it argues that the barefoot doctor program introduced Western medical knowledge into rural China at an unprecedented pace and therefore is responsible for the marginalization of Chinese medical knowledge.

Changing Ways of Knowing

In the social history of medicine in China up to the late imperial period, ways of transmitting medical knowledge are basically classified as either scholarly or nonscholarly.[1] Scholarly transmission refers to the ways that the literati or Confucian physicians obtained medical knowledge. Traditionally, there were three kinds of scholarly transmission: studying under masters, training within families, clans, and lineages, and self-study.[2] According to statistical data on physicians in Jiangsu, Zhejiang, and Anhui during the Ming dynasty, 101 healers obtained medical knowledge through self-study, 271 by studying under masters, and 769 through family training.[3] This evidence indicates that the family played the greatest role in the study of medicine in traditional Chinese society. Family medical tradition was also a key criterion of proficiency, as reflected in the proverb "Do not take medicine from a physician who is not a third-generation practitioner" (*yibu sanshi, bufu qiyao*). As a result, physicians emphasized their pedigrees through real or invented medical genealogies.[4] During the Ming and Qing dynasties, about 60 percent of practitioners with expertise in specific types or areas of healing came from families that had practiced medicine for at least two generations.[5] In turn, nonscholarly transmission describes the oral transmission of the medical knowledge of folk healers through practice within families, such as midwifery or the healing methods of religious and supernatural sects.[6] Villagers even believed that some healers obtained their skills from ghosts, the immortals, or unusual experiences. For example, fortune tellers in rural Hangzhou usually claimed to have gained mysterious powers following sudden accidents, like a serious illness.

Regardless of whether forms of learning were scholarly or nonscholarly, medical knowledge, techniques, recipes, and healing experiences were not readily shared.[7] Instead, they were often "jealously guarded and passed downed from generation to generation, because the monopoly on a cure ensured the continued patronage of patients, and thus a lucrative income."[8] Obviously, this greatly limited the recipients and scope of knowledge transmission, which was further limited because the various kinds of schools and lineages of Chinese medicine did not exchange knowledge or experience with each other in order to make progress. The founder of modern epidemic prevention in China was Wu Lien-Teh, known as the "plague fighter," who suppressed the pneumonic plague pandemic in Manchuria in 1911. A staunch advocate of modern medicine, Wu argued that the transmission feature of Chinese medicine was the main reason "the old-style Chinese medicine became more and more stagnant as time went on."[9]

However, great changes followed the beginning of formal education that resulted from China's broader move to modernize in the late nineteenth century. This development was particularly significant for the teaching and learning of Chinese medicine. In the 1930s, Chinese medicine schools appeared sporadically in the context of heated debate between practitioners of Chinese and Western medicine. The emergence of a professional association encouraged members to share private knowledge and break their ties to concepts of tradition and lineage to pursue collective goals.[10]

The different ways of knowing outlined thus far were reflected in the educational backgrounds of the healers in Jiang Village in the 1950s. Chen Hongting and three other founding members of the Jiang Village Union Clinic studied medicine under their fathers. Of the other founders, Chen Naixing had run a Chinese medicine shop called *Yinhetang* before liberation but was a doctor and had studied under the supervision of his master.[11] Sun Juzhuang was the only clinic founder to have graduated from the Chinese medicine school in Hangzhou. Folk healer Shen Fengxiang studied medicine under two masters: a monk who lived in the Autumn Snow Temple but was originally from a temple on Jiuhua Mountain, Anhui Province, and a Taoist from Tianjia Temple.[12]

The Communist regime disapproved on ideological grounds of teachers' private monopoly of knowledge.[13] Accordingly, the modes of medical knowledge dissemination in China entered a transition period after 1949, driven by the state's desire to increase the number and quality of practitioners. As part of these initiatives, in the early 1950s, granny midwives in Jiang Village were asked to take part in training classes on new delivery methods. Xu Aher, the granny midwife who had joined the village clinic, undertook the retraining program in the county seat in 1956. Meanwhile, the disciple system was integrated into the state-controlled education system in an effort to increase the total number of Chinese medicine doctors in the second half of the 1950s.[14] In 1955, four young men were selected to become Chinese medicine apprentices at the Jiang Village Union Clinic, but none of them were able to withstand the hardship this entailed. The first successful apprentice at the clinic was Chen Zhicheng, who was recruited in 1959 and started his training there in 1960 under Chinese medicine doctor Zheng Buying. Each day Chen Zhicheng got up at five o'clock, memorized textbooks, followed his master as he wrote prescriptions in the morning, and then read textbooks in the afternoon. After three years of this, he was permitted to treat patients alone. In the second half of 1963, Chen undertook an internship at Yuhang County No. 2 Hospital, where he studied under the supervision of an old Chinese physician.[15] Other newly recruited medical staff also received training in this way, like Zhu Shouhua, who was Chen Hongting's brother-in-law and the clinic's Chinese pharmacist. Although this style of training maintained the traditional master-apprentice relationship, it involved a significant shift in method, in that the trainees participated in hospital settings and had different mentors. Moreover, this model encouraged individuals to work with others in public, rather than private, learning modes. This apprenticeship method became the only way for union clinics to recruit medical staff by the early 1960s.

In 1965, Jiang Village Commune selected health workers for its twelve production brigades. They chose sixteen or seventeen students in total, usually two for each big brigade and one for each small one, and they attended two weeks of training classes in Chen Hongting's home.[16] This development in the selection and training of health workers was more significant than that of union clinic medical staff: it not only emphasized candidates' political origins but also adopted the classroom-based training method. As such, it changed traditional modes of knowledge transmission in the villages for the first time, though this work had still not been institutionalized by the late 1960s.

Chinese Medicine Doctors as
Agents of Western Medical Knowledge

Up to the mid-1960s, the medical knowledge structure within Chinese villages changed at a snail's pace. When Chinese medicine doctors had struggled against Western medicine doctors in a battle for state legitimacy in the 1930s, Western medicines were still largely unknown to most Chinese villagers. Even when the Nationalist government reluctantly granted Chinese medicine doctors legitimacy, they were still forbidden from using Western medical knowledge and techniques. The regulations for Chinese medicine doctors in 1933 stipulated that "Chinese medicine doctors shall not use scientific instruments, medicines, or injections."[17] The next year, the Nationalist government of Hangzhou City issued *Regulations for National Medicine Doctors*, which required that "national medicine doctors should not prescribe Western pharmaceuticals, should not use stethoscopes to diagnose patients, and should not give patients injections. Those who violate regulations should be punished by judicial organs, and their licenses should be revoked."[18] These measures were applauded at the time in an article from the medical journal of Guangji hospital, a missionary hospital established in Hangzhou in 1881: "the government cherishes human life and has strictly banned the use of Western medicine by Chinese medicine doctors. . . . Chinese medicine is Chinese medicine, while Western medicine is Western medicine. Chinese medical practitioners should not take the liberty of prescribing Western medicine and administering injection, just as Western medicine doctors should not currently serve as Chinese medicine doctors."[19]

Ironically, the People's Republic of China reiterated the same restriction in the early 1950s in, though it adopted "the unification of Chinese and Western medicine" (*tuanjiezhongxiyi*) in 1950 as one of the three health work principles at the First National Health Work Meeting with a goal of creating a single "new medicine." According to the Provisional Regulations Governing Doctors of Traditional Chinese Medicine implemented on May 1, 1951, a traditional Chinese medicine doctor was not allowed to prescribe chemically compounded medicines or give injections without scientific training in medical treatment, and under no circumstances was allowed to induce an abortion.[20] Chinese medicine was viewed as a "feudal society's feudal medicine that . . . needed to be transformed through strict controls on medical practice and reeducation of its practitioners."[21] Therefore, the new licensing regulations required Chinese medicine doctors to pass qualification examinations, which entailed extensive Western medical knowledge. Chinese medicine improvement schools were also established to improve Chinese medicine practitioners' political understanding and scientific techniques and disseminate theoretical and practical knowledge of Western medicine among them, in a program known as "Chinese medicine studying Western medicine."[22] Lecturers at these schools were usually doctors of Western medicine who offered a strong, condensed regimen of basic biomedicine (anatomic physiology, pathology, germs, medical history, and pharmacology).[23] Students also studied social sciences and preventive medicine (infectious medicine and public health), and they were encouraged to gradually develop toward preventive medicine and the scientificizing of Chinese medicine.[24]

The disadvantaged status of Chinese medicine was redressed with the initiation of "Western medicine studying Chinese medicine" in 1954.[25] All the same, daily epidemic prevention and treatment work, such as injections, rendered the dissemination of Western medical knowledge and techniques through Chinese villages irreversible. As the only available medical personnel, Chinese medicine doctors may have used some Western medicine techniques in daily medical practice and public health work. Therefore, traditional Chinese medicine doctors naturally became agents for the introduction of Western curative techniques and health education in Chinese villages.[26] Meanwhile, visiting mobile medical teams from urban areas also sporadically offered short training courses in particular areas of Western medicine to rural practitioners. Especially around 1965, these teams trained union clinic doctors as a kind of political task—that year, Zhejiang Health Department dispatched sixteen mobile medical teams to assist nineteen union clinics. For the first time, the young Chinese medicine doctors at these clinics learned first aid skills for the treatment of encephalitis, pneumonia, and dysentery, as well as how to make infusions, sterilize equipment, and operate on appendicitis.[27] All these modern techniques were quite new to the village medical world of the mid-1960s, and their instruction was effectively a process of dissemination of Western medical knowledge via students of Chinese medical colleges in urban areas.[28]

Interestingly, in contrast to the way in which doctors of Chinese medicine disseminated Western medical knowledge, Western medicine doctors were not particularly willing to study Chinese medicine. In 1958, this reluctance drew criticism from the Ministry of Health: "the majority of them [doctors of the first class of 'Western medicine studying Chinese medicine'] had been influenced by enslaving, bourgeois thoughts and were biased against Chinese medicine."[29] Furthermore, Chinese medicine doctors, particularly respected physicians, showed strong resistance to doctors of Western medicine expanding into Chinese medicine, as they felt that "the popularization of traditional medicine tended to degrade it" and "not anyone can be a traditional doctor."[30] The rapid demise of the private monopoly of medical knowledge after 1949 and the gradual introduction of Western medicine into Chinese villages formed the backdrop against which the barefoot doctors emerged.

Young, Gendered, and Educated Revolutionary Healers

The immediate source of candidates for the barefoot doctor program was the pool of former peasant health workers attached to the union clinics. When the barefoot doctor program and the cooperative medical service were first initiated around 1968 and 1969, former health workers were automatically redesignated as barefoot doctors in areas where health-care workers had been trained before the Cultural Revolution. In Jiang Village Commune, the group of health workers who had studied in Chen Hongting's union clinic in 1965—including Jiang Jingting (Mr. Cat-Dog), Shen Jinrong, and their peers from neighboring villages—were converted into barefoot doctors in 1968.[31]

However, the numbers of extant health workers was insufficient to meet the official directive that required each production brigade to have one or two barefoot doctors, so more needed to be selected. The family and personal political origins of potential barefoot doctors were particularly important: candidates were required to be healthy commune youths who were the indigenous sons and daughters of poor and lower-middle peasants. They had to have clean records and good political thoughts and be devoted to the collectivity and health work.[32] The selection procedure imparted a strong sense of revolutionary glamour in connection with these "newly emerged things." The official files for the Hangzhou area and other parts of China during the collective era of the 1970s record no significant changes to these selection criteria. The importance of maintaining the political purity and revolutionary sensitivity of the barefoot doctors was repeated again and again at all political levels.[33] When asked whether any sons and daughters of landlords and other "bad elements" could have been elected, Zhang Ahhua, a barefoot doctor of the Hejian Production Brigade inside Jiang Village, insisted that it was impossible. He explained that the five kinds of people with bad political backgrounds (landlords, rich peasants, counterrevolutionaries, bad elements, and rightists, all of whom had been the targets of political campaigns after 1949) lacked the correct social status to become barefoot doctors and added, "Anyway, I didn't know any barefoot doctors from these five elements."[34]

The selection procedure was set down in official instructions and included recommendation by a production brigade and approval by the communes. Young commune members who had just finished middle school were usually the ideal candidates to become barefoot doctors. The son of a former production brigade party secretary described the process as follows: "When we were given the order for every production brigade to select barefoot doctors, the brigades would send one or more of their members to study at the barefoot doctor training class. The brigade secretaries knew which guys had just graduated from school and seemed clever rather than stupid. So he decided that the brigade would send these guys to study medicine at the county hospital."[35] Shen Guanrong's experience was also quite dramatic:

> In the summer harvest and planting time in 1969, Doctor Chen, the director of the Jiang Village Commune Clinic, came to our village to do mobile medical services. One day, he said to me, "I find you clever and good at studying. I choose you to be a barefoot doctor. I will come to stay at your home. You will study medicine under me." He told our production brigade about this. He stayed and ate at my home for ten days. Then I studied for ten days under his guidance. Later, I followed Doctor Qie from the commune clinic doing mobile medical work for three months and studied medical books at the same time. Then I became a barefoot doctor in our village.[36]

Among these middle school graduates, young villagers who had some medical knowledge and skills were the perfect candidates for becoming barefoot doctors. Interestingly, villagers with physical disabilities or poor physical strength were also selected as candidates. During the 1970s, villagers engaged in agricultural labor were paid according to the daily work points (*gongfen*) they earned. As the work involved was strenuous manual labor, it was very difficult for disabled villagers to earn the normal work points, and life was obviously difficult for them. In contrast, barefoot doctors did less physical labor than those in the paddy fields, because they at least had time to sit down at medical stations. A barefoot doctor in Yuhang County admitted that "because my physical strength was poor, our brigade took care of me and arranged for me to come here to be a barefoot doctor."[37] During my fieldwork in Hangzhou Prefecture, I found three cases of people becoming barefoot doctors for this reason, including one in Jiang Village. The relative comfort of the job was also the reason priority was sometimes given to the relatives and friends of some production brigade cadres and villagers who had close relations with brigade-commune leaders or clinic doctors, instead of selecting barefoot doctors according to their abilities. Criticism of the unfair selection of barefoot doctors can be found in official files, particularly in the late 1970s.[38]

By 1970, Jiang Village Commune Clinic had selected a new batch of barefoot doctors, including Zhou Yonggan, Shen Guanrong, and Xu Shuilin. There was a revolutionary glamour to the selection procedure, which answered Mao's call to "stress rural areas in medical and health work," and demonstrated "clean political backgrounds for candidates participating in national programs." It further changed the traditional way of becoming a doctor or healer in China's villages and became the institutionalized mode of selecting health workers in the mid-1960s. The individual master-disciple relationship or family tradition no longer mattered. In Jiang Village, as Chen Zhicheng recalled, the Chinese medicine doctors who practiced before liberation were all from wealthy families. This was true of the five founding members of the Jiang Village Union Clinic. The Chen family was the most prominent family in Jiang Village: Chen's grandfather was an intellectual and had built a majestic house in the Tongzhi reign of the Qing dynasty. Likewise, Zheng Buying had been the secretary of Sandun District's Nationalist Party Committee, Shen Ahmei was a landlord, and Sun Juzhuang was nicknamed "Half-the-City Sun," as his family owned many shops and properties in urban Hangzhou. As Chen Zhicheng explained, the reason that doctors came from wealthy or elite families was that only they could afford medical training. After 1949, the literacy requirements for medical apprentices recruited by the union clinics were relatively high. Only well-off families could afford a school education for their children, while other villagers had to labor hard in the fields to earn work points to make a living. Chen Zhicheng came from the kind of family that could afford the "luxury" of medical study: his family owned a grocery store and was involved in business before 1949. After liberation, they were categorized as a "petty merchant" family, and their shop became the base for the Jiang Village Supply and Marketing Cooperative. Chen Zhicheng graduated from junior middle school in 1958 and studied for a year at senior middle school. At another time he might have continued his studies and become a doctor by the traditional route, but instead he dropped out because of the Great Leap Forward campaign.[39]

Compared with medical practitioners who started to practice medicine before 1949 and up to the late 1950s, the new selection criteria ensured that barefoot doctors came from ordinary rural families rather than the village elites as before. The scheme also quickly increased the number of people with medical knowledge in the villages, although it also lowered the threshold of medical education. Therefore, it remains a significant shift in the social history of medicine in both Jiang Village and China as a whole. The features that set barefoot doctors apart from existing professional Chinese medicine doctors and folk healers were their age, gender, and educational background, which are explored in detail in the following sections.

Age

When brigades selected commune members to be barefoot doctors, they wanted to ensure that these candidates would serve the brigades for as long as possible.[40] Surveys, interviews, and registration data for 156 barefoot doctors in Hangzhou Prefecture indicate that their ages when they became barefoot doctors ranged from 15 to 50 (see fig. 2.1). However, preference

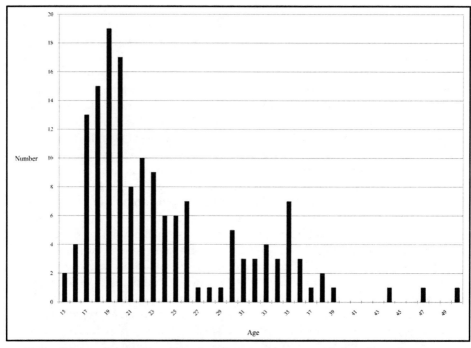

Figure 2.1 Age distribution of barefoot doctors (unit: person). Data from the barefoot doctor survey in Hangzhou Prefecture conducted from 2003 to 2005; Xiaoshanxian weishengju [Xiaoshan County Health Bureau], "1971 nian eryue tuijian qu hangwei xuexi mingdan" [The trainee list recommended to study in Hangzhou Health School in February 1971], XSA, vol. 25-1-38; Huanshan renmin yiyuan [Huanshan People's Hospital], "Fuyangxian chijiao yisheng fuxun dengjibiao" [Registration forms for Fuyang County barefoot doctor retraining class], October 1978, FYA, vol. 74-3-29; Gaoqiao renmin yiyuan [Gaoqiao People's Hospital], "Qingyunqu 1981 nian diyiqi chijiao yisheng peixunban huamingce" [Roster of the first barefoot doctor training class in Qingyun District in 1981], April 9, 1981, FYA, vol. 74-3-29; Sandunzhen zhongxiyi jiehe yiyuan [Sandun township of integrated Chinese and Western medicine], "Sandunzhen xiangcun yisheng qingkuangbiao" [Roster of village doctors in Sandun Township, Hangzhou City], January 17, 2005, SDA.

seems to have been given to young commune members aged between 17 and 20 who had just graduated from school and were not yet married and thus did not have as many family responsibilities as older members. The number of barefoot doctors surveyed that were from this age group was 60, amounting to about 41 percent of the total. The comparative youth of the barefoot doctors is revealed when these figures are compared with the ages of the union clinic doctors who had studied Chinese medicine before liberation and would go on to be trained in Western medicine. In Jiang Village, the founding members of the union clinic were mostly practicing Chinese medicine doctors in their mid forties, younger doctors who converted from apprenticeships like Chen Zhicheng were in their early thirties, but the barefoot doctors were only in their early twenties.

Gender

The selection of women as barefoot doctors was also significant. Women were in an inferior position relative to men as both healers and patients throughout the social history of medicine in China. The cohort of healers was male dominated in traditional Chinese society, particularly among professional healers.[41] There were some female physicians, but usually only in elite families.[42] In the villages, women healers were common, especially as midwives and practitioners of folk healing traditions. They were generally depicted as illiterate, ignorant, and unscrupulous in medical texts and in other writings (including novels), though in practice the importance of midwives during childbirth was widely acknowledged.[43] In Jiang Village, the founding members of the union clinic were all men and, though there were midwives in the village, they were not regarded as "doctors" by villagers.

As patients, women faced a number of sex-specific taboos in seeking treatment. Because of long-embedded traditions of sex segregation, a family member was expected to be present during a male doctor's consultation with a female patient. Male physicians were trained to deal modestly with female patients through diagnostic methods that included only limited physical contact.[44] It was extremely difficult for male physicians to communicate effectively with female patients, which hindered the possibility of correct diagnosis and treatment.[45] This phenomenon continued into the first half of the twentieth century. In an article about rural women's health, one author said, "if you had gone to the countryside, you would have met many women with pale faces and swollen eyes. All of them had gynecological diseases. . . . But they were constrained by traditional thoughts and believed that it is shameful to seek treatment. They would rather endure the infliction than struggle against the evils of their disease."[46] In the 1930s, when C. C. Chen was promoting a public health program in Ding County, he faced obstacles vaccinating girls and women, especially adolescents, who were ashamed of exposing their arms to a male vaccinator.[47] This continued to be a problem in villages during the 1960s and the 1970s, when women were too embarrassed to receive injections from male doctors or to let a male doctor press a stethoscope through their clothes and onto their chests. Gynecological checkups were simply unthinkable.

However, reproductive health was the most dangerous issue for women as a patient group. Both mothers and infants had high mortality rates before 1949. During the interviews I conducted, the old men often sighed when discussing this issue, saying that reproductive-age women in "the old society" always had one foot in the coffin. Some of the elderly women I talked to could not tell me how many babies they had given birth to, since the majority had died in infancy. Unassisted births were commonplace: as Granny He recalled, "I didn't need a midwife later. When my babies were due, I went upstairs and cut the umbilical cord myself."[48]

Reducing the high infant mortality rate caused by unhygienic and unscientific delivery methods was the first target the experimental rural health programs run by the Rural Construction School and the local Nationalist government, which therefore made the training of traditional birth attendants their key component. The reeducation of granny midwives was officially added to the agenda of the health-care program for the first time in the early 1950s to reduce maternal and child mortality.[49]

Women doctors were a powerful symbol of China's modernization and its aspiration since the early twentieth century of becoming a strong new nation.[50] However, large-scale training of female doctors was not initiated in the villages until the late 1960s. As described above, women villagers were extremely uncomfortable with being treated by male doctors, so training women doctors was important for the whole rural health program. From 1969 on, official instructions stipulated that each production brigade should have at least one female barefoot doctor. Besides basic general medical skills, these female barefoot doctors were taught new methods for delivering babies, family planning, and other obstetrical and gynecological work that was improper for male barefoot doctors to undertake.[51]

Despite official requirements, obstacles to women becoming barefoot doctors persisted, notably that the unwillingness of production brigades to send women to study medicine. In their opinion, since young female commune members would get married and move to their husband's villages sooner or later, their home brigade would not benefit from them in the long term. Married female commune members not only had to participate in labor, but they also were responsible for housework, so they did not have time to take on the extra work that barefoot doctoring entailed. As a result, there were generally fewer female than male barefoot doctors in the villages.[52] Nonetheless, women did begin to make some inroads into the barefoot doctor program. Seven women barefoot doctors were distributed over six of Jiang Village Commune's twelve production brigades in the 1970s, accounting for less than one-third of the total barefoot doctors. In addition to these female barefoot doctors, the health workers in Jiang Village production teams were mainly women.[53] In Hangzhou Prefecture, the percentage of female barefoot doctors ranged between 27.5 and 35.9 percent from 1974 to 1982 with an average of 33.3 percent.[54] Though men outnumbered women in the program, newly trained female barefoot doctors gradually replaced the aging granny midwives in delivering babies, while they also became the key force implementing the maternity and family planning programs in Chinese villages. In sum, the barefoot doctor program granted rural women equal rights to study medicine and facilitated the development of a fuller, broader public health program. The advent of female barefoot doctors also increased the number of women healers in the villages and transformed the gender balance of rural healers.[55] The frequent appearance of female barefoot doctors in revolutionary propaganda posters during the 1970s was a clear indication of the significant progress in gender and health, including the government's commitment and women barefoot doctors' roles.[56]

Educational Background

There is an old Chinese saying, *buwei liangxiang, bianwei liangyi,* which means "if a Confucian scholar cannot become a good official, he should become a good doctor." According to another old saying, *xiucai xueyi, longzhong zhuoji,* studying medicine is as easy for intellectuals as catching chickens in cages. The two sayings indicate the importance of educational background for elite medical practitioners. As reading texts was the main method of traditional instruction in medicine, trainees needed high literacy and educational levels, especially as traditional medical books were written in classical Chinese. Chen Zhicheng recalled that there were five textbooks: *Recipes in rhymes* (*Tangtouge*), *Drug properties in verse* (*Yaoxingfu*), *Rhymed formula for tongue* (*Shejue*), *Rhymed formula for pulse* (*Maijue*), and a text on anatomy. First he learned to recite them by heart, and then later he came to understand them little by little.[57] As such, the main obstacles to the wider dissemination of Chinese medicine in the villages were education and literacy levels. In contrast, these factors were not significant for the folk healers who dominated the rural medical world, as their medical knowledge was orally transmitted and their techniques were developed through practice.

However, within the new national health program, candidates' educational background and literacy levels directly determined the degree of medical proficiency they mastered and affected the medical service they provided. Educational qualifications also applied to other new and nonagricultural posts in the villages under the collectives, such as school teachers, tractor drivers, and members of the Experimental Team for Scientific Farming.[58] Education levels were therefore a practical issue considered by the production brigades when selecting candidates for barefoot doctor training: as the son of the production brigade party secretary explained, it was impossible to send a stupid or illiterate person to study medicine.[59] Luo Zhengfu, who became a health worker in 1965 and a Jiang Village Commune Clinic director in 1978, recalled that after the outbreak of the Cultural Revolution, educational background was emphasized as a selection criterion, primary education first and junior middle school later.[60] According to the registration data for of 144 barefoot doctors between 1978 and 1981 in Hangzhou Prefecture, 35.3 percent had completed only primary school while 65.6 percent went on to high school as well.[61] On average, these barefoot doctors had received seven years of education, roughly equivalent to a junior high school education, and none of them were illiterate. The barefoot doctors' levels of education may seem to have been very low in the hierarchy of the formal educational system by today's standards. However, as late as 1982, graduation rates for primary and middle school in the villages were 40.59 percent and 19.6 percent, respectively, while 39.58 percent of commune members in rural Zhejiang were illiterate.[62] In other words, barefoot doctors received far higher levels of education than their fellow villagers, including folk healers, who were basically illiterate, and former health workers (or half-peasant, half-doctors), who received only a primary education. The barefoot doctors' relatively advanced educational backgrounds determined their levels of success in absorbing Chinese and Western medicine.

Transgenerational Transmission of Medical Knowledge

The selection of barefoot doctors was in keeping with the proclamation in the People's Republic of China that medical study was no longer a personal or family matter, and this policy gradually increased the number of recipients of medical knowledge. Corresponding to the changes in candidate selection modes, knowledge transmission also followed a general trend whereby Western medicine was gradually introduced into China's villages and became increasingly embedded in village medical practitioners' knowledge base with each passing generation. So far this book has discussed the healers of Jiang Village beginning with Chen Hongting, a founding member of the Jiang Village Union Clinic, and continuing up to the arrival of a new batch of barefoot doctors in 1968–69. These healers can be categorized into four generations. Chen Hongting and the other four founding members of the clinic, including his father Chen Changfu, each studied Chinese medicine in traditional ways and started to practice medicine before 1949. The first generation of healers in Jiang Village, they absorbed Western medical knowledge into their daily practice after 1950. The director of the clinic after 1968, Chen Zhicheng, began studying medicine in 1959 by following his master, Zheng Buying. Chen Hongting's brother-in-law, Zhu Shouhua, started to work as a Chinese pharmacist disciple by following Chen in 1962. Chinese medical knowledge was transmitted within the clinic through the traditional master-disciple format, but Chen and Zhu's training differed from their masters' because Western medicine was also a compulsory subject. Anatomy was a key subject for

Chen Zhicheng, as indicated earlier, while Zhu learned to dispense Western medicine tablets in the pharmacy. Chen Zhicheng and Zhu Shouhua can be regarded as the second generation of healers.

As indicated earlier, the Jiang Village Union Clinic first undertook systematic health worker training in 1965, when the classroom training format replaced master-disciple knowledge transmission. These health workers were the third generation of Jiang Village healers. They absorbed Western medicine from Chinese medicine doctors in the union clinic, like director Chen Hongting, who had already acquired Western medical knowledge even though he was a Chinese medicine doctor. Chen Hongting gave lectures to these health workers on topics such as preventive medicine, endemic diseases, schistosomiasis, and malaria. Later, sources of medical knowledge for these healers diversified even further. As the best students of the first batch of sixteen to seventeen health workers trained in 1965, Luo Zhengfu and two other classmates were selected to study Western medicine for two years at Yuhang County Rural Doctor Training Class just after the outbreak of the Cultural Revolution in 1966. The three students then did one-year internships at Hangzhou City No. 1 Hospital in 1967, where they were required to familiarize themselves with each department. It is significant that this was the first time that Jiang Village healers had ever acquired medical knowledge in a modern hospital, outside the local community. More importantly, they studied Western medicine rather Chinese medicine. Upon completion of the course and their internships, the three returned to the commune clinic, where Luo worked in a surgical department, while his classmates worked in an internal medicine department and the department of obstetrics and gynecology, respectively. Luo Zhengfu recalled that they were asked to enhance the medical proficiency of the commune clinic.

As this first batch of health workers was not sufficient to serve the needs of the community, several young villagers were selected to join the barefoot doctor group in 1968–69.[63] These barefoot doctors became the fourth generation of Jiang Village healers. The sources and types of medical knowledge they received were radically diversified, as were the transmission modes. Zhou Yonggan started working as a barefoot doctor in 1968 and is still working in Jiang Village Township Hospital today. He recalled that "the training was made up of two parts: one was led by People's Liberation Army division no. 83013, quartered in nearby Liuxia Township, and one by Chen Zhicheng's commune clinic. Army doctors and health workers taught us. At that time, they answered Chairman Mao's call to 'stress rural areas in medical and health work.' In the commune clinic, Chen Zhicheng and Luo Zhengfu taught us."[64] According to Xu Shuilin, who studied medicine with Zhou Yonggan, "we studied simple theoretical knowledge and followed the military doctors, treating the soldiers. We learned medicine by putting it into practice. At the beginning, we had military training, followed by one or two weeks of medical study, including rural health knowledge and Western medical knowledge." He still remembers how Chen Zhicheng used white radishes to teach them acupuncture in the commune clinic.[65] Shen Guanrong started to work as a barefoot doctor somewhat later than Zhou and Xu. In contrast to their experiences, Shen mainly studied medicine in Jiang Village at the beginning of his training. As described above, he studied medicine for three months under the guidance of Doctor Qie, who had just returned to the commune clinic from Hangzhou with Luo Zhengfu.[66]

As such, up to 1970 barefoot doctors studied medicine in Jiang Village primarily through transgenerational transmission, though their instructors from the commune clinic had already started to leave the villages to absorb Western medical knowledge. After 1970, however, medical study was no longer confined to the local community. First, three barefoot doctors were selected to study at Yuhang County People's Hospital. Among them, Zhou Yonggan was required to study surgery, and other two learned about the five sense organs and internal medicine, respectively. Six months later, before they returned to the commune clinic, they each had to choose another person to take up the training positions they were vacating.[67] In the following years, new barefoot doctors filled these vacancies, and all of them went on to study at Yuhang County Health School or Yuhang County People's Hospital. According to Luo Zhengfu, they all studied Western medicine.[68]

In Hangzhou Prefecture, county barefoot doctor training classes took various forms, particularly in the early 1970s. However, they became more and more formal and standardized in the mid- to late 1970s. According to the training syllabi, there were basically three types of courses, which lasted three, six, and twelve months, respectively. Subjects fell into four categories: politics, labor, military training, and medical training. Each week, there were forty-two periods, including two periods for politics, two for military training (physical education), two for labor, five to seven for self-study, and twenty-eight to thirty-two for medical training, which accounted for about 70 percent of the total. Course lecturers were usually Western medicine doctors from county hospitals, health schools, and urban medical teams, so the barefoot doctors received systematic Western medicine training. By this point, commune clinics were no longer the source of medical knowledge for barefoot doctors. Instead, their role was to supply internship opportunities for barefoot doctors, while the medical staff became their mentors for their practice of medicine.

Compared with the introduction of Chinese and Western medical knowledge into the villages, the transmission of folk medical expertise continued to follow more traditional modes of learning. As indicated earlier, after the postliberation reshuffling of China's rural medical systems, folk healers were

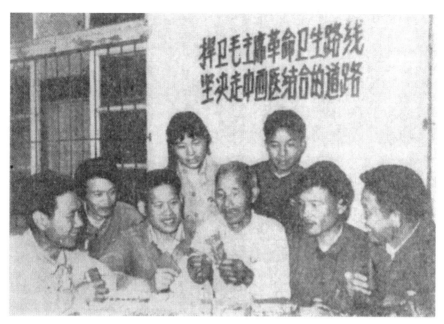

Figure 2.2. Barefoot doctors and a commune clinic doctor. The Chinese characters on the wall in the photo may be translated as "Defend Chairman Mao's revolutionary health route by resolutely following the path of the integration of Chinese and Western medicine." *ZJRB*, July 8, 1971. Reproduced with permission.

given legitimacy and incorporated into the medical stations. In Jiang Village Commune, Shen Jinrong the folk healer specializing in heat stroke and bonesetting became the barefoot doctor of his home village. He was also the only folk healer among the barefoot doctors of Jiang Village. Although he applied his special medical expertise when treating his fellow villagers as a barefoot doctor, he did not share this knowledge with his peers, as the revolutionary discourse incited barefoot doctors to do during this period. However, he did pass on his knowledge in a different way. On the Wulian Production Brigade was a young barefoot doctor named Hong Jinglin, who had been a classmate of Luo Zhengfu at the Jiang Village Union Clinic under Chen Hongting in 1965. Hong was in his early twenties in 1970, while Shen was already in his midforties. Shen's wife recalled that her husband regarded the young Hong Jinglin as an honest, hardworking, and reliable person, so he arranged for his daughter to marry Hong Jinglin. During daily practice, Shen unreservedly taught Hong the Shen family medical skills, including heat-stroke acupuncture, bonesetting, bloodletting, and techniques for treating injuries and fractures.[69] Though there is a proverb that says "teach the son rather than the daughter, and teach the daughter-in-law rather than the younger brother" (*chuanzi bu chuannü, chuanxi bu chuandi*), Shen Jinrong transmitted his specialist medical knowledge to an outsider who had been "converted" into a family member. This conservative transmission contrasted with the wide introduction of Western medicine into Chinese villages via school training and medical textbooks.

Unified Medical Readings and Contents

While the methods of knowledge transmission in villages had changed, medical publications became important channels for transmitting knowledge and sources for obtaining it. Indeed, scholars have argued that the emergence of medical publications signaled a change in the mode of transmission of medical knowledge, moving away from the ritualized initiation and apprenticeship of the master-disciple relationship toward published texts written for novice readers.[70] This expanded the range of people who had access to medical knowledge.[71] In the villages—regardless of whether we are talking about Chinese medicine doctors in union clinics with experience practicing medicine before 1949 or the Chinese medicine apprentices trained after the 1960s—medical books did play an important role in forming doctors' knowledge, as evidenced by Chen Zhicheng's list of compulsory reading described above. However, the supply and dissemination of such books was limited. Until the late 1950s, there were still no systems for publishing and distributing medical textbooks nationwide. Other kinds of healers, especially folk healers, relied almost entirely on experience to transmit their knowledge, and books played only an insignificant role, partly because so many of these healers were illiterate.[72]

Such informal dissemination methods were obviously unsuited to a nationwide program. This program needed a unified body of knowledge to promote a health program nationwide at the quickest possible pace. With the advent of the barefoot doctors, all of whom were at least partly literate, textbooks that specifically targeted them were soon widespread. At least eight such textbooks had been published and distributed nationwide by 1970,[73] and a total of twenty-one were published between 1969 and 1981, according to the catalogue of the National Library of China.[74] These numbers do not include texts published by prefectures or the counties. For example, in southern China, Jiangzhen Commune Health Clinic of Chuansha County, Shanghai Municipality, published four editions of *Training textbooks for barefoot doctors*, which were used for training, retraining, revision, and reference, though there were no significant variations to its contents over the four editions.[75] In rural Hangzhou Prefecture, at least one edition of this textbook was widely used by barefoot doctors during the 1970s. In addition, the Hangzhou Health Revolutionary Committee published *The manual for workers and peasants' medical and health care* and *The manual for barefoot doctors* shortly after the program was first promoted in 1969.[76] Meanwhile, national and provincial journals for barefoot doctors also appeared, such as the *Journal of Barefoot Doctors* and the *Journal of Zhejiang Barefoot Doctors*. Articles were usually written by physicians from urban hospitals, while some barefoot doctors exchanged their clinical experiences in medical practice.

Corresponding to the increasing range of medical publications for barefoot doctors, there were also special distribution methods for medical books. During the 1970s, the county health bureau issued one barefoot doctor training textbook free to each production brigade medical station and commune clinic. Meanwhile, county hospitals, county epidemic prevention stations, district clinics, commune clinics, and county worker-peasant-soldier schools were given barefoot doctor textbooks for training purposes.[77] The postal system enhanced the circulation of journals and ensured that they reached the barefoot doctors in a timely fashion.[78] The increasing variety and number of medical publications, as well as the distribution methods, were unprecedented in the social history of medicine in China's villages and greatly facilitated the dissemination and exchange of medical knowledge. The books and journals became an important source of the barefoot doctors' medical knowledge in addition to their brief stints of medical training.[79] They effectively became the barefoot doctors' "bibles" in their daily practice.[80]

The textbooks were comprehensive and covered all basic topics in medical education, including public health and epidemic prevention, first aid, family planning, basic surgical skills, and human anatomy. In *The manual for barefoot doctors*, the pages dealing with these matters accounted for one-third of the book. The remaining two-thirds of the book cover medicines and the prevention and treatment of common diseases. The section on medicines includes both Chinese herbal medicine and Western medicine. Within the Chinese medicine section are descriptions of each medicine's properties, a list of common Chinese medicines used to treat different diseases, and patent medicines.[81] The Western medicine section lists common medicines, basic techniques for using them, and basic clinical data.[82] In addition, new healing methods were introduced for the first time during the Cultural Revolution and publicized extensively through these textbooks, notably new acupuncture techniques (*xinzhen liaofa*). The sections on common disease prevention and treatment focused largely on drugs but also covered internal medicine, surgery, gynecology and obstetrics, the five sense organs, dermatology, and pediatrics. In each section, common diseases were listed, followed by descriptions of symptoms and explanations of methods of diagnosis. Different methods of treatment—both Chinese and Western—were then listed, followed by methods of prevention. In general, the content of these books and journals was oriented more toward Western medical knowledge, though this was combined with Chinese medicine to a certain degree, as previous scholarship has claimed.

The Westernized Structures of
Hybrid Medical Knowledge Transmission

Chinese herbal medicine had long traditions of knowledge transmission in China's villages before the advent of the barefoot doctors, who inherited this knowledge on the ground in largely ad hoc ways. In contrast, it was only with the arrival of the barefoot doctors that Western medical knowledge was systematically transmitted on a large scale in the Chinese countryside. The Western medical knowledge transmitted via the barefoot doctors can basically be divided into theory and practical techniques, with the latter being more significant. First, basic diagnosis techniques were disseminated to the barefoot doctors, which included the use of blood pressure meters, thermometers, and stethoscopes, known as the "three old instruments" (*lao sanjian*). Second, basic operational skills were rapidly popularized in villages, including administering injections, performing disinfection, and preparing intravenous drips. Third, as a result of the changed gender structure of healers discussed above, new techniques and technologies related to reproductive health were introduced into the villages on a large scale via women barefoot doctors, such as the use of IUDs. A series of factors determined the formation of the barefoot doctors' medical knowledge structures in the context of continuing Chinese medicine and introducing Western medicine, including literacy, training time, and self-study.

Educational levels affected the structure of medical knowledge, as indicated in official reports of barefoot doctors overcoming the difficulties posed by their low educational levels. As Wang Guizhen, the first woman barefoot doctor, said in a report:

> I began working as a barefoot doctor in 1965. Before then, I had only studied for a few years and attended a brief medical training course for three or four months. My educational level was low and my elementary knowledge was poor. It goes without saying that I could not understand much of the content of the medical books. I could not even read some common medical terms . . . and my family members and relatives were also worried about me.[83]

However, the barefoot doctors' low literacy levels did not impede them from developing practical operational skills, such as administering injections, preparing intravenous drips, and dispensing medicines according to the illustrated instruction labels on the medicine bottles or by digging up herbal medicines. An old Chinese pharmacist by the surname of Shao, who worked from the late 1940s to the mid-1990s, first at his home pharmacy and later at the commune clinic, observed that the barefoot doctors mainly studied Western medicine. Though some of them bought books to study Chinese medicine themselves, it was an individual choice rather than a systematic program. In his opinion, the main reason for this was that Western medicine was relatively easy to learn in comparison to Chinese medicine.[84] As Scheid found, even Chinese medicine college students and Western medicine doctors who were studying Chinese medicine in the mid-1950s did not have the intellectual skill and patience to study medical books written in classical Chinese.[85] This factor favored the dissemination of Western medical techniques or skills into the villages.

Training time was another influential factor. Whether barefoot doctors received training at county hospitals or health schools, district and commune clinics, or even from army doctors, their primary training during the 1970s was not long. Course lengths ranged from ten days to a year. In addition to attending primary training sessions when they were first selected as barefoot doctors, candidates also received retraining later when they worked on production brigades. Shen Guanrong was an ordinary barefoot doctor in Jiang Village Commune. He received a total of 375 days' training, including three months of theoretical studies under the guidance of one commune clinic doctor and ten days under that of Chen Zhicheng, six months at the Yuhang County Health School, and a three-month internship at the commune clinic when he was a barefoot doctor.[86] Shen's study record was basically consistent with that of his counterparts in suburban counties of Shanghai Municipality. By August 1979, about eleven years after the popularization of the barefoot doctor programs, there were 1,041 barefoot doctors in Chuansha County, where the barefoot doctor program was first initiated. Among them, the majority had studied for only two to four months at commune clinics, while only 271 (26 percent) had received six months to a year of medical training in the county.[87] In Shanghai County, there were 751 barefoot doctors by 1982. Among them, 447 doctors (59.5 percent) had received less than five months of training, 218 (29 percent) had studied for five to eleven months, while 86 (11.5 percent) had studied for more than one year.[88] It should be pointed out that this was Western medical training.

Short-term training made theoretical and practical self-study an alternative way for barefoot doctors to acquire medical knowledge. As far as theoretical study was concerned, barefoot doctor Xu Peichun of Chun'an County, Hangzhou Prefecture, saved all the books he read since he started work in 1969 after one year of study. These include the *Textbook for Rural Health Workers*; *Common Medicine for Children*; *Preventing Respiratory Infectious Diseases*; *Common Chinese Herbal Medicines in Zhejiang Province*; *Pesticide Use and Poisoning Prevention*; *Manual for Health and Epidemic Prevention*; *Common Medicines Used by Barefoot Doctors*; and *The Population Must Be Controlled.*[89] The composition of his readings indicates that Chinese herbal medicines were no

Table 2.1. The knowledge structure of candidates for the Excellent Village Doctor award in China, 2005 and 2010

	2005						2010	
	Time of becoming barefoot doctors							
	Before 1983		After 1983		Total		Total	
Category	Number	%	Number	%	Number	%	Number	%
Western	94	64.8	38	69	132	66	147	73.5
Chinese	36	24.8	15	27.2	51	25.5	51	25.5
Integrated	13	8.9	2	3.6	15	7.5	1	0.5
Mongolian	1	0.7	0	0	1	0.5	—	—
Tibetan	1	0.7	0	0	1	0.5	—	—
Chinese-Tibetan	—	—	—	—	—	—	1	0.5
Total	145	100	55	100	200	100	200	100

Source: Zhonghua renmin gongheguo weishengbu [The Ministry of Health of the People's Republic of China], accessed June 20, 2005, http://www.moh.gov.cn/moh; "2010 nian quanguo youxiu xiangcun yisheng houxuanren mingdan" [List of candidates for the Excellent Village Doctor award in 2010], *Jiankangbao* [Health Care Newspaper], November 30, 2010.

longer a dominant topic. Meanwhile, their short-term medical training allowed barefoot doctors to read these books to gain new knowledge for their daily work while developing practical operational skills more readily, which was particularly significant for the introduction of Western medical skills into the villages.

In this way, all these factors—Western medical training, medical textbooks, study through practice, and self-study—furthered the Westernization of barefoot doctors' medical knowledge. In Jiang Village, all the barefoot doctors interviewed claimed that they were Western medicine doctors rather Chinese medicine doctors from the very beginning, though they also claimed that in the 1970s they knew a little about Chinese medicine. By 1995, there were 297 barefoot doctors in Yuhang County specializing in Western medicine, while only 60 specialized in Chinese medicine.[90] Among two hundred of the candidates selected by the Ministry of Health for the Excellent Village Doctor award in 2005, Chinese medicine doctors accounted for only one-quarter of the total number of barefoot doctors.[91] The percentage of Western medicine doctors increased year by year and reached 73.5 percent in 2010 (see table 2.1). However, the actual proportion of Western medicine doctors was undoubtedly much higher than this, as the government had to guarantee certain awards for those specializing in Chinese medicine, Tibetan medicine, and Mongolian medicine to make sure of the award's representativeness.

The Transformation of the
Medical Knowledge Structure in Chinese Villages

To understand the evolution of the medical knowledge structure in Chinese villages, it may be helpful to contextualize the Westernized medical knowledge structure of barefoot doctors within the transformation of medical knowledge that has taken place in rural China since the early 1950s. As the basic medical units of the state medical system in the countryside, the union clinics existed in the context of the gradual confluence of Chinese and Western medicine from the 1950s. According to the statistical data for selected counties in Hangzhou Prefecture (see tables 2.2–2.4), there was an average of 5.3 doctors per clinic during the 1950s, 63.7 percent of whom were Chinese medicine doctors. During the development of union clinics, Chinese medicine apprentices were recruited and trained in each county, like Chen Zhicheng.[92] Meanwhile, medical graduates and professional secondary school graduates who majored in Western medicine also joined the clinics sporadically. However, the personnel numbers for the two types of medicine did not expand evenly, and the medical knowledge structure of the union clinics quickly changed. At the start of the 1960s, the average number of staff members of union clinics had gradually increased to 6.15, but the percentage of these who were Chinese medicine doctors had declined to 42.5 percent.

After the popularization of the barefoot doctor program, the rural medical knowledge structure changed completely. Starting in the late 1960s, the union clinics of Hangzhou Prefecture were changed into commune clinics. The average number of doctors per commune clinic increased to 10.3 in the 1970s, while the proportion who were Chinese medicine doctors dropped to just 30 percent (the remaining 70 percent were listed as Western medicine doctors). Compared with the 1950s and the 1960s, the actual number of union clinic doctors specializing in Western medicine was still not very large, though it was increasing. However, by the 1970s each commune had an average of 25.7 barefoot doctors, which was 2.5 times greater than that of the commune clinic doctors. These large numbers of barefoot doctors therefore became a key factor in the shift toward Western medicine. More importantly, as discussed earlier, the barefoot doctors were usually quite young when they were selected, which gave them the advantage of time in acquiring modern medical knowledge. Therefore, the knowledge of the healers working within the state medical systems in China's village communities quickly came to be dominated by Western medical knowledge. This trend was further accelerated by the advance of Western pharmaceuticals into the villages throughout the

Table 2.2. Average number of medical staff members in commune clinics (or union clinics) of selected counties within Hangzhou Prefecture (unit: person)

County	1950s	1960s	1970s	1980s
Fuyang	5.3	5.7	9.6	12.9
Xiaoshan	5.3	6.15	10.4	16.5
Lin'an	5.2	6.6	10.8	
Hangzhou Prefecture		6.12	12	
Average	5.3			14.7
National average		5.8	13.9	

Sources: Xu, *Fuyangxian weishengzhi*, 68–69; Xiaoshan weishengju, *Xiaoshan weishengzhi*, 54–56; Lin'anxian weishengzhi bianzhuan weiyuanhui, *Lin'anxian weishengzhi*, 107–16; Hangzhoushi weishengju [Hangzhou Prefecture Health Bureau], "1965 nian weisheng shiye zonghe baobiao" [Comprehensive statistical health work form in 1965], HZA, vol. 87-3-262; "Hangzhou diqu nongcun shengchan dadui shengchandui weisheng zuzhi qingkuang" [Survey of health organizations in production teams and production brigades in rural areas of Hangzhou Prefecture], 1975, HZA, vol. 87-3-302; "Hangzhou diqu nongcun shengchan dadui shengchandui weisheng zuzhi qingkuang" [Survey of health organizations in production teams and production brigades in rural areas of Hangzhou Prefecture], 1976, HZA, vol. 87-3-307; Zhongguo weisheng nianjian bianweihui [Editorial board of China health yearbook], ed., *Zhongguo weisheng nianjian 1983* [China health yearbook 1983] (Beijing: Renmin weisheng chubanshe, 1983), 57.

Table 2.3. Percentage of Chinese medicine doctors in commune clinics (or union clinics) of selected counties within Hangzhou Prefecture (unit: percentage)

County	1950s	1960s	1970s	1980s
Xiaoshan	59%	29.45%	29%	19.4%
Lin'an	60.6%	47.33%	26.4%	22.7%
Yuhang	71.5%	50.6%	34.9%	17.9%
Seven counties		48.6%		
Average	63.7%		30%	20%

Sources: Xiaoshan weishengju, *Xiaoshan weishengzhi*, 54–56; Lin'anxian weishengzhi bianzhuan weiyuanhui, *Lin'anxian weishengzhi*, 116; Yuhangxian weishengju weishengzhi bianzhuanzu, *Yuhangxian weishengzhi*, 80; Hangzhoushi weishengju [Hangzhou Prefecture Health Bureau], "1965 nian weisheng shiye zonghe baobiao" [Comprehensive statistical health work form in 1965], HZA, vol. 87-3-262.

Table 2.4. Average number of barefoot doctors per commune clinic in selected counties within Hangzhou Prefecture during the 1970s (unit: person)

County	Average	Maximum (Year)	Minimum (Year)
Fuyang	28.9	36.5 (1977)	23.5 (1973)
Chun'an	24.7	33.7 (1976)	16.0 (1973)
Jiande	23.5	53.0 (1970)	12.0 (1975)
Average	25.7	41.6	13.8

Sources: Xu, Fuyangxian weishengzhi, 73; Hangzhoushi weishengju Hangzhoushi weishengzhi bianji weiyuanhui, Hangzhoushi weishengzhi, 87; Chun'anxian jihua weiyuanhui [Chun'an County Planning Commission], Chun'anxian guomin jingji tongji ziliao, 1949–1978 [Statistical data of Chun'an County's national economy, 1949–1978] (Chun'an: Chun'anxian jihua weiyuanhui, 1980), 333–46; Yan, Jiandexian yiyao weishengzhi, 70.

1970s. In this sense, the barefoot doctors thoroughly transformed the knowledge structure of healing in the villages.

The barefoot doctors' Westernized medical knowledge was also significant in the context of the broader historical and urban-rural gap. When Chinese medicine doctors fought for state legitimacy and against the abolition of Chinese medicine in the early 1930s, they outnumbered Western medicine doctors, not only in rural China but also in the cities. A 1935 survey found that 1,182 Western medicine doctors were practicing in Shanghai, compared to 5,477 licensed Chinese medicine physicians, not counting unlicensed Chinese medicine doctors.[93] However, the situation was changing rapidly in urban areas even before 1949. In the urban area of Hangzhou, which was the provincial capital city of Zhejiang Province in the Nationalist era, the 446 registered Western medicine doctors already outnumbered the 380 Chinese medicine doctors by 1949. Though the data are not complete, the figures here indicate that the knowledge structure of physicians in the Hangzhou urban area had been Westernized by the end of the 1940s. The uneven ratio of Chinese and Western medicine doctors kept increasing in favor of the Western-style practitioners. By 1958, the number of Western medicine doctors was twice that of Chinese medicine doctors, according to a relatively complete data set generated by the implementation of more standardized registration systems.[94]

By 1977, there were a total of 2,858 doctors in urban Hangzhou, which broke down into 2,549 Western medicine doctors and 309 Chinese medicine doctors. In other words, the number of Western medicine doctors was 8.2 times that of Chinese medicine doctors. Indeed, only about twenty prestigious old Chinese medicine doctors (minglaozhongyi) remained, only seven of whom were able to work.[95] In China as a whole, there were 361,000 Chinese medicine doctors and 234,000 Western medicine doctors in 1959. By 1977, the numbers of Western medicine doctors had grown to 738,000, or 2.2 times more, while Chinese medicine doctors had decreased by one-third to 240,000.[96] The significance of the barefoot doctors is that the medical knowledge structures of the villages caught up with trends in the urban areas, albeit twenty years later. This had the effect of closing the medical gap between rural and urban areas and finally fulfilling the state's goal of transforming the knowledge structure of medicine in China. In the meantime, Chinese medicine faced real survival challenges. An official document pointed to the critical situation Chinese medicine was in: "no new forces of Chinese medicine are trained, and the academic experience of old Chinese medicine doctors is not being passed on. Chinese medicine and pharmaceuticals are declining steadily, and there are no qualified successors."[97]

This chapter argued that the traditional ways of acquiring medical knowledge and becoming medical practitioners in rural China started changing gradually after 1949. No longer was the transmission of medical knowledge a personal or family matter. Instead, the selection requirements for medical trainees emphasized political origins and basic literacy. Meanwhile, Western medical knowledge was initially introduced into the villages through Chinese medicine doctors who disseminated both Western and Chinese medical knowledge. The advent of barefoot doctors enhanced and magnified this trend. Not only did the barefoot doctor program lead to the complete abandonment of the traditional transmission mode, it also greatly expanded the geographic scope of medical studies. In other words, in contrast to the existing Chinese medical practitioners from union clinics and the traditional folk healers who gained their knowledge locally, the barefoot doctors actually went outside their local communities to absorb medical knowledge, which was mostly related to Western medicine.

During this process, the barefoot doctors played a variety of roles in the introduction of modern medicine into villages and in continuing the practice of traditional medicine. Because of the barefoot doctors' limited literacy and training time and the availability of suitable self-study materials, the medical skills and techniques they were able to develop were mainly Western. Meanwhile, as we will see in the chapters to follow, this process was influenced by the proliferation of Western pharmaceuticals, which allowed the barefoot doctors to develop a Western-influenced medical knowledge structure. This trend was also accompanied by the transformation of healers through their acquisition of modern medical knowledge in commune communities, which began in the early 1950s and coincided with the natural aging of folk healers within local communities. Ironically, although Chinese medicine doctors served as the first agents for the introduction of Western medical knowledge into the Chinese countryside, these doctors faded away as a result of the spread of the very knowledge that they helped introduce into their own communities.

Chapter Three

Pharmaceuticals Reach the Villages

Infectious diseases dominated the disease model of China's villages, just as they did in many other societies prior to the advent of modern medicine. The main pharmaceuticals consumed in rural China were herbal medicines that were mainly gathered from the fields, although traditional nonherbal pharmaceuticals were also used. Together, they comprised two of the basic features of the plural medical systems of traditional village life. However, beginning in the early 1950s, modern Western medicines, vaccines, and medical instruments were introduced into the villages as the newly formed state pharmaceutical sales network extended its national reach. This chapter shows that, contrary to common perceptions of the barefoot doctor program that emphasize its promotion of Chinese herbal medicine, the program was actually crucial to the expansion of Western medicine among villagers. Even though the national government legitimated and promoted Chinese herbal medicine, the barefoot doctor program proved ineffective in expanding the use of herbal medicine in the countryside. The first large-scale encounter of Chinese and Western medicines in rural China—which took place in the context of a modern, innovative, revolutionary health-care delivery program—proved to be a crucial juncture in the history of the use of traditional pharmaceuticals.

The Social Epidemiology of Rural Hangzhou

Diseases in Chinese villages were closely related to the natural environment and the labor and lifestyle practices of rural people. The environment of Hangzhou Prefecture is typical of the Yangtze delta area and has four main geographical features: delta, swamps, mountains, and hills. The terrain of Jiang Village, according to descriptions from the local gazetteer, is high in the south and low in the north, and it belongs to a "swampy plain." Seven rivers wind through the commune, with a total length of 24.17 km, and fishing ponds are densely concentrated. Arable land accounts for only 45.71 percent of the total area, while water areas comprise 50.29 percent.[1] Average temperatures and rainfall are generally mild, with a rainy season that begins in May or June, and very hot and rainy weather from July to September. These geographical and climatological features facilitated the spread of disease.[2]

The natural environment affected the spread of disease mainly through the water and human and livestock waste. In Jiang Village and other parts of rural Hangzhou, livestock feces were the main base fertilizers, while human feces were the main top dressing fertilizers in agricultural production prior to the introduction of chemical fertilizers in the 1950s. According to statistical data on neighboring Lin'an County in the 1930s, human and livestock feces accounted for 58 percent of the total fertilizers used, which also included green manures and plant ashes.[3] For the convenience of daily agricultural production, uncovered buckets of feces were left alongside rivers, ditches, ponds, and brooks. Fecal-borne parasites spread into the water supply when feces spilled out of these containers on rainy days and because villagers used to wash their chamber pots directly in the village rivers and ponds.[4] The frequent coming and going of fishing boats and fishermen led to cross infection.[5] A running water supply system was not constructed until the mid-1980s, so water for daily use had to be fetched from these contaminated areas. As a result, intestinal infections and parasitic diseases were common, particularly in summer and after serious floods.[6]

In addition, the villagers usually labored barefoot in the rice paddies or fields, where they came in direct contact with water, moist soil, and feces containing parasitic diseases such as schistosomiasis, hookworm, and filariasis.[7] For example, it was a common practice for villagers to fertilize the base of mulberry trees with human feces two to four weeks before harvest. Since mulberry leaves are usually picked in the rainy season, the barefoot villagers come into direct contact with hookworms when they walked on the moist soil under the trees.[8] To combat the problems caused by contaminated water and improper disposal of human and livestock waste, the Two Controls and Five Reforms campaign (*liangguan wugai*) was initiated in the villages of the Yangtze delta from the 1950s onward with the aim of cleaning up wells, toilets, barns, and the environment in general.[9]

In the meantime, from the 1950s to the late 1960s, changes in cultivation patterns increased peasants' exposure to contaminated water and mud. In these decades, agricultural production in Zhejiang Province expanded greatly as dry land was turned into paddy fields and as single-cropping of rice was replaced by double-cropping, so that a total of three crops (two of rice and one of rapeseed or wheat) were grown each year. These changes in farming techniques increased peasants' contact with water, which in turn increased their vulnerability to certain kinds of diseases.[10] In 1965, Huang Yuguang, then director of the Hangzhou City No. 2 Hospital, went to the countryside to provide medical services with the urban medical team. Within seven months, he had operated on 107 infected legs and feet, including chronic cases of villagers who had suffered from their symptoms for more than twenty years.[11]

Besides labor styles, poor living conditions also contributed to the spread of diseases in the villages. Mosquitoes were commonplace in rural Zhejiang in the 1950s and 1960s. As a local gazetteer explained in the 1980s, "the living conditions of the masses are very poor. There are many mosquitoes and no mosquito nets."[12] According to the 1954 Zhejiang Province Mosquito Nets Survey, the 281 households surveyed had an average of only 0.84 mosquito nets each.[13] Moreover, Chinese peasants had very poor habits of hygiene and sanitation. Li Jinghan's survey of Ding County in northern China in the 1930s found the following depressing results: "They [the villagers] are not only the poorest people but also the dirtiest and weakest people in the world. You go to the villages and open your eyes, and you can see everything without needing a detailed survey. . . . Their yards, bedrooms, and toilets are very dirty. There is no clean food or water. . . . The peasants live in such a dirty environment apparently comfortably without giving any attention to the filth around them."[14] Li's description of the unsanitary habits of villagers in northern China was also true of villages in the Yangtze delta in the 1950s. Though the situation had improved somewhat by the 1950s because of hygiene education and the Patriotic Hygiene campaign, villagers' habits regarding food, water, and personal hygiene were inadequate. For example, it was still quite common for villagers to drink water without boiling it first.[15] Likewise, in the Yangtze delta, food rots quickly in the hot summer months and is easily contaminated by flies and mosquitoes. However, summer was the busiest time for villagers, as they had to harvest the first rice crop and plant the second within the half of a month between the "great heat" (dashu) and "the beginning of autumn" (liqiu), according to the twenty-four solar terms of the Chinese agricultural calendar. This process was called quick harvesting and quick planting (shuangqiang), and during it they had less time to pay attention to food hygiene. As late as the mid-1970s, a medical team from the Hangzhou Liberation Army Hospital found that Jiang Village commune members still did not pay adequate attention to dietary hygiene during these busy agricultural periods.[16] Because of these habits, intestinal tract diseases were rampant, especially dysentery, in the summer months.[17]

Even basic personal hygiene habits such as washing were not widespread. This was particularly unhealthy for children, who often played in the dirt inside houses, in yards, or in villages. As many did not wash their hands before eating or collecting food, worms entered their bodies easily.[18] As a result, intestinal tract diseases and ascariasis diseases were rampant among children.[19] As late as the 1950s, it was common for several family members to use the same towel and bowl of water to wash their faces in the morning, and some old villagers only did so once every four to five days.[20] The situation had only improved slightly by the 1960s and 1970s, when favus of the scalp, which was due to poor washing habits, was still common among the villagers.

All these factors contributed to the rampant spread of infectious diseases in rural Hangzhou and other parts of the Yangtze delta in the 1950s and 1960s. From 1950 to 1969, twenty-one acute infectious diseases were reported in Hangzhou Prefecture.[21] Smallpox was the first of these to be eradicated, in 1953, while kala-azar (visceral leishmaniasis) and relapsing fever were eradicated in 1955 and 1956 respectively.[22] Thus, by the time the barefoot doctors were popularized in the villages, 18 infectious diseases remained, five of which accounted for 97.1 percent of the total patients from infectious diseases in the 1950s and 92.6 percent in the 1960s (see tables 3.1 and 3.2). Of these five diseases, measles, malaria, dysentery, and pertussis (whooping cough) were the four most common in both decades, while the fifth most common was influenza in the 1950s and epidemic cerebrospinal meningitis in the 1960s.[23] As Chen Hongting described, four parasitic diseases—schistosomiasis, malaria, filariasis, and hookworm—were also rampant.

For the state, the identification, control, and eradication of disease were key to the nation-building process. In a Communist regime, the health of peasants was hugely important: agricultural production depended on them, and they were also the main sources of labor for factories and recruits for the army.[24] Great efforts were therefore made to contain the most serious infectious diseases.

Continuous large-scale public health campaigns meant that infectious diseases no longer posed serious danger to villagers by the early 1970s, just after the advent of barefoot doctors in the villages. According to a retrospective investigation into causes of death conducted in Yuhang County by the Zhejiang Province Health Department in 1977, acute infectious diseases ranked ninth among causes of death in 1974–76, with victims accounting for only 2.9 percent of the total death toll. In contrast, the first three causes of death were cardiovascular diseases (16.23 percent), malignant tumors (16.09 percent), and respiratory diseases (14.52 percent).[25] Similar changes also occurred in four other counties in Hangzhou prefecture for which disease data are available.[26] The actual percentages for all chronic diseases should be much higher. As a former production brigade accountant of Jiang Village put it, "Science was not as developed as it is today. A lot of illnesses could not be diagnosed."[27] Another production brigade party secretary was frank: "Life wasn't worth much in the old days. When patients were seriously ill and could not eat anymore, they simply died. People just took it for granted."[28] The situation regarding parasitic diseases also improved greatly from the mid-1950s to the advent of barefoot doctors in the late 1960s, as is illustrated by the case of schistosomiasis. Yuhang County was listed as one of the counties most seriously infected with schistosomiasis in the 1930s. By the end of 1954, forty-six of its fifty-five communes and 376 of its 574 production brigades were infected with schistosomiasis, or about 83.6 percent and 64.7 percent, respectively.[29] Entering the 1960s, the number of acute schistosomiasis patients decreased year by year, dropping from 462 cases in 1962 to 130 in 1965, and then to just 7 in 1968 before reaching 0 in 1969.[30] In this sense, the disease model of rural China (at least in rural Hangzhou) under

Table 3.1. The five major acute infectious diseases in Hangzhou Prefecture, 1950–59

Rank	Diseases	Patients Number	%	Deaths Number	Incidence (1/100,000)	Mortality (1/100,000)	Fatality (%)
1	measles	321,100	42.7	6,420	1,059.77	21.99	2.00
2	malaria	263,987	35.1	205	794.48	0.62	0.08
3	dysentery	82,470	11.0	432	248.20	1.30	0.52
4	pertussis	46,084	6.1	173	218.97	0.82	0.38
5	flu	15,984	2.1	20	75.95	0.10	0.13
Total		729,625	97.1	7,250			

Sources: Ren, Hangzhou shizhi, 1: 462; Hangzhoushi weisheng fangyizhan, Yiqing ziliao huibian, 1950–1979, 18–20.

Table 3.2. The five major acute infectious diseases in Hangzhou Prefecture, 1960–69

Rank	Diseases	Patients Number	%	Deaths Number	Incidence (1/100,000)	Mortality (1/100,000)	Fatality (%)
1	malaria	490,743	40.5	28	1,158.78	0.07	0.01
2	measles	397,710	32.8	1,834	939.10	4.33	0.46
3	dysentery	128,617	10.6	130	303.70	0.31	0.10
4	pertussis	60,700	5.0	45	143.33	0.11	0.07
5	epidemic cerebrospinal meningitis	44,969	3.7	2,183	106.18	5.15	4.85
Total		1,122,739	92.7	4120			

Sources: Ren, Hangzhou shizhi, 1: 462; Hangzhoushi weisheng fangyizhan, Yiqing ziliao huibian, 1950–1979, 18–20.

went the epidemiologic transition from infectious and parasitic diseases to chronic diseases in the early 1970s, not the early 1980s, as current scholarship widely argues.[31]

While the health campaigns of the new socialist regime brought about this drastic epidemiologic transition within slightly more than two decades, its social and political institutions also had an unexpected impact on the social epidemiology of rural China, notably in connection with women. Prior to the Communist victory, women in rural areas of Hangzhou Prefecture rarely labored in rice paddy fields because of the gender-based production mode ("Men till, women weave") and the physical constraints of bound feet. As a result, they were rarely victims of schistosomiasis, the main intermediate hosts of which are snails which thrive in rice paddy fields—this channel of infection accounted for 70.7 percent of total schistosomiasis victims.[32] As women (and their children) often outlived husbands who died of schistosomiasis, the disease was often associated with widows and widows remarrying in local gazetteers and old villagers' memories.[33] However, the socialist revolution's "liberation" of women led to their participation in agricultural production outside the home.[34] Their involvement increased further because of the shortage of male laborers, who were transferred to irrigation work, construction projects, and to industrial undertakings.[35] As such, women had to labor in the paddy fields to earn work points (gongfen) from dawn to dusk regardless of the weather, while also undertaking heavy housework, such as cooking food and raising pigs.[36] This strenuous manual labor caused widespread gynecological and obstetric diseases among women, though the dangers posed by parasitic diseases greatly decreased throughout the whole collective era from the late 1950s to the early 1980s.

Traditional Ways of Accessing Pharmaceuticals

Wherever there are diseases, people try to find pharmaceuticals to treat them. In the plural medical systems of traditional Chinese villages, diseases were defined in different ways and treated using different pharmaceuticals by the professional, folk, and popular traditions. Among these, Chinese medicine shops were one of the main sources of pharmaceuticals for villagers. According to Chen Zhicheng, there were three Chinese medicine shops in Jiang Village before 1949, one of which was in the center of the village, and the other two at its eastern and western ends. Customers could buy medicines on credit and would be given their bills (jingzhe) at the end of each year. They would clear their debts for the early months of each year when the bamboo shoots and silkworm cocoons were collected in March and April. Payments in the second half of the year were made when the persimmons were harvested and fish were caught for sale in September and October. Any remaining debts would be paid at the end of the year. As the customers who were given credit usually had land and property, pharmacy incomes in Jiang Village were quite stable.[37] The owners usually had some basic medical knowledge and dispensed medicines themselves, as they did not usually hire staff or only had one or two apprentices. The shops were generally small and were usually located inside owners' homes.[38] Correspondingly, trading hours were very flexible, and owners were available to dispense medicine if someone knocked on the pharmacy doors at night. Many medicine shops advertised that they dispensed "authentic medicine,

[and] never cheated old men or little boys," a common saying. The quality of medicine was also monitored by the Chinese medicine doctors who prescribed it, since poor-quality medicine would affect treatment and compromise doctors' reputations.[39] Therefore, medical practitioners would suggest which pharmacy patient families should buy medicine from, a practice which, to some extent, exerted pressure on the pharmacy. Before 1949, these private Chinese medicine shops had their own medicine supply sources and networks.[40] For example, those in Jiang Village and neighboring villages usually went to urban Hangzhou to purchase medicines from bigger medicine shops.

Despite the existence of medicine shops, with their relatively convenient service, and a pharmaceutical sales network, villagers did not necessarily enjoy easy access to Chinese *materia medica* and patent medicines.[41] In fact, villagers' consumption of pharmaceuticals was quite limited. In the summer of 1932, the Department of Agricultural Economics at Jinling University in Nanjing and the Central Health Commission conducted a joint survey of 298 rural households in twenty villages in Liangzhu Township, Hang County, which is only sixteen km from Jiang Village. According to this report, "Rural households are poor. Thus, they spend little on medicine. The medicine that they bought was usually *xingjunsan* (for treatment of heatstroke, diarrhea, stomachache, and internal heat), *biwendan* (for treatment of heatstroke, acute gastroenteritis, and diarrhea), and *shayao* (for treatment of heatstroke)."[42] The so-called pharmaceuticals that villagers consumed were actually herbal medicines. For example, villagers gathered loquat leaves and decocted them to drink as cold remedies, and they gathered particular herbal grasses and mashed them into a paste to apply to infected wounds and sores. Ordinary villagers either had this basic knowledge or consulted their neighbors, friends, and relatives if they did not. Local folk healers knew where and how to gather slightly more sophisticated herbal medicines. In some cases, alternatives to pharmaceuticals were used. For example, villagers knew how to treat heatstroke through a form of acupressure. Although this treatment resulted in the patient being covered with many unsightly red dots, it was quite effective. In many cases, villagers simply took it for granted that no pharmaceuticals were available.

Compared with Chinese medicine, the amount of Western pharmaceuticals consumed in rural China was negligible, even though they had first appeared in the Hangzhou area in 1871. They were introduced by Dr. Meadows, a British missionary doctor of the Church Missionary Society, which was the first Western medical practice in the history of the city.[43] But it was not until 1905 that the first Western medicine retail shop, the Shanghai Chinese-English drug store, set up a branch in Hangzhou.[44] Local gazetteers make no record of the exact time that Western medicine shops appeared in rural Hangzhou, but, judging by the time at which Western medicine and hospitals emerged, it was probably much later than urban Hangzhou. Of the seven counties in the Hangzhou area, Xiaoshan County (near urban Hangzhou) was the first to operate a Western hospital, which opened in the 1910s. In the remaining six counties, new-style hospitals only emerged in the 1920s, but their numbers were limited.[45] By 1949, the average ratio of Chinese medicine shops (*guoyaodian*) to Western medicine shops in the seven counties of Hangzhou Prefecture was 17.5:1. In Yuhang County, there were 147 Chinese medicine shops but only 24 Western medicine shops.[46] Furthermore, the majority of the hospitals and medicine shops were located in county seats and big towns and were not accessible to villagers.

Another more important factor affecting villagers' access to Western medicines was their scarcity. Even though after World War II Western medicine could be imported more easily and there were seven or eight kinds in circulation—including quinine and headache powder—supplies were still quite limited and prices were high. For example, a bottle of penicillin was worth 50 kg of rice before 1949.[47] According to the old Chinese pharmacist called Shao, even if villagers were prescribed these medicines, they were rarely actually used.[48] Therefore, while scholarly debates have raged over the position of Western medicine since the 1930s, it was meaningless to most villagers, who—as late as the early 1950s—were still largely dependent on local knowledge and traditional practices for medical treatment.[49]

The Preliminary Formation of a Pharmaceutical Sales Network

For thousands of years, China's doctors and pharmacies operated separately from one another, with the exception of the "doctors who sit in the pharmacy," who used the premises as consulting rooms. Village pharmacies were part of limited networks, confined to certain geographic scopes by transport issues. After liberation, village pharmacies underwent a series of changes that would lead to the integration of doctors and pharmacies and the formation of a new state pharmaceutical network based on the pharmaceutical networks and private Chinese medicine shops already in existence during the early years of the Communist regime. The main purposes of these initiatives were to allocate, supply, and sell both Western and Chinese pharmaceuticals to villages efficiently and economically, while meeting the growing demands of various medical and health campaigns. After 1953, as part of the campaign to transform capitalist enterprises into socialist ones, private Chinese medicine shops were gradually incorporated into local union clinics or supply and marketing cooperatives.[50] In Jiang Village, two of the three medicine shops were incorporated into the supply and marketing cooperative in 1955. One private medicine shop, run by Chen Naixing, continued to operate, but it was eventually annexed by the union clinic, which Chen himself also joined in 1956.[51] From 1958 to 1960, during the Great Leap Forward campaign, all the remaining medicine shops in Zhejiang Province were incorporated into local union clinics, as it was thought that combining the two would be convenient for patients' families because they would no longer need to travel between doctors and pharmacies. It was also expected that doctors would bring more monitoring of pharmaceuticals and guarantee their quality. This brought an end to the separation of doctors and pharmacies that had existed for thousands of years and gave way to the integration of doctors and pharmacies (yiyao heyi) in hospitals, which continues to the present day.[52]

When rural pharmacies were incorporated into clinics or rural supply and marketing cooperatives, the pharmaceutical sales network was gradually established. County pharmaceutical companies were first set up in the early 1950s, with the aims of managing the wholesale and supplies of medicines within the county through the union clinic pharmacies, supply and marketing cooperatives, and medicine shops at district and commune levels, as well as some medicine peddlers. In addition to the normal pharmaceutical supplies, the government also initiated a series of programs sending medicines out into the countryside.[53] At the end of 1953, the Hangzhou Pharmaceutical Company established the Hangzhou-Chun'an line sales team to send medicine to the countryside and conduct experimental work in eight counties along the road from Hangzhou to Chun'an. Twenty-eight medicines were promoted, including children's fever-relieving pills and diarrhea-stopping tablets. As the pharmacist Shao recalled, after 1956 more and more Western medicines gradually came into in circulation.[54] Meanwhile, the county pharmaceutical companies dispatched cadres to the countryside to publicize commonsense healthcare and introduce general knowledge of pharmaceuticals among the peasants.[55] As part of this broad program, medical kits were also supplied to the villages in 1955, but this effort was less successful.

The distribution of medicines in the countryside expanded even further in 1965, which saw the start of the urban mobile medical program described in chapter 1. Yuhang County started by sending twenty-two types of Chinese patent medicines and thirty-eight types of Western medicines as the first batch of medicines to the countryside.[56] From September to October that year, the County Pharmaceutical Company organized seventeen staff members into four teams to deliver these medicines to the countryside, and dispatched them to eleven production brigades and eleven production teams. The teams conducted experimental work in which they trained health workers to use medicines and supplied medicines to production teams.[57] Meanwhile, empty medical kit boxes were once again distributed to each county pharmaceutical company, which in turn allocated them to villages and left the villagers to buy the medicines themselves.[58] Following official instructions,

Table 3.3. List of over-the-counter (OTC) medicine in rural areas of Hangzhou Prefecture, August 1965 (unit: RMB)

Name	Specification	Unit	Retail Price
Fever-reducing tablets and painkillers	10 tablets	bottle	0.10
Gastropin tablets	48 tablets	box	0.14
Fever-reducing and pain-relieving powder	10 bags	bundle	0.15
Anti-inflammatory tablets	10 tablets	bottle	0.15
Berberine tablets	10 tablets	bottle	0.20
Sodium bicarbonate tablets	100 tablets	bottle	0.15
Antidysentery tablets	10 tablets	bottle	0.15
Painkiller tablets	10 tablets	bottle	
Children's fever-reducing tablets	10 tablets	bottle	0.20
Children's Sulfadimidine powder	3 packs	bag	0.07
Cough relief tablets	100 tablets	bottle	0.30
Antimalarial tablets		bottle	
Children's cough syrup	100 ml	bottle	0.39
Precious Pagoda lozenges	100 tablets	bottle	1.50
Ascarid-repelling tablets	6 tablets	bag	0.12
Chlortetracycline eye ointment	2.5 g	tin	0.13
Eye drops	10 ml	bottle	0.10
Toothache drops	5 ml	bottle	0.14
Anti-itch lotion	20 ml	bottle	0.23
Paste for sores	20 g	piece	0.14
Paste for chilblains	20 g	tube	0.24
Mercurochrome solution	20 ml	bottle	0.16
Iodine	20 ml	bottle	0.20
Gentian violet	20 ml	bottle	0.16
Beriberi-clearing liquid	20 ml	bottle	0.20

Note: These were among fifty-two pharmaceuticals—which also included a few Chinese patent medicines—that the state designated to be sent to the countryside in August 1965.

Source: Hangzhou yiyao shangyezhi bianzhuan weiyuanhui, *Hangzhou yiyao shangyezhi*, 126–27.

Jiang Village Union Clinic distributed a total of seventy-nine wooden medical kits, one to each production team.[59] According to Luo Zhengfu, the wooden medical kits mainly contained sulfonamide medicines, fever-relieving medicines, cooling ointments, and *rendan* (for treating heatstroke and vomiting). Production team health workers carried medical kits to the field every day.[60] One health worker said, "After the medical kit was distributed to the villages, the villagers were very happy. At midnight, people would knock on the door complaining of stomachache and asking for medicine. When I was laboring in the fields, people would come to look for me and ask for medicine."[61] Therefore, by the mid-1960s, ordinary villagers were much more familiar with the cheapest, most common Western medicines than they had been in the early 1950s (see table 3.3 for a list of these medicines). This trend also started to gradually change the rural pharmaceutical structure, in that villagers no longer depended solely on medicinal herbs gathered from the fields. However, the sending of medical kits and common medicines to the countryside was still not popularized by the late 1960s. In the majority of rural areas, this pharmaceutical sales network only reached the commune level, the second level of the two-tier medical system that then prevailed (that is, the county hospitals and the commune union clinics).

Medical Stations and the March of Western Pharmaceuticals into China's Villages

Communes and production brigades started to establish cooperative medical stations with the popularization of barefoot doctors in rural China after 1968. Their varied locations included the rooms next to the brigade party committee rooms and village meeting halls. A barefoot doctor with a medical kit presided over each, as established in the new official instructions. The medical stations and kits extended the pharmaceutical sales network throughout rural China at a rapid pace and were thus highly significant in the social history of medicine in Chinese villages. Meanwhile, the wholesale pharmaceutical network was further extended to the commune level. The people's disease prevention and treatment hospital (formerly known as the county people's hospital) of each county commissioned each commune clinic to serve as a medicine wholesaler. The cooperative medical stations run by the commune clinics or production brigades could buy Chinese and Western medicines and medical instruments at wholesale prices,[62] which were 15 percent below the retail price.[63] The 1974 release of a manual by the Ministry of Commerce entitled *Instructions on Strengthening the Work of Medicine Supply to Rural Areas* further strengthened the medicine wholesale and supply network.[64] Barefoot doctors were responsible for replenishing their own medical supplies to meet the demands for prescription and distribution of medicine in daily practice, and, thanks to these improved supply chains, they could reach suppliers and return home in a day. In addition to the downward extension of the pharmaceutical network, pharmaceutical companies and health bureaus also held sporadic medicine and medical instrument exhibitions during the 1970s.[65] All these factors contributed to the increase in the supply of medicines to the countryside.

With regard to villagers' access to pharmaceuticals, however, network, prices, and quantity were all crucial factors. In the 1950s and 1960s, pharmaceutical prices were still high compared with villagers' incomes. For example, in 1957, bottles (100 × 2.5g tablets) of tetracycline and Terramycin cost RMB 170.13 and RMB 177.88 respectively, yet the average annual income of villagers that year was less than RMB 50.[66] In other words, villagers would have to work for three years to buy a single bottle of tetracycline or Terramycin.[67] Another broad-spectrum antibiotic, Chloromycetin, was regarded as an especially effective medicine during the 1960s, but it, too, was well beyond the ordinary villager's reach. As a report criticizing doctors for their lack of consideration of the actual situations of poor and lower-middle peasants pointed out, "Things like this always happen in the villages: the *yang* (foreign or modern) doctors from the cities who come to the villages often write prescriptions which usually cost several yuan, but ordinary people cannot afford to pay so much money. Doctors prescribe patient-specific medicines for whooping cough, such as Chloromycetin, but most peasants found it was too expensive and left unhappy."[68]

As such, the reduction of prices was a crucial factor for villagers. On August 1, 1969, pharmaceutical prices were reduced nationwide "in obedience to the great leader Chairman Mao's glorious instructions to 'stress rural areas in medical and health work.'"[69] Prices for 1,230 kinds of antibiotics, sulphanilamides, fever-reducing medicines, pain-relieving medicines, vitamins, hormones, and other medicines were reduced by 37.2 percent.[70] These products constituted about 72.1 percent of the total pharmaceuticals available at the time. By 1971, medicine retail prices were only one-fifth what they had been in 1949 (see table 3.4).[71] Moreover, prices of Western pharmaceuticals were unified nationwide in an attempt to standardize prices throughout the provinces. This also removed the difference in prices between urban and rural localities and dramatically lightened the burden that medicine prices represented for villagers in mountainous areas, in the countryside, and in border areas.[72]

In Jiang Village, Shen Xianbing, the commune clinic accountant, recalled this moment: "After the Cultural Revolution broke out, on the one hand, propaganda work was conducted, such as singing 'Citation Songs' [*yulu ge*, quotations of Chairman Mao set to music], like 'Sailing on the Sea Depends on the Helmsman.' On the other hand, the Hangzhou Pharmaceutical Company started supplying medicines to the countryside."[73] Because Jiang

Table 3.4. Prices for major Western medicines in Hangzhou Prefecture, 1953–84
(unit: RMB)

Medicines	Specification	Unit	1953	1957	1965	1969	1984
Penicillin	0.2 million	bottle	1.12	0.83	0.31	0.25	0.14
Streptomycin	1 million	bottle	2.84	2.15	0.62	0.43	0.28
Antondin	10×2 ml	box	0.94	0.78	0.80	0.61	0.69
Analgin	100×0.5 g	bottle		10.66	5.54	2.50	2.30
Tetracycline	100×0.25 g	bottle		170.13	18.13	6.00	3.50
Terramycin	100×0.25 g	bottle		177.88	10.25	4.38	2.50
Chloromycetin	100×250 mg	bottle		74.56	20.72	6.72	5.00
Sulfapyridine	1000×0.5 g	bottle	73.73	72.87	74.16	34.80	28.0
Sulphaguanidine	1000×0.5 g	bottle	17.00	16.72	15.00	14.17	13.0

Sources: Hangzhou yiyao shangyezhi bianzhuan weiyuanhui, *Hangzhou yiyao shangyezhi*, 254;
Zhongguo yiyao gongsi, *Zhongguo yiyao shangye shigao*, 274.

Village had implemented the commune-wide cooperative medical service,
money was submitted to the management committee from each production
team. A total of RMB 2 was submitted for each commune member, half of
which they paid themselves and half of which the production team paid on
their behalf. The production team usually deducted these fees at the end of
each year, when production team accountants came to the credit cooperatives to draw money and distribute the profits earned by production teams
to the commune members. Shen and his colleagues waited for them at the
credit cooperative and asked them to transfer the money into the cooperative medical service account directly.[74] They then went to buy medicines
from the Hangzhou Prefecture Pharmaceutical Company, as Jiang Village
is not far from the Hangzhou urban area. Luo Zhengfu said, "We rode the
tricycle there in order to save money. The production brigade cooperative
medical stations later collected the medicine from our commune clinic.
When they had used up their supply, the barefoot doctors replenished their
medical kits with medicines from the commune clinic during our regular
meetings."[75] Hong Jinglin remembered the first time he collected medicine
from the commune clinic. His brigade had submitted RMB 180, and he then
rowed a small boat of medicine back to the brigade, thereby establishing
Jiang Village Commune's first brigade medical station.[76]

Like Western pharmaceuticals for common diseases, vaccines (or biological products) were of great significance for combating acute epidemic diseases.

As late as the 1930s and 1940s, ordinary Chinese were still not able to afford the basic cholera vaccine. When cholera broke out in neighboring Xiaoshan County in 1931, local newspapers suggested residents receive intravenous injections of normal saline solution to stop serious vomiting and diarrhea. However, ordinary families could not afford the fees for this, as one bottle of saline solution cost 50 kg of rice.[77] More seriously, there were no vaccines for the majority of epidemic diseases. Herbal therapy was the only solution, and usually dozens of prescriptions were put forward as being the most efficacious in treating a given disease. However, the *materia medica* for these prescriptions were often difficult to obtain and usually became extremely expensive during epidemics.[78] For example, in the case of epidemic cerebrospinal meningitis, doctors prescribed only antelope and rhinoceros horn, which were beyond the means of ordinary families. Furthermore, patients in a critical condition could not take Chinese medicine decoctions, because they were unable to swallow them.[79]

From the early 1950s on, basic vaccines for diseases such as cholera and plague were soon applied to inoculation work, while the range of available vaccines increased gradually thereafter. By the time the barefoot doctor program was instigated in Hangzhou Prefecture in 1970, fifteen vaccines had already been administered there. These vaccines covered all eighteen of the epidemic diseases that had occurred regularly in the rural Hangzhou area during the late 1960s (see table 3.5). The vaccines for the most serious epidemic diseases—measles and epidemic cerebrospinal meningitis—were invented and applied between 1967 and 1970.[80] Before the introduction of measles vaccines into Hangzhou Prefecture in 1967, the local gazetteer records how "various kinds of folk prevention measures were tried in the villages, such as urine-soaked eggs. However, these methods could not curb the outbreak of disease or reduce its seriousness."[81] The situation was similar for epidemic cerebrospinal meningitis: "The masses tried gargling different medicines or taking Chinese herbal medicine soup and sulphanilamides as they looked for efficient ways to reduce the incidence of infection. However, all of these efforts ultimately failed."[82] The rampant spread of epidemic cerebrospinal meningitis was curbed only after the application of vaccines through inoculation. The local gazetteer claimed "the prevention efforts were changed from passive to active efforts from then on."[83]

As the mortality rates of measles and epidemic cerebrospinal meningitis were the highest of all the infectious diseases affecting rural China, the invention and application of their vaccines were of great significance.[84] The mortality rates of infectious disease started declining after 1968 and dropped to their lowest ever levels by 1970, where they have remained ever since (see fig. 3.1). The incidence rates of infectious diseases in the seven counties of Hangzhou Prefecture declined by 68 percent between 1968 and 1983. When the barefoot doctors were reclassified as village doctors in 1985, the incidences

Table 3.5. Vaccines in four selected counties in Hangzhou Prefecture, 1949–70

Vaccine	Year of first inoculation
Smallpox	1950
Typhoid, paratyphoid	1950
Bubonic plague	1952
BCG	1952–57
Diphtheria toxin	1952–54
Pertussis	1954
Epidemic Japanese B encephalitis	1957–58
Anthracnose	1960
Diphtheria, Pertussis, Tetanus (DPT)	1961
Dysentery bacteriophage	1961
Polio	1962
Paracholera	1962
Leptospirosis	1961–66
Measles	1967–70
Epidemic cerebrospinal meningitis	1970

Sources: Yan, Jiandexian yiyao weishengzhi, 141–42; Lin'anxian weishengzhi bianzhuan wei-yuanhui, Lin'anxian weishengzhi, 257; Xu, Fuyangxian weishengzhi, 15–16, 173–77; Xiaoshan weishengju, Xiaoshan weishengzhi, 139–79; Qian Xinzhong, Zhongguo weisheng shiye fazhan yu juece [Health development and decision making in China] (Beijing: Zhongguo yiyao keji chu-banshe, 1992), 850–86; Huang Shuze and Lin Shixiao, eds., Dangdai zhongguo de weisheng shiye [Health development in contemporary China], vol. 2 (Beijing: Zhongguo shehui kexue chu-banshe, 1986), 291–343.

of infectious disease had dropped to the lowest levels in history and have remained there until the present day (see fig. 3.2).

Vaccines and other epidemic prevention medicines were provided free of charge. Furthermore, their distribution was strictly conducted by medi-cal practitioners, who delivered medicine to the door of each household and watched them being taken (songyao shangmen, kanyao luodu). As clinic accountant Shen Xianbing recalled,

In the old days, we had to work very hard, since the higher-ups always came to our village to check on our work. When they came to our village and told the local people that some medicine was too bitter and sour to be swallowed [in

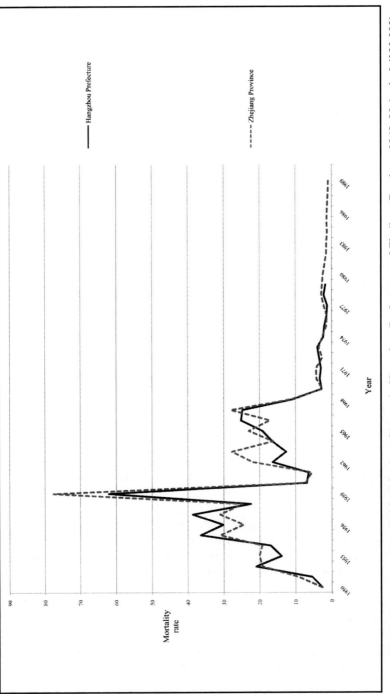

Figure 3.1. Mortality rates of notifiable infectious diseases in Hangzhou Prefecture and Zhejiang Province, 1949–90 (unit: 1/100,000). Data from Hangzhoushi weisheng fangyizhan, *Yiqing ziliao huibian, 1950–1979*, 12; Zhejiangsheng weisheng fangyizhan [Zhejiang Province Sanitation and Epidemic-Prevention Station], ed., *Zhejiangsheng yiqing ziliao huibian, 1950–1979* [Compiled data of epidemic diseases in Zhejiang Province, 1950–1979] (Hangzhou: Zhejiangsheng weisheng fangyizhan, 1982), 1–4; Zhejiangsheng weisheng fangyizhan [Zhejiang Province Sanitation and Epidemic-Prevention Station], ed., *Zhejiangsheng yiqing ziliao huibian, 1980–1989* [Compiled data of epidemic diseases in Zhejiang Province, 1980–1989] (Hangzhou: Zhejiangsheng weisheng fangyizhan, 1994), 7.

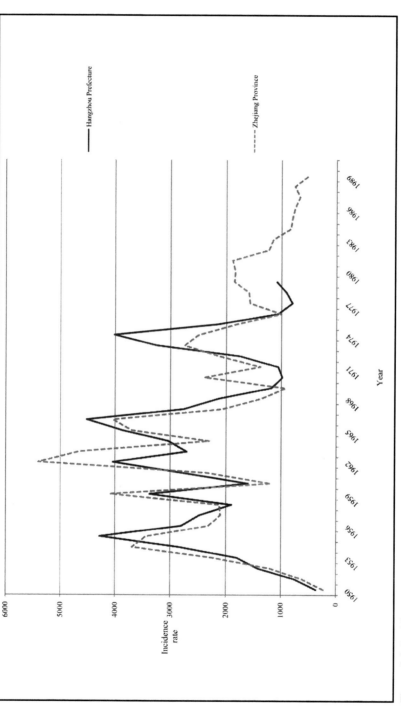

Figure 3.2. Incidence rates of notifiable infectious diseases in Hangzhou Prefecture and Zhejiang Province, 1949–90 (unit: 1/100,000). Data from Hangzhoushi weisheng fangyizhan, *Yiqing ziliao huibian, 1950–1979*, 12; Zhejiangsheng weisheng fangyizhan, *Zhejiangsheng yiqing ziliao huibian, 1950–1979*, 1–4; Zhejiangsheng weisheng fangyizhan, *Zhejiangsheng yiqing ziliao huibian, 1980–1989*, 7.

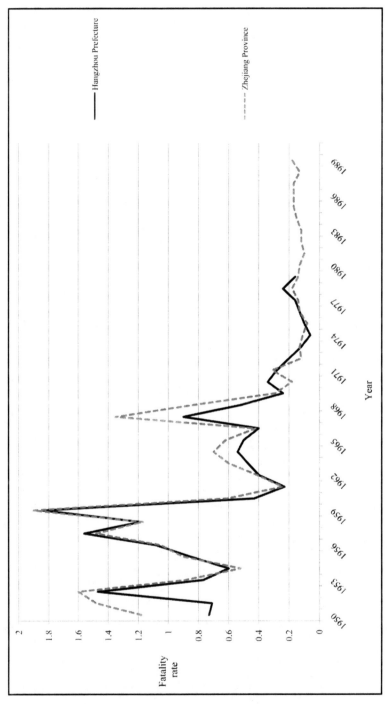

Figure 3.3. Fatality rates of notifiable infectious diseases in Hangzhou Prefecture and Zhejiang Province, 1949–90 (unit: percentage). Data from Hangzhoushi weisheng fangyizhan, *Yiqing ziliao huibian, 1950–1979*, 12; Zhejiangsheng weisheng fangyizhan, *Zhejiangsheng yiqing ziliao huibian, 1950–1979*, 1–4; Zhejiangsheng weisheng fangyizhan, *Zhejiangsheng yiqing ziliao huibian, 1980–1989*, 7.

order to get the local people to say what they really thought about the medicine], some stupid guys in the village told the higher-ups that they never took the medicine. We were criticized because of this.[85]

At the same time, beginning on January 20, 1974, barefoot doctors supplied their patients with prophylactic and contraceptive medicines and devices for free, although some villagers were too shy to ask for them.[86] Basic medical instruments were also popularized rapidly, notably stethoscopes, thermometers, and blood pressure meters. Instruments for inserting and removing IUDs were also issued to female barefoot doctors after they completed their IUD training.[87]

The Legitimization and Promotion of Chinese Herbal Medicines

Other researchers have already highlighted the application of Chinese herbal medicine campaigns within the barefoot doctor program, arguing that its aim was to reduce costs.[88] "Popularizing new needles and medicinal herbs," "popularizing the rural cooperative medical service," and "training revolutionary medical staff groups" were claimed to be the three pillars of the rural health revolution.[89] However, Chinese herbal medicines were not promoted at the beginning of the program. When the first cooperative medical service program in Changyang County, Hubei Province, was reported on in the *People's Daily* on December 5, 1968, no mention was made of Chinese herbal medicines.[90] The increase in Chinese medicine use came only when reduced pharmaceutical prices began to have a negative impact on the state's coffers.[91] The Hangzhou Chinese and Western Pharmaceutical Station lost RMB 3,746,000 because of the reduction in medicine prices, while seven counties under the jurisdiction of Hangzhou Prefecture lost RMB 567,000.[92] The state's loss was also closely linked to international situations, such as the Sino-Soviet conflicts that dragged on throughout the 1960s. The official media announced that "in view of the international situation, it is believed that war is inescapable," and propaganda units circulated the slogan "Be prepared for war, be prepared for natural disasters, and serve the people whole-heartedly" (*beizhan, beihuang, wei renmin*). As a result, all medical agencies from the central government to the local level began stockpiling medicines, which affected the market supply.[93] As one villager recalled, "In the beginning, the use of Western medicine was reduced in preparation for war. [Because of this preparation] it would be easy to use Chinese herbal medicines if war broke out."[94]

Under these circumstances, Chinese herbal medicines and folk medical practices were promoted to meet the demands of the national health program.

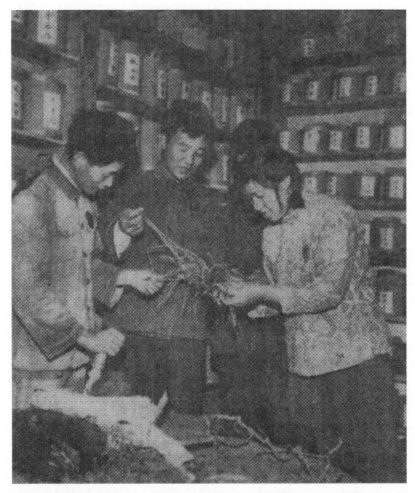

Figure 3.4. Barefoot doctors and herbal medicine processing room. *ZJRB*, June 25, 1970. Reproduced with permission.

Chinese herbal medicine sources are very abundant and widely distributed. The keeping, processing, and usage of Chinese medicinal herbs are relatively simple and easily mastered. Our masses have a lot of experience. Hence, fully employing the functions of Chinese herbal medicines could meet the demands for medicine among the poor and lower-middle peasants, further strengthen and develop the cooperative medical service, and promote the development of socialist health and medicine. Meanwhile, it answers the demand for combat readiness and fulfills Chairman Mao's great strategic guidelines to "be prepared for war, be prepared for natural disasters, and serve the people whole-heartedly."[95]

From January 1970 to January 1972, the Health Bureau of the Zhejiang Province Revolutionary Committee compiled *Common Chinese Herbal Medicines of Zhejiang Province*, based on investigations into Chinese herbal medicines for rural diseases commonly found in the whole province. Its three volumes recorded 433 types of Chinese medicinal plants in Zhejiang.[96] Herbal medicine resources were abundant in every county within Hangzhou Prefecture, albeit to different extents. In general, more medicinal plants were available in mountainous counties, such as Chun'an and Lin'an, for which the book records 1,510 and 1,200, respectively. Relatively few medicinal plants grew on the plains: only 300 types were recorded in the flatland county of Xiaoshan. In Fuyang and Jiande, counties with a mix of plains and mountains, 742 and 767 Chinese medicinal plants were available, respectively.[97]

In Jiang Village, Chen Zhicheng recalled that "at the beginning [of the medical cooperative], we used both Chinese and Western medicines, and nonmedical staff were prohibited from prescribing medicines. Usually there were no more than two kinds of medicines with dosages for less than three days in one prescription. By 1972, we could no longer continue to prescribe medicines."[98] At that point, the second year that the cooperative medical service had been operating, the commune clinic launched the Chinese herbal medicine campaign. The clinic appointed a staff member to take charge of this work, which included planting, gathering, and processing. A small piece of land was allocated for the cultivation of medicinal plants, and a special room was set aside for processing. According to barefoot doctor Xu Shuilin, they planted a few common medicinal herbs but not very many. Instead, they mainly gathered the plants they needed locally under the leadership of Chen Zhicheng, although the clinic once sent the barefoot doctors to Changxing County in northern Zhejiang Province. After gathering the medicinal herbs, the clinic staff would process, slice, and dry them, which required relatively high levels of skill and technical ability. These herbal medicines had beneficial effects for some particular diseases. For example, *Plantago asiatica* (Chinese plantain, *cheqiancao*) helped discharge urine, *Solidago Virga-aurea Linn* (goldenrod, *yizhihuanghua*) cleared "heat" and dispelled toxins, and *Paris polyphylla Smith* (Rhizoma paridis, *qiyeyizhihua*) for treating snake bites. In order to teach villagers to recognize these common herbal medicines, the clinic made small signs and put them next to examples of the plants along the roadside. Meanwhile, the clinic established a pharmaceutical manufacturing laboratory. Chen Hongting's brother-in-law the pharmacist Zhu Shouhua was put in charge of the laboratory and went to Shanghai to study manufacturing techniques, while another pharmacist learned how to make distilled water at Hangzhou City No. 5 Hospital. According to Zhu, they also made Codonopsis tissue fluid, placenta tissue fluid, and other solutions used for injections. With this knowledge they were able to guarantee the quality of the medicines used in their own clinic, and, more importantly, they aimed to sell these medicines to neighboring commune clinics in order to cover the daily operation costs of their own clinic and the commune cooperative medical service.[99]

For the most part, the commune clinic medical staff carried out the technical aspects of the Chinese herbal medicine campaign in Jiang Village, and the barefoot doctors in each production brigade simply followed them. Nonetheless, official discourse praised the barefoot doctors' performance in the Chinese herbal medicine campaign: according to the propaganda of the time, many "hundred-herb gardens" (*baicaoyuan*) and "folk medicine factories" sprouted in villages everywhere. Barefoot doctors searched for many folk prescriptions and proven recipes that offered good curative effects with low costs. They greatly reduced the cooperative medical service fund expenses and alleviated the burden on collective and commune members.[100]

Dilemmas of Chinese and Western Pharmaceuticals

The advent of the barefoot doctors and the establishment of medical stations created the context within which Western medicines and Chinese herbal medicines circulated together in Chinese villages for the first time in the social history of medicine in China. On the one hand, the availability of Western pharmaceuticals meant that villagers did not solely depend on local vegetation for their medicines. On the other hand, the state legitimized these same Chinese herbal medicines in order to meet the demands of national health programs. However, new dilemmas were associated with both types of pharmaceuticals in the villages during the early 1970s.

With regard to Western pharmaceuticals, the extension of the medicine wholesale and supply network down to the commune level did increase the types of pharmaceuticals available to the villagers and reduce medicine prices by enabling medical stations and villagers to buy Western medicines conveniently and relatively cheaply, yet there were still problems in terms of supplies and prices. The goal of having sufficient supplies to meet the demands of the huge number of Chinese villagers who comprised the majority of China's population depended on the pharmaceutical production capacity. Chen Zhicheng recalled that since barefoot doctors had been present to treat patients, demand for pharmaceuticals had increased and could not be met by the existing Western pharmaceutical supply.[101] Additionally, the funds available to cooperative medical services were limited. If barefoot doctors had kept prescribing Western medicines, these funds would quickly have been exhausted, and this, in turn, would lead to the collapse of the medical services as a whole. In Jiang Village, the payments made by individual commune members were deducted at the time of dividend allocation at the end of the year. However, some production teams did not have sufficient money to submit their part of the fees, while some were reluctant to do so in later years. This caused a shortfall in the medical fund, which correspondingly led to the shortage of pharmaceuticals. Chen Zhicheng described how the brigade medical station pharmacies did not have many pharmaceuticals, and the commune members and barefoot doctors became unhappy. Later he decided to allocate pharmaceuticals according to the patient numbers of each brigade medical station, which still bought medicines from the commune clinic but in limited quantities.[102] However, insufficient pharmaceutical supplies and limited funding continued to pose severe practical problems for the daily operation of the cooperative medical service in Jiang Village throughout the 1970s.

In contrast, the legitimization of Chinese herbal medicine was supposed to reduce the cost of the medical stations over which the barefoot doctors presided. This also made the barefoot doctors distinct because, in theory, part of their daily work was to gather, plant, and process medicines. However, a key problem for the regular use of Chinese herbal medicines was that their supply was unstable. The immediate problem for individual barefoot doctors in gathering herbs was that not all wild Chinese medicinal plants were always available in each geographic location, particularly in mountainous areas. Barefoot doctors therefore devoted a lot of time to trying to gather the right plants.[103] Identifying these correctly was not easy, however: recognizing the right plant species required both knowledge and experience, which could only be accumulated with time and practice. Even if the barefoot doctors were capable of searching for and gathering the herbal medicines, there was the additional problem of whether barefoot doctors were willing to engage in such hard work. One barefoot doctor in neighboring Fuyang County still remembers the hardship of gathering herbal medicines following the old herbal medicine man of the brigade: "We gathered a lot of herbal medicines. There was an old man who gathered herbal medicines, chopped, and dried them. Otherwise, they would rot. . . . It was very hard work when we gathered the herbal medicines. We carried our lunch boxes up into the mountains."[104]

The time at which medicinal plants were gathered was also very critical.[105] The roots, stalks, leaves, and fruits of the same plant can have different medical functions at different times of the year.[106] If medicinal plants were gathered in the wrong season, they would be useless. For example, according to a local proverb, "*Herba artemisiae scopariae* (capillary wormwood herb, *yinchen*) should be gathered in March and April. If they are gathered in May and June, they can only be used for firewood as they will be useless as medicine."[107] After the herbal medicines were gathered, there was still the problem of what to do with them next—that is, how to process and preserve them for use. Usually they needed to be washed and dried, and some needed special additional processing. However, because of poor processing techniques, official documents pointed out that "it was a common phenomenon to gather a batch of herbal medicines, only for the medicine to become rotten and have to be discarded."[108]

Planting Chinese medicinal herbs turned out to be even more problematic than gathering them from the wild. Soil conditions were the first problem. Jiang Jingting, the barefoot doctor nicknamed "Mr. Cat-Dog" in Jiang Village, recalled that they planted medicinal herbs, but that the soil in Jiang Village was too wet and too different from the soil in the mountains for the plants to thrive. To solve this problem, they had to dig up soil from the mountains and carry it back to the village to plant the medicinal herbs in.[109] Even if the soil was suitable, planting and growing herbs still took skills, experience, and good judgment as to whether to plant herbs deep or shallow, dense or sparse, and to use garden or wild varieties. Anxi Commune, twenty-four kilometers from Jiang Village, was declared a model for the cultivation of Chinese medicinal herbs in Zhejiang Province when the cooperative medical service was implemented in the 1970s. However, the summary written by the Anxi Commune Party Committee pointed out that a lot of problems arose in the cultivation of medicinal herbs because of lack of experience. First, although each "hundred-herb garden" contained many kinds of medicinal herbs, these gardens did not produce sufficient quantities of any single herb. Second, although many herbs were planted, the gardens were not properly tended or cultivated, which resulted in poor yields. Third, for some kinds of medicinal herbs, such as Chinese plantain and goldenrod, cultivation was not as economically efficient as gathering them from the wild. Fourth, yields were too low when attempts were made to cultivate wild medicinal herbs in gardens. For example, Anxi commune planted *Andrographis paniculata* (Herba andrographitis, *chuanxinlian*), which usually produced sprouts 50 to 60 days after planting, but none ever grew to maturity, so they pulled them up and threw them away. As to rare and expensive medicinal herbs, they had to be transplanted from other localities. In Anxi Commune, they transplanted *Codonopsispilosula* (Radix Codonopsis Pilosulae, *dangshen*) from other provinces, but all of the plants died before the hot season within the first two years.[110]

Even when herbs had been successfully gathered from the wild or grown in gardens, producing medicines from them proved even more complicated. In one report summarizing how barefoot doctors overcame the difficulties of processing medicines, the production brigade party secretary made a detailed description.

> In the beginning, we could only make some *yinpian* (small amounts of prepared medicinal herbs ready for decoction). But the poor and lower-middle peasants said, "What a big bag of medicinal herbs! It is too hard to decoct them." We discussed this with the barefoot doctors. They proposed a change

to the system of processing the herbs and we immediately supported them. The first difficulty we encountered was that no one knew the techniques. At the time, the commune clinic dispatched medical staff to come to the brigade and guide us in making some pills and *miwan* (honey pills). Because we had no experience, the pills we made were very coarse. The adults felt they were too coarse for their throats. It was completely impossible for children to take them, and the cost of the honey boluses was too high. It was a heavy burden for poor and lower-middle peasants and not good for the consolidation of the cooperative medical service. Then they thought these two problems could be solved if *shuiwan* (water-honey boluses) could be made, so they began making water-honey boluses. However, the barefoot doctors were not proficient at these techniques, and the water-honey boluses they made were not consistent in size—some were big and others were small.[111]

As for the preparation of herbal injections, the inconsistent quality resulted in side effects that were often extreme, resulting in many accidents.[112] Storing herbal medicines also presented problems, since, in order to be effective, they needed to be stored in dry, well-ventilated places, and the individual barrels or jars needed to have lime (calcium oxide) at the bottom to prevent moisture from entering them.

Each of these factors resulted in uncertainty in Chinese herbal medicines supplies. It also caused health departments to waiver in their support for the Chinese herbal medicine campaign. In 1974, a report written by a few Chinese medicine doctors complained that "the county health bureau did not actively support the herbal medicine reforms conducted by the rural clinics. They never actively supplied the necessary equipment and solutions for herbal medicine reforms, and they did not pay enough attention to the training of future generations of Chinese medicine doctors and pharmacists. The so-called plans and blueprints only existed on paper and were never implemented."[113] Nor was the situation good in Jiang Village. As Luo Zhengfu said, "We once did it [used Chinese herbal medicines] for a few years, about two years. The energy, money, and efforts we spent planting and gathering medicinal herbs was not as good as buying the medicine. It involves experience, land, processing, slicing, and so on. Relatively speaking, however, we were not too badly off. Other communes were much worse off than us."[114] Yan Shengyu of Longzhang Production Brigade joined the barefoot doctor group in Jiang Village Commune in 1978. He recalled that he gathered medicinal herbs only twice from 1978 to 1983. The first occasion was during his internship, when he studied at a county health school. The second was when the Jiang Village Commune Clinic arranged for the barefoot doctors to gather herbs in Chaoshan Township, twenty-three kilometers from Jiang Village. The aim was to teach barefoot doctors to recognize the medicinal herbs in the wild. In Yan Shengyu's words, "it was merely a symbolic gesture."[115]

Table 3.6. Gathering and planting of medicinal herbs in cooperative medical stations in Hangzhou Prefecture, 1976

	Production Brigades					
	Brigades with a cooperative medical service					
			Gathering and planting of medicinal herbs		Area of medicinal herb fields	
County	Total number	Total number	Total number	%	mu	per brigade
Xiaoshan	750	736	165	22.41%	212	1.28
Yuhang	550	550	165	30.00%	473	2.87
Lin'an	636	581	180	30.98%	80	0.44
Tonglu	407	407	163	40.04%	98.90	0.61
Fuyang	589	451	292	64.75%	60.47	0.21
Jiande	515	492	281	57.11%	200	0.71
Chun'an	852	815	463	56.80%	307	0.66
Average				43.16%		0.97

Source: Hangzhoushi weishengju [Hangzhou Prefectural Health Bureau], "Nongcun chijiao yisheng weishengyuan jieshengyuan qingkuang" [Statistical data of rural barefoot doctors, health workers and midwives], 1976, HZA, vol. 87-3-307.

As a result, the general situation for Chinese herbal medicines was not opportune in Hangzhou Prefecture. The best year for the barefoot doctor program was 1976, in terms of the percentage of the production brigades implementing the cooperative medical service. During that year, however, only 43.16 percent of the total number of production brigades implementing the cooperative medical service also gathered and planted Chinese medicinal herbs themselves (see table 3.6). The percentages in other years must be much lower than this figure. The limited availability of the Chinese herbal medicines consumed by villagers for thousands of years contrasted the increasing availability of Western pharmaceuticals year by year throughout the 1970s. From 1977 onward, the Chinese herbal medicine campaign abated and eventually faded out of the village medical world because of increasing supplies of Western medicine and the decline of a supportive ideological context, although Chinese herbal medicines were still compulsory components of the training and programs for the cooperative medical service. On May 22, 1981, the State Council issued its *Instructions on Strengthening Medicine Management.* Though the publication aimed to regulate and standardize Chinese herbal medicines, the strict requirements it included eventually pushed herbal medicine out of the daily medical practice of barefoot doctors. After the May 1981 directive, medical units other than county hospitals were prohibited from making Chinese medicinal herb injections.[116] Moreover, if accidents happened, the individual doctor was forced to take responsibility for the error, so no one dared to use these techniques any longer in Jiang Village.[117] As a result, the herbal medicine movement rapidly lost momentum while, at the same time, Western medicinal products were marching into the villages on the strength of a more developed pharmaceutical network and the cheaper prices that emerged in the economic reform era.[118]

During the barefoot doctor program, Chinese herbal medicines were given official legitimacy because of economic factors, even though they were ostensibly promoted in the name of political exigencies and ideology. In theory, the revival of Chinese herbal medicines had two basic advantages. On the one hand, the incorporation of herbal medicine men into the medical stations gave the barefoot doctors a source of knowledge and guidance in the gathering, cultivation, and preparation of medicinal herbs. On the other hand, herbal medicines could be made more easily available than Western pharmaceuticals in the villages to cure various diseases. The government legitimization and promotion of herbal medicines led to their use being transferred from individual and family practices to a mass campaign that was supposed to fit into a nationwide health program.

The encounter of Chinese herbal medicines with Western pharmaceuticals through the barefoot doctors had great significance for the development of the pharmaceutical structure in the villages. Their intermingling reveals that the intellectual and theoretical controversy over Chinese and Western medicines—in terms of the conferral of state legitimacy—started to shift toward real contestation for the first and last time in the social history of medicine in the Chinese countryside. During this process, Chinese herbal medicines, which had enjoyed popular acceptance and practical legitimacy before the arrival of the barefoot doctors in the villages, were seriously challenged by Western medicines, the spread of which was facilitated by their steadily increasing availability combined with their steadily decreasing prices. This situation also illustrates the dilemmas inherent in the implementation of Chinese herbal medicine use when it was expanded from sporadic, small-scale use to regular, large-scale use within a national health program. In this sense, the barefoot doctor program provided the first real context in which Chinese and Western medicines would compete in the village medical arenas. The competition resulted in a rapid rise in the use of Western medicines and the onset of a progressive marginalization of Chinese medicines in daily medical practice.

Chapter Four

Healing Styles and Medical Beliefs

The Consumption of Chinese and Western Medicines

Together with medical knowledge and pharmaceuticals, the healing techniques of Western medicine gradually entered the village medical domain from early the 1950s onward.[1] These new healing methods emerged gradually among village healers, particularly among the union clinic doctors. In Jiang Village, Chen Hongting, who had practiced as a Chinese medicine doctor in his father's footsteps, was already prescribing a few tablets of aspirin before liberation.[2] After 1949, he learned to administer injections, to obtain a blood sample, and to hatch schistosomes from human feces in order to diagnose schistosomiasis. After 1958, Chen Zhicheng recalled, "We carried medical kits during prevention work and provided mobile medical services. We bought quite a bit of Western medicine and used a lot." In 1961, when he followed his master Zheng Buying to study Chinese medicine, they were already using thermometers, blood pressure meters, and stethoscopes for diagnosis. He said, "We were Chinese medicine doctors, but we used thermometers to measure body temperature."[3]

As early as 1953, official documents had already criticized some Chinese medicine doctors for misunderstanding Chinese medicine's great contribution to public health: "they had the incorrect understanding that Chinese medicine was not scientific, that it could not treat illnesses, and that it had no future. [They believed that] it was not acceptable to prescribe Chinese medicine. In these circumstances, the majority of Chinese medicine doctors started to use Western medicine and stopped using Chinese medicine."[4] Many students who graduated from the advanced Chinese medicine training schools also abandoned Chinese medicine.[5] Prescribing Western medicine also became an important way of making money for rural medical practitioners, both private medical practitioners and union clinic doctors.[6] Some union clinics faced criticism for treating patients with an injection of amidopyrine (a nonopioid analgesic, antipyretic, and anti-inflammatory) no matter the illness, and a few administered Western medicine injections and powders. It was very common for Chinese medicine doctors to prescribe streptomycin, penicillin, and anesthetics, regardless of the disease.[7] Although Western pharmaceuticals were scarce in the mid-1960s, some doctors were already overprescribing them. The neighboring Lin'an County

Health Bureau suggested in 1966 that "to improve the efficiency of our medical services, we need to take very seriously the problems [of doctors] disregarding proper diagnostic techniques and proper principles for prescribing medicine in order to make money."[8] Despite official criticism, the advent of Western medicine became an irreversible trend. The barefoot doctors' healing styles were formed against this complex background and served to further transform the villager's comparative medical beliefs, with the result that there was a fundamental change in the pharmaceutical consumption structure.

The Spectrum of Healing Styles in Revolutionary Discourse and Daily Practice

During the 1970s, the barefoot doctors were described as "newly emerged things" of the Great Proletarian Cultural Revolution. In particular, acupuncture and Chinese herbal medicines were described as playing a heroic role in rural medicine. Equipped with the silver needle and bunch of herbs that symbolized these two practices, barefoot doctors became the official representations of rural revolutionary health. These revolutionary images were portrayed in different kinds of media, including newspapers, radio broadcasts, and films.[9] During the 1970s, two propaganda films, *Chunmiao* (1975) and *Hongyu* (1975), focused on barefoot doctors and showed them struggling against "witches (*wupo*)" and "reactionary doctors." *Chunmiao* is about a barefoot doctor named Tian Chunmiao practicing medicine in a rice paddy village in Southern China. The film was based on the story of Wang Guizhen, from Jiangzhen Commune, Shanghai, who was reportedly the first woman barefoot doctor in China.[10] Actually, the name Tian Chunmiao was a metaphor for these "newly emerged things": *Tian* means "soil," while *Chunmiao* means "the sprout of spring" in Chinese. This name alluded to the barefoot doctors' emergence from amidst the pressures of old reactionary doctors in the villages.[11] Similarly, the film *Hongyu* is about a sixteen-year-old boy who became a barefoot doctor in a mountainous village in northern China.

Regardless of the political labels applied to them, the healers other than barefoot doctors portrayed in these two films represented the gradual change in medical knowledge and healing styles in villages dating back to before liberation. In the film *Chunmiao*, the first of the barefoot doctors' enemies is an old woman named Jia Yuexian, who was labeled a "witch." She did not work in the fields with the production brigade but instead hung a yellow banner with the character *Yi* (doctor) outside her house and provided treatment for her fellow villagers. Another antagonist is Qian Jiren, the medical team leader of the commune clinic and the son of a former landlord and Chinese medicine doctor. The clinic director Du Wenjie had likely been a Chinese medicine apprentice, as he said, "I worked hard

and suffered a lot of hardship starting out as an apprentice prior to liberation." On the revolutionary side is the young and handsome commune
clinic doctor Fang Ming, who had just graduated from a medical university.
Additional characters included nurses and technicians in the commune
clinic, wearing white uniforms and caps and assisting the doctors. A scene
in a village located high on a mountain includes an herbal medicinal man.
In the film *Hongyu*, the title character's village is much simpler. Sun Tianfu
is the only doctor and the son of the owner of a Chinese medicine shop
before liberation. In addition, there is an old Chinese medicine doctor in
a neighboring county.

The barefoot doctors in the films *Chunmiao* and *Hongyu* obtain their
medical knowledge against this background. Hongyu train at a county hospital, where Chinese and Western methods are integrated. Three scenes in
the film indicate his sources and structures of knowledge. In the first, an
old man holding a bunch of herbal medicines is shown lecturing to barefoot doctor students. On the blackboard is information about two medicinal herbs, *Rhizoma coptidis* (coptis root, *huanglian*) and *Herba menthae* (mint,
bohe), and Mao's instruction "Chinese medicines are great treasures" hangs
on the wall. In the second scene, a middle-aged doctor is shown teaching
Hongyu how to use a microscope. Finally, a teacher is shown teaching the
barefoot doctor students how to perform acupuncture treatments.

The struggles between barefoot doctors and their enemies are reflected
not only in the barefoot doctors' attitudes toward the poor and lower-middle peasants but also in their healing styles (see tables 4.1 and 4.2). The benefits and effectiveness of acupuncture and herbal medicine are emphasized,
and they form the main treatment in the case of a boy named Little Dragon,
who has acute tuberculosis, as well as the cases of Uncle Shuichang's backache and Xiaolian's mother's serious cold. The commune clinic leader in
Chunmiao looks down on these healing methods, arguing, "Did anyone use
grasses and sticks (*caocao bangbang*) to treat illnesses in the past?" Likewise,
Sun Tianfu openly sneers at Hongyu for daring to administer acupuncture:
"I, Sun Tianfu, have been practicing medicine for thirty years. I have never
dared to administer acupuncture. But Hongyu, a little guy, dares to do so."
In contrast, the revolutionary healers are the barefoot doctors' firm allies.
When the revolutionary doctor Fang Ming arrives in a hurry to treat Little
Dragon, he finds that Chunmiao has cured him. Fang Ming is very curious
and asks Little Dragon's mother which medicines Chunmiao prescribed.
The boy's mother tells him with pride, "What Chunmiao used was just a silver needle and a bunch of herbal medicines." In the next scene, Chunmiao
is shown walking through the gate of the yard with a basket of herbal medicines in her hand, her bare feet covered with mud, while the village folk are
waiting for her. The brigade party secretary proudly exclaims, "This is the
doctor for us, the poor and lower-middle peasants: a barefoot doctor!"

Table 4.1. The healing styles of Hongyu and Chunmiao

Barefoot doctor	Patients	Illnesses	Diagnostic technique	Medicines
Hongyu	Xiaolian's mother	serious cold	stethoscope	fever-reducing injection; a dose of herbal medicines
	Old stone mason	chronic leg pain		herbal medicines
		poisoning from *Semen Crotonis Pulveratum* (croton seed powder, *badoushuang*)	stethoscope	green bean soup
	Zhao Laohuan	chronic leg pain		acupuncture
Tian Chunmiao	Wang Laoqing's son	poison indigestion	stethoscope	eight bottles of glucose injections
	Little kid	cough	stethoscope	one pill three times a day
	Villager			acupuncture, poultices
	Uncle Shuichang	backache		acupuncture, herbal medicines
	Little Dragon	acute tuberculosis and high fever	put ear on chest	herbal medicines
	Old granny			acupuncture

Sources: The films *Chunmiao* and *Hongyu.*

Table 4.2. The healing styles of "reactionary doctors," "bad doctors," and "witches"

Healers	Patients	Illnesses	Diagnostic technique	Medicines
Jia Yuexian				incense ashes
Qian Jiren	Xiaomei	high fever	puts on a gauze mask, and a stethoscope	none, referred to county hospital
Jia Yuexian	Little Dragon	acute tuberculosis	takes pulse while claiming he is scared	soda, burn paper
Qian Jiren	Uncle Shuichang	backache	presses and kicks the back	none, patient told to eat and sleep
Sun Tianfu	Xiaolian's mother	serious cold	takes pulse	pilose antler, rhinoceros horn

Sources: The films *Chunmiao* and *Hongyu.*

These revolutionary films reflected the government's preferred healing styles, foregrounding Chinese medical practices but showing them to be supplemented by Western (modern) medical methods, such as stethoscopes. This indicated that the barefoot doctors, like the new village healers, were different from the extant healers. However, the healing styles used by barefoot doctors in daily practice were different from those images constructed in revolutionary discourse. The recollections of two barefoot doctors—Yan Shengyu of Jiang Village and Xu Peichun of Chun'an County—offer us glimpses of the barefoot doctors' actual healing styles. Jiang Village and Chun'an County are representative of the different types of places where barefoot doctors practiced medicine, since Yuhang County (including Jiang Village) is on the plains, whereas Chun'an County belongs to a mountainous area. On the other hand, the two doctors came from different backgrounds and started to work at different stages of the barefoot doctor program. Xu attended a junior middle school and studied medicine for a year at a county worker-peasant-soldier school. He started practicing medicine in the early days of the barefoot doctor program in 1969, when he was 19. By contrast, Yan had a secondary school education and studied in a county health school for a year, half in theoretical study and half as an intern in a commune clinic. He joined the medical station in 1978, when he was 20. The following sections describe in more detail their recollections of barefoot doctor treatment styles with regard to diagnostic techniques and the use of Chinese medicine, Western medicine, and acupuncture.

Diagnosis

Physicians in premodern society relied on three techniques to determine the nature of an illness: the patient's own descriptions, the physician's observation of the patient's physical appearance and behavior, and, in rare cases, the physician's manual examination of the patient's body.[12] Chinese doctors looked at their patients' complexion (*wang*), listened to their breathing (and smelled their breath and other bodily odors) (*wen*), asked questions to elicit their account of their disorder (*wen*), and touched their wrist during the complex procedure of taking the pulse (*qie*).[13] Of these procedures, checking the pulse was regarded as the key technique. According to popular Chinese medical beliefs, the skills of a clinician are demonstrated by the ability to ascertain what is wrong with the patient from the pulse and a few short questions—usually the fewer questions the better.[14] By contrast, Western medicine depended on the use of a stethoscope to diagnose illnesses. Therefore, manual pulse-taking and the use of the stethoscope represented the basic diagnostic techniques of Chinese and Western medicine, respectively, in the villages from the 1950s onward.

As a barefoot doctor in the 1970s, Xu Peichun recalled that he mainly used the Western method of "look, touch, knock, and listen"(*wang, chu, kou, ting*), rather than the Chinese medicine method of "look, smell, ask, and check the pulse"(*wang, wen, wen, qie*). He mainly used a stethoscope to diagnose illnesses. One of his medical station colleagues could make a pulse diagnosis because his family had a tradition of practicing Chinese medicine. However, in Xu's opinion this technique was not as "advanced" as the stethoscope, because his colleague nearly caused a few incidents of medical malpractice.[15] Yan Shengyu used the same method as Xu, emphasizing the role of "listening" and "knocking" to make a diagnosis using a stethoscope.[16] Both Xu and Yan knew the basic theory of pulsetaking. According to Yan, the other two colleagues at his medical station, who did not have family traditions of Chinese medicine, claimed they could carry out a diagnosis by pulse-taking. But Xu and Yan also admitted that they did not do so very often because it was quite difficult and less accurate than using a stethoscope.

Chinese Herbal Medicines

Xu started prescribing Western medicines after his graduation from the county worker-peasant-soldier school in 1969, but he recalled that, around

1971 or 1972, the higher-level authorities called for the use of herbal medicines. In the mountainous county where Xu lived, a few brigades were skilled in using Chinese herbal medicines, so Xu and his colleague went to these model brigades to study from them. The county published three volumes of herbal medicine recipes, and Xu basically prescribed herbal medicines for the villagers according to these recipes. However, he recalled that "the situation changed later" when the higher-ups ceased emphasizing Chinese herbal medicine. As to *materia medica*, he claimed that he knew how to prescribe them.[17] In contrast, Yan did not generally prescribe *materia medica* and herbal medicine after he returned to the village from the county health school in 1978. But he admitted that they bought some *materia medica* from the Hangzhou Pharmaceutical Company in urban Hangzhou. Likewise, they sometimes took a big pot out into the fields and gathered *Flos Loniceraejaponicae* (honeysuckle flowers, *jinyinhua*), *Radix Glycyrrhizae* (licorice root, *gancao*), *Herba Senecionis scandentis* (climbing groundsel herb, *qianliguang*) and goldenrod. They decocted this to make a medicine which they distributed to the commune members who were laboring in the fields.[18]

Acupuncture

Traditionally, acupuncture was a major method through which folk physicians, especially itinerant healers, cured illnesses. As they usually did not stay in one place for a long time, they depended on speedy results to make a livelihood.[19] However, the practice of acupuncture had already declined in the late imperial era in China.[20] Up to the early 1950s, it was apparently still not very popular, at least not in Yuhang County, where a Chinese medicine representative meeting was held in December of 1954 to promote acupuncture. According to the survey, only 28 Chinese medicine doctors could practice acupuncture.[21] By 1955, there were still only 55 Chinese medicine doctors who could practice acupuncture in the whole county, which had a total population of 490,400. The ratio of Chinese medicine doctors practicing acupuncture to the general county population in 1955 was thus 1:8,916.[22] However, in the 1970s, the practice of acupuncture was listed as one of the key medical techniques of the barefoot doctors. As mentioned in chapter 2, Chen Zhicheng taught acupuncture to barefoot doctor students by having them practice poking needles into white radishes. In practice, both Xu and Yan followed "four-character formulas" to treat common rural illnesses: for a headache, look for the *lieque* point; for a toothache, the *hegu* point; for a stomachache, the *zusanli* point; and for a backache, the *weizhong* point (*toutong xun lieque, yatong hegushou, dufu sanli liu, yaobei weizhong qiu*).[23] However, in old pharmacist Shao's eyes, the barefoot doctors only knew how to perform very elementary, unscientific acupuncture. The villagers did not have much faith in the barefoot doctors' acupuncture skills, because it is hard to find acupuncture points accurately, and acupuncture is useless if the points are not correctly targeted.[24]

Western Medicines

Xu and Yan recalled that most of the medicines they prescribed were Western, such as streptomycin, Analgin, tetracycline, and Terramycin. However, Xu particularly mentioned the lack of special medicines for children. In his words, "The science was as not highly developed as it is today. We had to prescribe adult medicine for children. For example, for adults, we prescribed two tablets of Analgin per dose, while a two-year-old child would be given one-twelfth of the adult dosage. So I would crush the tablet into powder and then divide it."[25]

Injections were already very popular among barefoot doctors. Xu described the procedure as follows: "Since there was no tap water in the village to sterilize the injection needles, we had to use well water. We put many needles into an aluminum lunch box, and then we put the lunch box on the stove and let the water boil for 15 minutes. It is really amazing that no accidents ever occurred at that time. You would never dare to do that now."[26] Meanwhile, the use of saline and glucose intravenous drips was introduced into China's villages by the barefoot doctors after 1970, though these were performed using quite simple procedures. In Jiang Village, saline intravenous drips were first used in 1970. Initially, Chen Zhicheng dared not administer them because the intravenous line had to be sterilized by boiling, and the treatment had strong side effects, causing the patients to feel hot and cold. The barefoot doctor by the surname of Zhou recalled that Chen did not know what to do about this reaction.[27] Even as late as the mid-1970s, intravenous glucose drips were still only rarely administered in the village medical stations. But the barefoot doctors eventually started to administer intravenous drips in their daily medical practices, and, by the end of the 1970s, both Yan and Xu claimed that they had become skilled in the administration of intravenous medication. Elderly villagers who were seriously ill or who had become unable to eat were given glucose intravenous drips. The barefoot doctors usually sterilized the needles and the rubber intravenous tubes by boiling them in aluminum lunch boxes. The same needles and tubes were used again and again. There was also a "four-character formula" for the use of intravenous drips: use salt first, then glucose; quickness first, slowness later; add potassium chloride upon seeing urine; a low dose is better than an overdose (*xianyan houtang, xiankuai houman, jianniao bujia, ningqian wuguo*).[28]

Antibiotic Tablets or Herbal Decoctions

The preceding discussion indicates that barefoot doctors applied a variety of different methods. However, the key question here is how often each healing method was applied in their daily practice. The barefoot doctors whom I interviewed provided different answers to this question. Xu recalled that he started practicing Western medicine after 1969. Even after he and his colleagues started to practice herbal medicine and acupuncture around 1972, as required by the higher authorities, Western medicines continued to account for more than half of the medicines he prescribed for several years. His use of Chinese herbal medicines and acupuncture later declined, and he made a more complete shift to Western medicine after 1982.[29] By contrast, Yan recalled that when he returned to the brigade medical station in 1978, more than 80 percent of the pharmaceuticals he prescribed were Western medicines.[30]

These accounts by the barefoot doctors interviewed in Hangzhou Prefecture indicate a general trend toward the adoption of Westernized healing styles and great popularity of the prescription of Western pharmaceuticals. This was confirmed in a critical report issued by the Yuhang County Health Bureau in 1975, according to which "a few medical personnel in our medical units are suspicious of the 'newly emerged things.' Influenced by this trend, the use of Chinese herbal medicines suffered a serious setback and declined dramatically. Some doctors in hospitals readily prescribe a host of different kinds of antibiotics."[31] This report criticized these practices for "favoring Western medicines and neglecting folk medicines (*zhongyang qingtu*)."[32]

Barefoot doctors preferred Western medicine because of practical considerations. As chapter 2 indicated, barefoot doctors' medical knowledge was basically oriented toward Western medicine. Though the government called for the barefoot doctors to use Chinese herbal medicines in daily practice, in reality, there were limits to their application of Chinese *materia medica* and herbal medicines. Barefoot doctors Xu Peichun and Yan Shengyu attributed the problem to the difficulties in studying Chinese medicine and prescribing *materia medica*, as it required high levels of literacy, particularly the ability to understand ancient Chinese texts and expressions.[33] A villager argued that many barefoot doctors did not know how to prescribe *materia medica*: "It was very hard to master Chinese medicine skills; so the majority of the barefoot doctors still used Western medicines. The reason for the unpopularity of Chinese medicines lay in the fact that the barefoot doctors' medical skills were insufficient."[34] For Chinese herbal medicine to be effective, multiple combinations and mixtures needed to be prescribed.[35] In contrast, the prescription of Western medicines did not require much medical knowledge, as the functions of the medicines were clearly listed on the medicine bottles and boxes. Since any barefoot doctor, even one with only basic literacy skills, could read and understand these instructions, it was easy to just prescribe a few tablets or administer an injection.

Besides being easier to prescribe, Western medicine was also considered much safer than Chinese herbal medicines. One villager recalled that the villagers used to take herbal medicines because of local customs, which had been handed down through the generations. But, since it was difficult to master the precise amount to be taken, outcomes ranged from good to disastrous—sometimes the medicines cured the illness, but in other cases the patients lost their hearing ability.[36] As one official report complained, since some medical staff believed that it was dangerous to use Chinese herbal medicines and safer to use Western medicines, they did not dare to go ahead and prescribe Chinese medicinal herbs.[37]

In addition to the issues of knowledge structure and fears about safety, the relatively rapid effect of Western medicine in curing diseases was another important reason for barefoot doctors' preference. Yan Shengyu made it clear why he used Western medicines: "The villagers usually didn't come to see the doctors when they got sick. When they finally did come in to see us, it usually meant that the illness had become serious, with symptoms such as a high fever and diarrhea. Western medicines were used in these cases because they could cure the illness quickly."[38] Another barefoot doctor by the surname of Fang was not willing to talk about the percentages of different pharmaceuticals he prescribed, but he admitted that if the illness was somewhat serious, he first used Western medicines, including injections and intravenous therapy, to bring it under control.[39] The barefoot doctors all attributed the "magic effects" of Western medicine to the lack of antibiotics before the 1970s. Xu Peichun compared the treatment of illnesses with the methods of killing the insects that attacked the rice crops: "It was easy to treat a person's illness back then. Let me give you a comparison. When we planted rice back then, we only needed to use lime to kill the insects. But now, even the chemical pesticides are not enough, because the insects have become resistant to them. This is the same reason that the people's illnesses have now become difficult to cure."[40]

For this reason, the official report complained that many barefoot doctors believed that using Chinese herbal medicines and acupuncture was very outdated,[41] while more and more medical stations only used Western medicines.[42] The memories of villagers confirm this trend. As one villager explained, "In our village, the barefoot doctors studied for about a year at the health school in the county seat. . . . They knew both Chinese and Western medicine. In the early 1970s, whenever they prescribed medicines, they would ask the patient which [type of] medicine he or she would prefer, but basically they were Western medicine doctors. After 1975, they began using Western medicines more and more."[43] Visitors to Chinese villages during this period also observed this phenomenon. A few professors from the Chinese University of Hong Kong who visited Doushan Commune in Taishan County in 1978 reported that "if our impressions were correct, although the Chinese and Western medicines operated together in the commune, it was the latter that was more prevalent."[44]

The barefoot doctors developed healing styles that were significant in two ways. On the one hand, the comparison of the percentage of Western medicine prescribed by barefoot doctors as opposed to other doctors in the three-tier medical network reveals an interesting phenomenon. According to Yan Shengyu, more than 80 percent of the medicines he prescribed since 1978 were Western medicines. If the villagers wanted to see Chinese medicine doctors, they had to go to Chen Hongting's commune clinic, where Chen Hongting and Chen Zhicheng specialized in Chinese surgical and internal medicine, respectively. According to Yan's estimate, around half the medicines Chen Hongting and his colleagues prescribed in the mid-1970s were Chinese medicines. During the same period, the doctors at the district clinics and county hospitals were constantly criticized because they practically never prescribed herbal medicines or *materia medica*, according to a report of the Yuhang County Health Bureau.[45] As to the proportion of Western medicine prescribed within each level of the three-tier medical network, the commune clinics (former union clinics) had the lowest percentages. This was because the union clinics were basically staffed by doctors trained in Chinese medical traditions before the early 1950s, though they sometimes recruited students from medical schools to join their clinics. District and county hospitals, particularly the latter, could recruit medical students who had received modern (Western) medical educations and were reluctant to serve in the countryside. Barefoot doctors received their Western medical educations at county schools, though they also had some knowledge of Chinese medicines. In this sense, around the time that the barefoot doctors were gaining Western medical knowledge and putting it into practice, the commune clinics became the last venues where Chinese medicines were being prescribed in the rural medical world.

Nonetheless, the formation of the barefoot doctors' healing styles also followed a general transformation of village healers' medical culture through the confluence of Chinese and Western medicine.[46] As noted at the start of this chapter, Chinese medicine doctors already knew how to prescribe Western medicine before 1949, but not all of them did so—some still maintained their traditional practices. However, even the most conservative Chinese medicine doctors started to prescribe Western medicine in the 1970s. Luo Aijuan, a commune clinic pharmacist in Chun'an County recalled that there were four medical personnel in the commune when she started work in the pharmacy in 1972. One of them was an old Chinese medicine doctor who was famous in the area and whose private clinic had been the basis for the commune clinic. He was still mainly using Chinese medicine when Luo joined the clinic but also gradually began to prescribe Western medicines after 1975. To make a treatment safer, he would add some Western medicines as the last items of the otherwise Chinese medicine prescription, but with dosages that were half the normal quantity.[47]

The gradual change in healing methods was also growing more apparent among folk healers, who were increasingly interested in acquiring new skills and using certain "modern" treatments or technologies in their own work.[48] This is reflected in the film *Chunmiao* when Qian Jiren, the commune clinic director, takes many Western medicines from the clinic and gives them to the "witch" Jia Yuexian, telling her, "You should learn how to use this modern, foreign medicine (*yang yao*) and treat the villagers with it. You should give out something. Don't just think about making money." When Jia Yuexian treats Little Dragon's acute tuberculosis, she gives Little Dragon's grandmother a few tablets of soda. Meanwhile, Jia asks her to burn some paper, and she charged RMB 5 for her services. In other words, she adopts both Western and traditional medical techniques, while trying to maintain her identity as traditional healer. In real life, folk healer Shen Fengxiang in Jiang Village knew by the early 1970s how to take a patient's temperature by putting a thermometer into the patient's mouth or rectum. He also prescribed merbromin and gentian violet, and he used bandages, acupuncture, firecupping, a stethoscope, and plaster casts.[49] The behavior of both the fictional healer Jia and the real-life healer Shen can essentially be interpreted as traditional healers adapting to the challenge of Western medicine, a phenomenon well understood in medical anthropology.[50]

Being "Quick" or "Slow," Treating "Roots" or "Symptoms"

According to current scholarship, the responses of Chinese people to Western medicine over the course of the history of modern China have ranged from resistance to receptiveness.[51] However, these responses mainly reflected the attitudes of urban Chinese who had access to Western medicine. For Chinese villagers, the rarity of Western medicine in rural China and rural economic crises precluded opportunities to experience or believe in Western medicine.[52] The understanding of Western medicine among ordinary villagers was therefore far behind that of their urban compatriots, even though Western medicines, injections, and surgery were available in rural areas by the early 1950s. Villagers thought it was very strange how the "iron wire" (syringes)could penetrate the skin of their arms.[53] In 1965, in the summary report on the experimental work on sending Chinese and Western medicine to rural areas, the Yuhang County Health Bureau claimed that poor and lower-middle peasants welcomed this work. The report mentioned that one villager's swollen foot healed in two days after he took a small pack of antiphlogistic powder, which he bought for RMB 0.06 together with two other villagers. A vice brigade director who was bedridden with diarrhea for two days recovered after taking a tablet, bought for RMB 0.02, that the village health workers gave him.[54]

After 1969, Western pharmaceuticals marched into the villages to an extent unprecedented in China's history, facilitated by the reduction in medicine prices, the extension of the supply-marketing network, and the founding of the cooperative medical service, as described in chapter 3. Consequently, villagers gained access to more Western medicines than ever before and no longer had to rely solely on the fields and mountains for their medicines.[55] The possibility of comparing Chinese pharmaceuticals with these new Western ones brought about a change in villagers' attitudes toward both. First of all, compared with Western medicines, villagers found the large volumes of Chinese *materia medica* and medicinal herbs that had to be taken to be less convenient. The *Hangzhou Pharmaceutical Commerce Gazetteer* described the problems in promoting Chinese herbal medicine in the Hangzhou Chinese and Western Pharmaceutical Station, which was in charge of pharmaceutical wholesaling for the counties under the jurisdiction of Hangzhou and a few counties in neighboring Anhui Province: "for Chinese medicinal herbs, you have to carry a big bag full of herbs, decoct a big pot full, and drink a whole, big bowlful (*lingling yi dabao, jianjian yi daguo, hehe yi dawan*)." This presented serious practical problems for patients: for example, when one peasant bought thirty doses of Chinese herbal medicines, he had to use a long wooden pole to carry them back to his home.[56] The cooperative medical service of Anxi Commune, Yuhang County, mentioned in the previous chapter, was regarded as a model in Zhejiang Province for its production of Chinese herbal medicines. But even there it was reported that people complained that "herbal medicine is good, but usually it comes in a big bag, and you need a big bowl for boiling it, so it is not convenient."[57] This inconvenience contributed to the promotion of Chinese patent medicines, of which only small quantities needed to be taken. These were medicines extracted and processed from raw herbal medicines and produced in various formats, including pills, liquids, syrups, powders, granules, instant teas, and capsules.

Effectiveness was another key factor that contributed to the formation of comparative medical beliefs. When the cooperative medical service was first implemented, ideas about Chinese and Western medicines were rather diverse among different age groups of villagers: young and middle-aged villagers often preferred to take Western medicines, while the few elderly villagers still favored Chinese herbal medicines. The elderly thought that Western medicines would cure the symptoms, while Chinese medicines would cure the roots of the illnesses (*xiyao zhibiao, zhongyao zhiben*). As a villager recounted, "A few elderly men complained to the barefoot doctors for always prescribing Western medicines, saying, 'You should dig up some herbal medicines.' These old men believed that diseases could only be completely cured by taking herbal medicines (*duangen*)."[58] However, as a general trend, the villagers gradually shifted their preferences from herbal to Western medicines, because they came to believe that Western medicines cured diseases quickly, while Chinese medicines cured diseases slowly (*xiyao lai de kuai, zhongyao lai de man*). This belief was further influenced by the barefoot doctors' preference for prescribing Western medicine in their daily practices.

In view of this situation, the Yuhang County Party Committee criticized some commune members who thought that since the cooperative medical service had been established, they should be given "good" medicines, which in their eyes were Western medicines. Some villagers complained that it was acceptable to use Chinese herbal medicines to treat chronic diseases, but that they were useless for acute diseases. Their motivation was practical, in that they depended on work points to feed themselves, and so they could not afford to delay their treatment. This preference for Western medicine was even evident in mountainous areas, where appropriate medicinal herbs were available and where villagers had more recent experiences with taking herbal medicines. A local newspaper in Lin'an County in a mountainous area reported that some people had adopted new attitudes toward Chinese herbal medicine as a result of changing views about safety, money, and collectivization. According to this report, villagers thought that Western medicines must be safe, since they were purchased with money, while Chinese medicinal herbs were said to be dangerous, since they were collected from the mountains.[59] Criticism in an official report best summarized the villagers' preferences and the government's stand on this, while simultaneously taking a swipe at the recently deposed chairman of the People's Republic of China, Liu Shaoqi: "the reason for the preference for Western medicine is that we didn't criticize Liu Shaoqi's 'revisionist health route' deeply and completely. Pernicious ideas, such as the idea that 'Chinese herbal medicine is not scientific' and 'Western medicines will definitely replace Chinese herbal medicines' were not sufficiently repudiated."[60]

Interviews with former barefoot doctors confirmed what official reports said about villagers' growing preference for Western medicine. As a barefoot doctor who started practicing medicine in Fuyang County in 1969 explained, "In our area, villagers didn't believe in herbal medicines. At that time, people always discarded the bags of herbal medicines along the roads and near the fences when they walked out of the clinics."[61] Therefore, barefoot doctors sometimes needed to persuade villagers to take Chinese herbal medicines. Financial factors also came into play: villagers thought that they were entitled to Western medicines because they had already submitted money to fund the cooperative medical service.[62] By contrast, medicinal herbs were available for free in the fields and mountains, which led one villager to complain, "if we're going to use medicinal herbs, then why should we join the cooperative medical service?"[63] In a similar case, when an elderly woman with a mild case of diarrhea was given herbal medicine by a barefoot doctor, she became very angry and said, "I paid two yuan [to the cooperative medical service], so why do you ask me to take herbal medicine?"[64] Her anger is understandable, as RMB 2 was a significant sum for villagers during the 1970s. For example, in the western mountainous area of Hangzhou Prefecture, Chun'an County, the villagers' annual savings were only RMB 3.22 per capita in 1971 and RMB 6.55 in 1977.[65]

Villagers' new medical beliefs did not stop there. They also believed that Western medicine, though strong and fast-acting, could cause severe side effects and often only relieve superficial symptoms. Chinese medicine, on the other hand, was regarded as gentle and gradual; although it might fail to cure the illness, at least it would not harm the patient.[66] With regard to this issue of side effects, Arthur Kleinman found that in Taiwan's Chinese society during the late 1970s, popular ideology asserted that Chinese medicines have no side effects, and, even if patients do experience side effects from taking Chinese medicines, they do not complain. By contrast, if a Western medicine so much as tastes bad, patients believe that they are experiencing side effects.[67] Nonetheless, these beliefs did not affect the general trend of villagers' increasing preference for Western medicine. As Felix Mann found in the mid-1960s, the tendency among Chinese to rate Western medicine more highly than their own traditional medical system was probably due to the fact that Western medicine, particularly since the advent of antibiotics, can cure quite a number of diseases that the Chinese medical system cannot.[68] Villagers therefore developed a particular mode of seeking health care and medicines in which they would choose Western medicines to treat the symptoms of serious illnesses, while they would choose either Chinese or Western medicines for minor illnesses. In general, they either tried Western medicine first followed by Chinese medicine, or took Chinese and Western medicine at the same time.[69]

Self-medication also became more popular among villagers than before. For common headaches, fever, and diarrhea, villagers knew which tablets they should take, despite their lack of medical education. The increasing popularity of self-medication was unhampered by over-the-counter medicine regulation laws, because they had not yet been implemented. In this way, the comparative medical beliefs about Chinese and Western medicines gradually became normalized.[70] In a survey of villagers' attitudes toward traditional Chinese and Western medicines in Linping and Bolu townships, Yuhang County, in 1999, it was found that respondents in both towns strongly favored the use of Western medicines. The main reasons given for this preference continued to echo those explored above: greater convenience, perceived effectiveness, and efficiency in rapidly relieving symptoms and curing ailments.[71]

However, villagers' attitudes toward doctors from the two different medical traditions were different from their attitudes toward pharmaceuticals. Edward Shorter discusses the impact of technologies on the authority and status of physicians in the social history of medicine. He argues that advanced technologies not only controlled physicians; they also helped to reduce the physicians' authority over their patients because patients knew that much of the diagnostic work was done by technology and technicians.[72] However, Chinese villagers not only respected newly arrived medical technologies, pharmaceuticals, and doctors, they also continued to appreciate traditional techniques and old Chinese medicine doctors (*laozhongyi*). Yan Shengyu's recollections of villagers regard for doctors trained in Chinese medicine during the 1970s supports this position: in their opinion, accurate diagnoses and Chinese medicine prescriptions required a high degree of proficiency.[73] Even today, the former barefoot doctor Xu Shuilin still admires Chen Zhicheng for the accuracy of his pulse-taking.[74]

Fluctuations in the Fortunes of the Cooperative Medical Services

Starting in 1969, the barefoot doctors and the cooperative medical services had been quickly popularized nationwide as part of a new socialist medical program that was successfully implemented through a political campaign.[75] However, just as official discourse claimed that "every 'newly emerged thing' will definitely encounter difficulties and fluctuate during their growth process," the cooperative medical services indeed experienced fluctuations in fortune.[76] In May 1969, half a year after the cooperative medical services were initiated nationwide, a report in the *People's Daily* pointed out some serious problems: "the first is the increasing number of patients visiting clinics. The second is poor funding. The third is that the barefoot doctors have no experience in prescribing medicines. The fourth is those old doctors who have not cast off the old habits of blindly believing that only good medicine can cure diseases."[77] As a result, official instructions during the 1970s repeatedly emphasized that the key to running the cooperative medical services successfully was to focus on the use of acupuncture and Chinese herbal medicines, as only in this way could the cooperative medical services be strengthened. In contrast, dependence on tetracycline and Chloromycetin would weaken the system, since these medicines cost money.[78] However, no matter how many pages of official instructions they issued, they were unable to reverse the decline of Chinese herbal medicine and the advance of Western medicine because of the barefoot doctors' healing styles and the villagers' comparative medical beliefs. These also became the main factors behind the constant fluctuations in the implementation of the cooperative medical services from their beginnings in 1969–70.

By 1973, only four years after the cooperative medical services had been implemented nationwide, the percentage of production brigades implementing them had dropped to the lowest levels in the history of the program. In Hangzhou Prefecture and Zhejiang Province, the proportion of brigades implementing cooperative medical services dropped to 38.55 and 29.10 percent respectively,[79] and the situation was similar in the neighboring provinces of Shanghai, Fujian, and Jiangsu, data for which is also available.[80] The Yuhang County Cooperative Medical Service was the most successful not only among the seven counties of Hangzhou Prefecture, but also in Zhejiang Province as a whole during the 1970s. But the cooperative medical service also went through a serious decline in this county. By July 1974, the percentage of the production brigades implementing the cooperative medical services had declined by 20 percent across the whole county. The official report claimed that a group of class enemies cursed that "it was too early to run the cooperative medical service . . . [which] was badly run." This group cursed the barefoot doctors, saying that they "only knew how to smear mercurochrome" and that "the tails of rabbits cannot grow longer," meaning that the program could not develop any further, and attempted to kill the "newly emerged things" in the cradle.[81] The percentage of production brigades implementing the cooperative medical service only increased again in 1976, as the result of political pressure from above. Although in this same year implementation reached the highest level of the 1970s, it soon started to decline again.[82] The main difficulties encountered by the cooperative medical services throughout the 1970s continued to be financial problems resulting from overuse, unfair use, and poor management.[83] Chen Zhicheng recalled that when he was the director of Jiang Village Commune Clinic, he was always trying to find ways to reduce the clinic deficit and supplement the budget of cooperative medical service, for example, by trying to prescribe more medicines to free medical service beneficiaries, drawing the money from the government's investment in public health, and selling distilled water to neighboring communes.[84] For production brigades without such solutions, the cooperative medical service had very a fragile basis, as its implementation depended solely on the collective economy. When the collective economy met with difficulties, cooperative medical services could easily face decline or simply cease operation.[85]

However, even after the cooperative medical services were discontinued, medical stations and barefoot doctors continued to exist within the production brigades, thereby maintaining some degree of stability in health care from 1968 to 1983. As the barefoot doctor Fang recalled, "Our brigade's cooperative medical service collapsed around 1975, yet there was no interruption in the operation of our brigade medical station. It was maintained by our brigade. . . . The villagers paid the fees for the medicines they needed when they came here. In the beginning, the brigade put in some money. As long as the money didn't decrease, it was okay."[86] Therefore, the percentage of brigades with medical stations and barefoot doctors was higher than that of the brigades with cooperative medical services.[87] In the Hangzhou area, only 63.08 percent of production brigades implemented the cooperative medical services in 1975, whereas 97.8 percent of brigades had barefoot doctors, so there were 1.88 barefoot doctors per brigade.[88] Thus, when the cooperative medical service ceased to function, the medical stations supplied medicines and medical services to the villagers based on fees for services, while some medical stations operated as medicine retailing shops.[89] In production brigades without medical stations, the medical kits the barefoot doctors carried were the main channels through which medicines were dispensed to villagers.

Structural Changes in Pharmaceutical Consumption

Because of the long-term stability of medical stations and kits in villages, the structure of pharmaceutical consumption there underwent a significant change during the 1970s. An analysis of the quantity, types, and sales income of various pharmaceuticals may reflect the structural changes brought about by the advent of barefoot doctors and the establishment of the cooperative medical stations. However, research exploring these issues faces a major problem, namely the unavailability of documentary sources. The majority of the brigade barefoot doctors, who were usually accountants for the medical stations, did not record the incomes and expenditures of the cooperative medical services in detail during the 1970s. When barefoot doctors did keep records, they usually discarded them after some time, seeing them as nothing more than useless waste. The few barefoot doctors who did not dispose of their records refused to show them to others, as a few villagers believed that the accounts were not accurate. Fortunately, Hong Jinglin of Wulian Brigade saved some incomplete account books for the commune and brigade levels. The expenditure breakdown of the Jiang Village Cooperative Medical Service in 1971, the first year of the program, indicated that the consumption of Western pharmaceuticals already slightly exceeded the consumption of Chinese pharmaceuticals (see table 4.3). However, recorded expenditures on pharmaceuticals should not be taken as exact indications of the amount of Chinese and Western pharmaceuticals that villagers consumed. Barefoot doctor Xu Shuilin claimed that the key turning point in the consumption of Western pharmaceuticals in Jiang Village was around the year 1974. As Xu put it, "It [the choice between Chinese and Western pharmaceuticals] was not emphasized as much as before. There were more and more Western medicines. Chinese medicine was less and less emphasized. We felt the effects of Chinese medicine were not as good as those of Western medicine. Though the higher-ups still called for us to use it, less attention was paid to Chinese medicine."[90] Though incomplete, pharmaceutical inventories from 1975 to 1979 indicate that the consumption of Chinese pharmaceuticals was almost negligible in Jiang Village during those years.

Table 4.3. Breakdown of the pharmaceutical consumption of Jiang Village
Cooperative Medical Service, 1971 (unit: RMB)

Category	Jiang Village Headquarters	Sanshen Branch	Luojiazhuang Branch	Total	100%
Type I: Chinese medicine					
Materia medica	9313.96	2265.57	3171.93	14751.46	41.5
Decoction	76.71		44.8	121.51	0.3
Sub-total				14872.97	41.8
Type II: Western medicine					
Western pharmaceuticals	12336.33	2397.79	3540.83	18274.95	51.4
Surgery	5.47	0.8	0.1	6.37	0.0
Injection	99.9	0.3	12.95	113.15	0.3
Sub-total				18394.47	51.7
Type III: Others					
Outpatient	72.9	0.2	11.8	84.9	0.2
Birth	27.5		2.5	30	0.1
Dressing	653.98	110.32	142.75	907.05	2.6
Registration	795.98	21.2	447.41	1264.59	3.6
Subtotal				2286.54	6.4
Total	23382.73	4796.18	7375.07	35553.98	100

Source: "Jiangcun hezuo yiliao kaizhi mingxibiao" [Expenditure breakdown of Jiang Village
Cooperative Medical Service, 1971], supplied by barefoot doctor Hong Jinglin, Jiang Village.

The data from Jiang Village presents a fragmented picture of pharmaceutical consumption. Fortunately, Jiande County Health Bureau saved complete, detailed data from 1961 to 1983, which provides a more convincing picture. Cooperative medical stations and the barefoot doctor program were instigated nationwide in 1970, which can therefore be seen as a watershed year in terms of medicine consumption. The first crucial issue to be explored is medicine expenditure, both in total and per capita. By 1970, the total medicine expenditure in Jiande County remained RMB 1 million, which did not include the cost of medical instruments and chemical solutions. However, total medicine expenditure increased to RMB 1.2 million in the second year (1971) and continued to increase year by year from then onward (see fig. 4.1). In the same

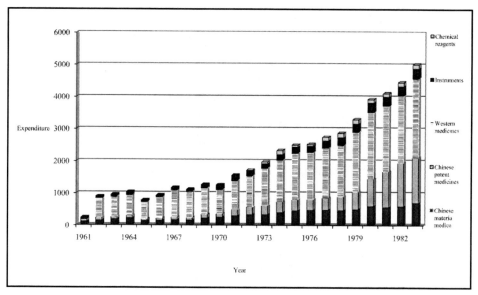

Figure 4.1. Expenditures on different kinds of pharmaceuticals in Jiande County, 1961–83 (unit: RMB 1000). Data from Yan, *Jiandexian yiyao weishengzhi*, 110–11.

way, medicine expenditure per capita in Jiande County was kept under RMB 3 before 1970, grew to around RMB 4 in 1971, and has continued to increase steadily ever since. As state employees enjoyed free medical services, subtracting the total free medical service expenditure per capita from the per capita medicine expenditure of the county reveals villagers' medicine expenditure per capita. This was roughly the same as that of the per capita consumption for the whole county.[91] This data indicates that the establishment of the medical stations and the presence of the barefoot doctors increased pharmaceutical consumption significantly.

A second critical issue was the different kinds of pharmaceuticals being consumed during this period. What was the consumption of Chinese *materia medica* like when the Chinese herbal medicine campaign was promoted in villages during the 1970s? According to the statistical data concerning thirty kinds of common Chinese *materia medica* in Jiande County, the average consumption rate per capita was under 0.06 *jin* (approximately 30g) before 1969. The consumption rate stayed the same in 1970 but suddenly increased to 0.08 *jin* (40g) in 1971, before settling at between 0.08 and 0.1 *jin* (40 and 50g) from 1971 to 1982 (see fig. 4.2). This means that the average consumption rate of Chinese *materia medica* saw no significant change in conjunction with the Chinese herbal medicine campaign and the foundation of the cooperative medical stations. The amounts of Chinese *materia medica* consumed therefore remained relatively stable until 1983, though their total

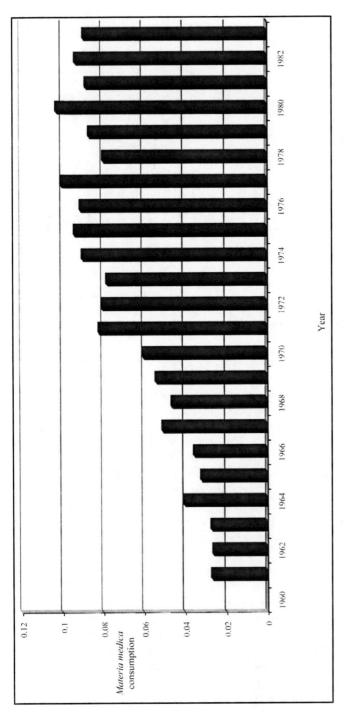

Figure 4.2. *Materia medica* consumption per capita in Jiande County, 1960–83 (unit: *jin* or 500g). Data from Yan, *Jiandexian yiyao weishengzhi*, 110–11.

Table 4.4. *Materia medica* and Chinese patent medicine consumptions in three counties of Zhejiang Province, 1961–89

	Jiande County							Comparison of three counties				
	Materia medica and Chinese patent medicine							Pharmaceutical consumption per capita (unit: RMB)			Percentage of *materia medica* and patent medicine	
		Materia medica and Chinese patent medicine		*Materia medica*		Chinese patent medicine						
Year	Total sales of Chinese and Western medicine (unit: RMB1000)	Total (unit: RMB1000)	Percentage of total sales (unit: %)	Sales (unit: RMB1000)	Percentage of total sales (unit: %)	Sales (unit: RMB1000)	Percentage of total sales (unit: %)	Jiande	Wuyi	Jinyun	Wuyi (unit: %)	Jinyun (unit: %)
1961–69												
1961	1,009	183.3	18.2	111.7	11.1	71.6	7.1	2.9				
1962	898	245	27.3	148	16.5	97	10.8	2.5	1.6		27.9/9.0	
1963	956	261	27.3	190	19.9	71	7.4	2.5	2.1	1.8	25.9/8.6	25.3/8.4
1964	1,031	300	29.1	222	21.5	78	7.6	2.7	2.4	1.8	27.7/8	27.9/6.7
1965	782	191	24.4	133	17.0	58	7.4	2.0	2.1	1.6	23.2/8.7	22.0/7.1
1966	937	214	22.8	149	15.9	65	6.9	2.3	2.2	1.7	20.7/9.4	17.0/7.2
1967	1,174	249	21.2	168	14.3	81	6.9	2.8	2.9	1.9	16.9/9	17.2/7.1
1968	1,116	237	21.2	157	14.1	80	7.2	2.7	2.5	1.7	18.4/9.3	16.9/7.7
1969	1,268	339	26.7	222	17.5	117	9.2	3.3	2.7	1.8	18.1/8.9	15.8/7.8
Average	1,019	246.6	24.2	166.7	16.4	79.8	7.8	2.6	2.3	1.8	22.4/8.9	20.3/7.4

Table 4.4. *Materia medica* and Chinese patent medicine consumptions in three counties of Zhejiang Province, 1961–89—*(concluded)*

	Jiande County							Comparison of three counties				
		Materia medica and Chinese patent medicine										
				Materia medica		Chinese patent medicine		Pharmaceutical consumption per capita (unit: RMB)			Percentage of *materia medica* and patent medicine	
Year	Total sales of Chinese and Western medicine (unit: RMB1000)	Total (unit: RMB1000)	Percentage of total sales (unit: %)	Sales (unit: RMB1000)	Percentage of total sales (unit: %)	Sales (unit: RMB1000)	Percentage of total sales (unit: %)	Jiande	Wuyi	Jinyun	Wuyi (unit: %)	Jinyun (unit: %)
1970–78												
1970	1,260	360	28.6	251	19.9	109	8.7	3.2	2.7	2.2	19.3/8.5	18.6/6.6
1971	1,550	491	31.7	294	19.0	197	12.7	3.9	3.0	2.3	21.6/9.9	21.2/9.7
1972	1,710	570	33.3	336	19.6	234	13.7	4.3	3.9	2.5	19.4/10.6	19.4/10.1
1973	1,970	621	31.5	336	17.1	285	14.5	4.9	4.9	3.3	17.2/10.8	17.4/10.1
1974	2,326	733	31.5	404	17.4	329	14.1	5.7	5.3	3.7	16.7/11.2	17.1/12.2
1975	2,496	810	32.5	458	18.3	352	14.1	6.0	5.6	4.0	17.4/12.6	16.2/12.5
1976	2,513	813	32.4	476	18.9	337	13.4	6.0	5.7	3.7	16.2/12.5	16.5/14
1977	2,740	858	31.3	484	17.7	374	13.6	6.5	6.1	4.2	16.3/13.7	17.4/11.3
1978	2,872	901	31.4	470	16.4	431	15.0	6.7	6.5	4.7	18.7/11.5	17.2/12.7
Average	2,159.7	648.1	31.6	389.9	18.3	294.2	13.3	5.2	4.9	3.4	18.1/11.3	17.9/11.0

1979–83											
1979	3,289	1,060	32.2	503	15.3	557	16.9	7.7	6.9	4.8	18.5/13.4 23.3/9.5
1980	3,923	1,436	36.6	604	15.4	832	21.2	9.1	7.6	6.2	19.6/10.9 21.0/10.6
1981	4,106	1,674	40.8	569	13.9	1105	26.9	9.5	8.4	6.5	18.0/18.7 16.6/13.6
1982	4,451	1,950	43.8	594	13.3	1356	30.5	10.1	9.8	7.8	17.7/21.5 16.8/17.9
1983	5,009	2,111	42.1	704	14.1	1407	28.1	11.3	11.4	11.2	17.7/22.9 15.718.9
Average	4,155.6	1,646.2	39.1	594.8	14.4	1051.4	24.7	9.5	8.8	7.3	18.3/17.5 18.7/14.1
1984–89											
1984	—	—	—	—	—	—	—	—	11.4	9.3	17.5/24.6 18.9/20.2
1985	—	—	—	—	—	—	—	—	13.0	8.8	16.8/28.4 22.0/22.5
1986	—	—	—	—	—	—	—	—	14.0	10.8	18.3/27.3 16.8/20.1
1987	—	—	—	—	—	—	—	—	15.8	13.5	17.7/25.3 15.7/21.7
1988	—	—	—	—	—	—	—	—	17.5	17.9	23.0/25 17.6/22.4
1989	—	—	—	—	—	—	—	—	16.1	14.8	19.2/21.1 15.1/21.0
Average	—	—	—	—	—	—	—	—	14.6	12.5	18.8/25.3 17.7/21.3

Sources: Yan, *Jiandexian yiyao weishengzhi,* 116; Ying Yiping, ed., *Wuyixian weishengzhi* [Wuyi County Health Gazetteer] (Wuyi: Wuyixian weishengju, 1992), 205; Jinyunxian yiyaozhi bianzhuan xiaozu [Editorial Team of Jinyun County Medical and Pharmaceutical Gazetteer], ed., *Jinyunxian yiyaozhi* [Jinyun County Medical and Pharmaceutical Gazetteer] (Jinyun: Jinyunxian yinshuachang, 1990), 226–30. No data available for Jiande County for the period 1984–89.

sales income slowly increased as prices increased.[92] As a percentage of total sales of all pharmaceuticals, Chinese *materia medica* increased from 16.4 percent in 1961–69 to 18.3 percent in 1970–78 before declining to 14.4 percent in 1979–83. The Jiande County trend was paralleled in Wuyi and Jinyun counties, the only two for which data are available in Zhejiang Province (see table 4.4).

While consumption of Chinese *materia medica* declined, that of Chinese patent medicines increased steadily. As mentioned in the previous chapter, some Chinese patent medicines—such as *xingjunsan*, *biwendan*, and *shayao* for treating heatstroke—were sold as common medicines at rural medicine shops by the 1940s. After the late 1950s, the kinds of Chinese patent medicines available increased slowly, while production technologies and packaging also improved. As prepared medicines, Chinese patent medicines solved the inconvenience of collecting and drying fresh herbal medicine and decocting *materia medica*. As former commune clinic pharmacist Luo said, "If we prescribed *materia medica*, patients would have to carry many bags of it and decoct the medicine themselves. For those chronic patients who needed to take medicines quite often, patent medicines were more convenient than *materia medica*. But in terms of effects, *materia medica* was much better than patent medicine because decoctions were extracted directly from the *materia medica*."[93] In Jiang Village, barefoot doctor Yan Shengyu recalled that, by 1978, "there were already some Chinese patent medicines, such as cow bezoar tablets (*niuhuang jiedupian*) for clearing away heat and toxic materials and *Fructus Forsythiae* tablets (*yinqiao jiedupian*) for treating colds and flu. They were not expensive. But there were not many brands. Later there were more and more Chinese patent medicines because many Chinese medicine factories were established."[94] Meanwhile, the increasing promotional activity by pharmaceutical companies, the state's efforts to standardize compound prescriptions, and patients' preference for easily consumable (and acceptable-tasting) medicine also contributed to the increase of Chinese patent medicines on the market.[95]

These changes were reflected in the sales volumes of Chinese patent medicines. In Jiande County, Chinese patent medicines accounted for only 7.8 percent of the total sales income of various pharmaceuticals in 1961–69 (see table 4.4), before rising to 8.7 percent in 1970, 12.7 percent in 1971, and 13.3 percent in 1971–78. The proportion of patent medicines to total pharmaceutical sales incomes only exceeded that of Chinese *materia medica* for the first time in 1979. When the barefoot doctor program for all intents and purposes stopped running in 1983, this percentage jumped to 24.7 percent in Jiande County. In the wholesale areas of the Hangzhou Chinese and Western Pharmaceutical Station, which included both rural and urban areas, sales of Chinese patent medicines increased by only 62.2 percent from 1959 to 1979, but these figures soared to 317.3 percent in 1983 and 624.1 percent in 1987.[96]

However, this increase came mainly from sales of nutritional and tonic medicines rather than curative pharmaceuticals.[97] In the words of a local gazetteer, "after the late 1960s, nutritional and tonic medicines were believed to serve 'bourgeois lifestyles.' This resulted in their long-term subordinate position. With the improvement in urban and rural residents' living conditions after 1979, they started to pay attention to their own health." As an old villager put it, "In the Collective Era (before 1983), what we wanted was to have full meals. Later, economic conditions improved greatly. Villagers had money to take tonics. A few families even took tonic products throughout the year!"[98] In the meantime, nutritional and tonic medicines also became indispensable gifts when villagers visited sick relatives and friends. According to the statistic data for seventeen major Chinese patent medicines in the wholesale areas supplied by the Hangzhou Chinese and Western Pharmaceutical Station, the sales incomes for nutritional and tonic medicines increased steeply, as did their percentage share of total Chinese patent medicines sales, growing from 33.29 percent in 1979 to 38.32 percent in 1980. Tonic sales eventually surpassed those of curative Chinese patent medicines, representing an average of 51.77 percent of total sales between 1981 and 1985.[99]

Interestingly, villagers have their own classifications and interpretations of pharmaceuticals. When asked what Chinese patent medicine was, an old villager was confused by the term and said, "The barefoot doctor gave me a few tablets once and told me, 'this is Chinese patent medicine,' at the time the household contract responsibility was implemented. But I really don't know."[100] When asked the same question, an eighty-six-year-old villager who served as the brigade party secretary from the late 1950s to the early 1980s gave a different interpretation: "Herbal medicine refers to fresh medicinal plants dug from the mountains without processing. *Materia medica* refers to processed herbal medicine. Chinese patent medicine refers to important *materia medica*. Western medicines are chemical products. Young guys who can recognize characters on medicine bottles should know which medicines are Chinese patent medicines."[101] But both villagers insisted that nutritional "medicines" and tonics are definitely not medicines.

No matter how Chinese patent medicine is classified and interpreted, the increase in its sales volumes became the sole factor behind the increased percentage of Chinese medicine (including *materia medica* and patent medicines) over total pharmaceutical sales. In Jiande County, the average percentage of Chinese medicine over total pharmaceuticals increased from 24.2 percent in 1961–69 to 31.6 percent in 1970–78 before soaring to 40.8 percent in 1979–83. Though this increasing percentage of the sales income represented by Chinese medicine does indicate a decrease in the percentage represented by Western pharmaceuticals, the actual quantity of Western medicine consumed increased steadily year by year. As discussed earlier, Western pharmaceutical prices were reduced by about 37 percent in 1969, and there were further reductions in 1974 and 1984. Therefore, increasing expenditure and decreasing prices resulted in a significant increase of

Western pharmaceutical consumption throughout the 1970s in villages. Antibiotics predominated these Western medicines: in Jiande County, the top ten medicines consumed per capita throughout the 1970s were tetracycline, penicillin, Terramycin, Gastropin, piperazine citrate (for repelling ascarids), antipyretics, painkiller tablets, Anlagin, ephedrine tablets, and syntomycin.[102] These medicines were particularly effective for treating the most common of villagers' diseases during the 1970s, as discussed in chapter 3. Meanwhile, instruments and disposable materials, including syringes, needles, cotton, and bandages, were used on a large scale.[103] This also represented a great change: in 1949, there was only one thermometer per eighteen thousand people in China,[104] but after 1968, each brigade generally had a thermometer, a blood pressure meter, and a stethoscope.

Partly as a result of this influx of Western pharmaceuticals and medical suppliers, the way in which Chinese medicine was used began to change. In 1985, an official from China's Ministry of Health admitted in a report delivered at a WHO seminar that "generally speaking, traditional medicine is used to the greatest extent (about 40 percent of the cases) in primary health care and much less in hospital practice, except in the traditional hospitals and wards. Most of the general hospitals use modern medicine and add some traditional medicine."[105] However, the Chinese medicines to which the official referred were mainly Chinese patent medicines. From the early 1980s on, it became increasingly rare to see patients' families decocting *materia medica* for them, at least in rural Hangzhou. However, Chinese patent medicines do still account for a part of total pharmaceutical consumption, albeit a minor one. According to Yan Shengyu, who is currently working at the Jiang Village medical station, he and his colleagues prescribe Chinese patent medicines to 60 percent of total patients. For these patients, Chinese patent medicines account for 25 percent of total prescribed medicines, mainly as supplements to Western medicines.[106]

The advent of the barefoot doctors and the establishment of medical stations led to villagers forming comparative ideas about medicines, had a huge impact on Chinese medicine in terms of its standardization, and led to a radical revolution in pharmaceutical consumption in Chinese villages. These changes to rural medical ideas and consumption patterns necessarily imply the transformation of pharmaceutical consumption across China, given that China's rural population accounts for the majority of its citizens, even though those in rural areas still consumed vastly fewer pharmaceuticals than their urban compatriots.[107]

Overuse of Western Pharmaceuticals

Villagers gradually came to prefer Western medicine, and this preference brought with it a considerable problem of overuse. Yan Xiaocheng was a Chinese medicine doctor from the Research Institute for Chinese Medicine in Beijing. He followed urban medical teams in Beijing, Henan, Shanxi, and Tibet from 1964 to 1974. In a letter written to the *Journal of Barefoot Doctors* in 1978, Yan warned that "the abuse of Western medicine among barefoot doctors and other medical staff in rural areas is very serious, particularly the overuse of injections. Injections are being given regardless of which diseases are being treated." He suggested that the journal should emphasize teaching barefoot doctors how to prescribe medicines properly.[108] C. C. Chen, the leader of the rural experimental medical program in Ding County in the 1930s, also noted in the late 1970s that barefoot doctors in Sichuan Province were legally entitled to prescribe drugs without restriction, with little or no supervision.[109]

When rural reform was initiated in the early 1980s, barefoot doctors became private medical practitioners. Because no fees were usually charged for consultations and examinations, village clinics came to depend on profits from pharmaceutical sales to maintain daily operations.[110] Prescribing Western medicines became even more popular. According to the statistical data, 89.1 percent of village clinic profits were from prescribing medicines.[111] The former barefoot doctor Fang frankly acknowledged that he prescribed Western medicine in order to make money:

> We needed the money to support ourselves, as we were not paid by the government. We could make money by prescribing Western medicine. This is known as 'supporting doctors by selling medicines'(*yiyao yangyi*). As to the herbal medicines, how could you charge money for them? For a bunch of herbal medicines, can you charge the villagers RMB 5 or 6? No one would accept it. I belonged to the Western medicine category of village doctors. We could not survive by prescribing only Chinese herbal medicines.[112]

Another barefoot doctor said, "After the [economic] reforms and opening up, it was more and more convenient and flexible than before. All you had to do was to call the pharmaceutical company, and the company would deliver right to your door."[113]

Western healing methods therefore achieved even greater dominance in the villages when the barefoot doctor program came to an end in the early 1980s. According to medical anthropologist Sydney White's work in the Lijiang basin in Yunnan Province in 1989 and 1990, Western medicine had already triumphed in terms of healing styles, though she concluded that by this time Chinese and Western medicine had been integrated:

> Many of the medicines of systematic correspondence afflictions just outlined were treated by Lijiang basin village practitioners primarily with injections of antibiotics, IV infusions of glucose water, vitamins, and/or antibiotics, or tablets of WM (Western medicine) pharmaceuticals. Some of the afflictions were treated primarily with Chinese medicine pharmaceuticals (which could be

administered through injections or IV infusions as well as in ways more con-ventional historically to Chinese medicine). And some of the afflictions were treated with a combination of both Western medicine and Chinese medicine pharmaceuticals and techniques.[114]

By the late 1990s, there were still no regulations for or limits to the prescription of medicines by barefoot doctors. The distinction between prescription medicine and over-the-counter medicine was not followed rigorously. Meanwhile, the villagers were becoming more and more famil-iar with common medicines and usually asked for particular drugs. More significantly, patients themselves asked for glucose intravenous drips. Even in cases of strained lumbar muscles, they would still demand vitamins and amino acids because it made them feel good, so they believed they were effective.[115] Barefoot doctors rarely declined requests of this nature. In late 2009, Yan Shengyu, who was the last to join the Jiang Village barefoot doc-tor group in 1978, complained, "now, I treat about 70 patients per day, and every day at least 20 of them demand that I give them intravenous drips."[116] In a later interview, he said, "patients just sit down and before I have even made a diagnosis for them, they say immediately, 'Doctor, I have a cold, so please give me two bottles of drips.' Patients would like [medicines] to take effect quickly. Today I have flu and go on a drip, so tomorrow I will be able to go to work. Nowadays people believe firmly in intravenous drips."[117] To a certain extent, drip therapy became a kind of panacea or placebo for villag-ers.[118] Because of this, clinics and hospital infusion rooms in today's China are always full of patients on intravenous drips, often for minor complaints. The prevalence of the practice has given rise to the term named "drip bottle forest" (*diaoping senlin*) to describe the common scene of bottles and long tubes trailing over infusion frames in hospital infusion rooms.[119]

These phenomena also occur in the relatively remote border areas where Western medicine and even Chinese medicine arrived quite a long time after 1949. According to Liu Xiaoxing's anthropological study in Yunnan during the 1990s, self-medication was commonplace among vil-lagers, who had also become proficient at other medical techniques, such as giving themselves injections. People could go to the township hospital or health station if they felt they needed to. Otherwise they simply used the medicine they bought from the township hospital or farmers' market. Most families had their own medical kits, and most of the medicines they used were Western biomedicines.[120]

The barefoot doctors' unlimited prescription powers and villagers' self-medication practices resulted in an overuse of pharmaceuticals (both West-ern and Chinese patent medicines), as also happened in other developing countries.[121] In a study of households in central China in the late 1990s, it was found that 75 percent of the individuals interviewed had bought modern medicines without prescriptions during the previous two weeks.[122] According to Liu Yuanli's statistical data, 20–36 percent of the prescriptions given by village practitioners in 1998 unnecessarily contained corticosteroids. The percentage of children receiving intramuscular injections for treatment of the common cold was as high as 46–64 percent.[123]

The overuse of medicines aroused the attention of the government. In Hangzhou Prefecture, *The Basic Catalogue of Medicines Prescribed by Village Doctors of Zhejiang Province* was put into effect until May 2006. According to the regulations it contained, village doctors could prescribe 277 kinds of medicines in seventeen categories but were forbidden from prescribing medicines and preparing herbal remedies (*yinpian*) with strong or toxic side effects.[124] In spite of this, the abuse of Western medicine is still rampant under the market economy of twenty-first century China.[125] According to the February 2010 edition of *Economy Survey China* issued by the Organization for Economic Co-operation and Development (OECD), this overuse is particularly common among village doctors, who have an incentive to over-prescribe, given that they rely on sales of medicines for part of their income. For nearly three-quarters of the patients surveyed, the medicine prescribed was an antibiotic, while one-fifth were prescribed two or more drugs. The risks of pharmaceutical overuse were further increased because most medicines were given by injection, mainly intravenously.[126] For all these reasons, pharmaceuticals account for 45 percent of China's health-care expenditure (or 1.6 percent of its GDP),[127] far above other countries, where pharmaceuticals usually account for one-quarter of total health-related spending.[128]

Scholars once argued that the practice of integrating Chinese and Western medicine that emerged after the Cultural Revolution was a natural hybrid in which Chinese medical discourse occupied a position that was by no means subordinate to Western medicine.[129] However, the merger was actually far from equal. No Western medicine doctors used any traditional Chinese medicine techniques for diagnosis or treatment, while all traditional Chinese medicine doctors mentioned that they used both Western and traditional Chinese techniques to diagnose and treat their patients.[130] This was the context within which the barefoot doctors developed their own healing styles. Though in many ways barefoot doctors represented an integration of Chinese and Western medicine, in reality they expressed obvious preferences for Western medicine, which affected villagers significantly. As barefoot doctors introduced new healing styles and a host of Western medicines to rural China, villagers, in turn, developed a preference for Western medicine. Interestingly, as Farquhar found in the early 1990s, urban Chinese "are these days much more enthusiastic users of Chinese medicine than rural people."[131] Her findings have been increasingly verified during the first decade of the twenty-first century. As former commune clinic pharmacist, Luo, who is now living in urban Hangzhou, said, "Nowadays villagers basically take Western medicines. On the contrary, those big hospitals in Hangzhou would prescribe Chinese medicine and decoct *materia medica* for patients because they have decoction machines."[132] Together, the barefoot doctors' healing styles and the villagers' medical preferences led to a steady increase in pharmaceuticals consumption in China, while fundamentally changing the structure of consumption by tipping the balance in favor of Western medicine from then on. Although the overall consumption of Chinese medicine (both *materia medica* and patent medicines) also increased to some extent, it was marginalized as the medicine of "last resort" for chronic, incurable diseases, undesirable insufficiencies, and even acute infectious diseases like SARS.[133]

Chapter Five

Relocating Illness

The Shift from Home Bedside to Hospital Ward

For ordinary Chinese villagers, seeking treatment in a hospital was completely unheard of until the middle of the twentieth century. Until about the mid-1960s, most medical encounters between doctors and patients in the professional medical sector in Chinese villages had changed little since the times of those villagers' distant ancestors. Hospitalization, wards, referrals, and medical consultations were all still remote and strange ideas to the majority of villagers. This pattern would change in the early 1980s. As the odors of decocted medicinal herbs gradually ceased to fill the village skies, medical encounters were no longer confined to villagers' homes. Instead, China's rural residents increasingly left their villages to seek treatment in clinics or hospitals outside their local communities, sometimes through referrals and sometimes on their own initiative. From this point on, hospitalization—including the patient experiences of hospital stays and formal medical consultation—became increasingly common in the lives of villagers. Barefoot doctors were instrumental in bringing these radical changes to the rural population because of their integral role in the process of implanting medical institutionalization in Chinese villages through the establishment of a hierarchical medical system, the formalization of medical encounters, and the codification of the medical community.

Home-Based Medical Encounters in an Isolated Medical World

The previous chapters have discussed the individual, fragmented, and independent nature of professional medical practice in Chinese villages up to the late 1940s. The so-called home-based clinics were usually one-person operations. Chen Hongting's clinic was unusual in that two practitioners worked there (Chen and his father). However, these home-based clinics lacked many of the features we associate with modern medical clinics, such as the basic layout of a medical building and departmental divisions. Moreover, each clinic basically limited itself to practicing within its community, mainly the township in which it was located. Furthermore, unlike today, there was no clear spatial demarcation of daily medical practice. Medical encounters between doctors and patients mainly occurred in the patients' homes. There were certain advantages to this method, since seeing the patient's home enabled doctors to contextualize illness more accurately, integrate this information with the patient's description of symptoms, and tailor diagnosis and treatment to the patient's environment. For example, doctors could not only make sure that patients were looked after, they could also observe evidence of strained relationships between family members that might obstruct patients' recovery. While visiting patients' homes, doctors could ask relatives and others to offer assistance and could provide authoritative advice directly to them about their roles in the patients' recovery.[1]

The individualized nature of medical service delivery in the countryside was typified by the absence of any coordination among doctors throughout the entire process of diagnosis, treatment, and recovery, both within the local community and outside of it. Patients would commonly see a single practitioner exclusively, which contrasts with contemporary norms of patients interacting with a hierarchy of practitioners within a modern hospital setting.[2] In contrast, within the plural medical world of rural China, consultations with multiple physicians were interpreted as territorial encroachment and could lead to fierce disputes.[3] When asked about patient referrals among peer physicians, Chen Zhicheng answered immediately that "it was impossible in the 'old society.'"[4] An elderly pharmacist confirmed this, saying, "doctors never recommended other doctors to their patients."[5] The main reason for this was that making a profit was the sole aim of medical practice for these professional practitioners.[6] Only in very rare circumstances did networks emerge in which practitioners shared knowledge and patients, and even in circumstances such as these "the members of this network were also related to each other, and to other local elites, by means of intersecting ties of kinship, discipleship, and participation in joint social activities."[7]

By the late 1940s, the Nationalist government had begun to encourage the formation of a medical community in the countryside. The first step was the establishment of a subbranch of the Chinese Medicine Doctor Guild in the late 1940s. As chapter 1 noted, according to the structure designed by the County Social Department, Jiang Village belonged to the sixth branch office and was under the leadership of Zheng Buying, who would become one of the founding members of the Jiang Village Union Clinic in 1952.[8] The sixth branch had twenty-two internal medicine clinics (twenty-two doctors) and three surgery clinics (four doctors).[9] However, the implementation of this policy of medical administrative mapping did not change the status of private medical practice, nor did it have an impact on the actual scope of the medical community. At the same time, the county seats of rural Hangzhou already had hospitals with specialist divisions, proficiency hierarchies, and coordinated delivery services. However, these hospitals did not play meaningful roles in the medical lives of villagers.[10] The absence of a "hospital consciousness" among rural dwellers at this time was mainly due to the scarcity of hospitals, medical staff, and facilities. It was not related to fears of high hospital death rates associated with pauperism or to patients' reluctance to lose the right to choose their doctors, features that had inhibited hospital attendance in Western European and North American societies.[11] Hospital-phobic behavior manifested elsewhere was often due to a collision of cultures, but this does not appear to have been a problem in rural China.

The Medical Community, Minihospitals, and Medical Coordination

The individual, independent, and scattered practice of medicine in an isolated medical world continued to characterize locations like Jiang Village until 1952 and the birth of the union clinics, which marked the formation of a fixed medical venue in communities. From that point onward, the new socialist government made an effort to demarcate acceptable geographical jurisdictional boundaries for the medical community. As was explored in the previous chapters, some union clinics signed contracts with agricultural cooperatives, which paid a fixed amount on behalf of their members in exchange for treatment and medicine for cooperative members.[12] In addition to the establishment of fixed medical venues, regular mobile medical services became part of the union clinics' daily duties. The government declared these to be "an important measure for delivering medicine and doctors to peoples' doors, and this directly serves agricultural production. In the busy summer harvesting and planting time, the clinics should actively organize mobile medical services."[13] As part of their daily duties, union clinics were also commissioned to undertake public health work in their townships. These three daily tasks (treatment at the clinic, irregular mobile services, and public health works), provided constant work for the union clinics and enhanced the formation of a medical community for the first time in China.

At the same time, the administration of private medical practitioners was further tightened. The county government issued licenses based on an investigation into the practitioner's medical proficiency. Licenses were also issued by health bureaus, which organized independent medical practitioners into separate geographical areas for the delivery of medical services.[14] An attempt was made to regulate itinerant doctors and herbal medicine peddlers, who were given "letters of introduction" with designated expiry dates. When they left a particular area, the local union clinics wrote comments on the back of these letters.[15] Further restrictions and regulations resulted in a gradual reduction of the geographic scope of their services. For example, in

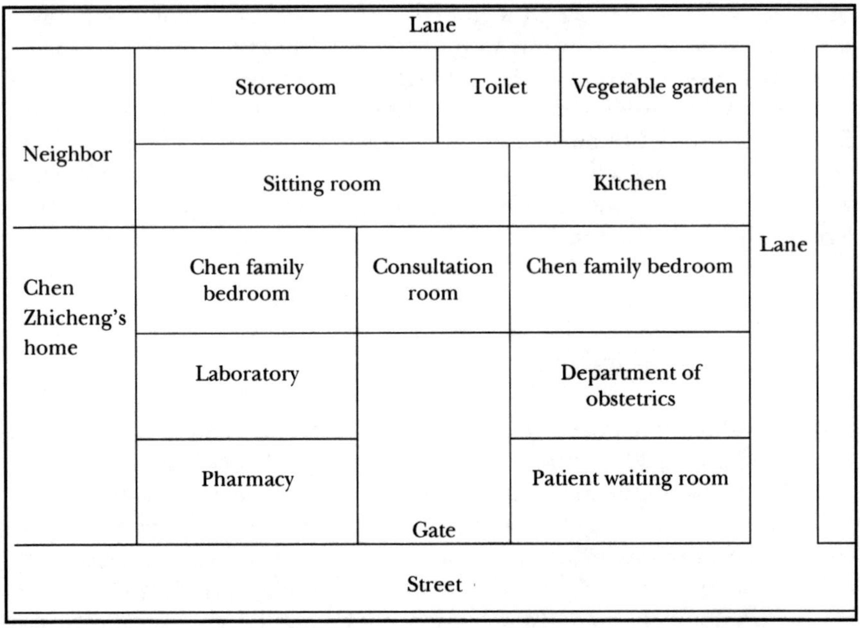

Lane				
Neighbor	Storeroom	Toilet	Vegetable garden	Lane
	Sitting room		Kitchen	
Chen Zhicheng's home	Chen family bedroom	Consultation room	Chen family bedroom	
	Laboratory		Department of obstetrics	
	Pharmacy		Patient waiting room	
		Gate		
Street				

Figure 5.1. Layout of Jiang Village Union Clinic and Commune Clinic, 1952–73. Information from Chen Hongting, interviews, November 2003–June 2004.

1962, itinerant doctors and herbal medicine peddlers were required not to cross provincial borders; in the first half of 1963, they were forbidden from crossing prefectural borders; in the second half of 1963, they were forbidden from crossing county lines; and by 1964, they were totally restricted to operating only in their own home counties.[16] If private medical practitioners disobeyed these rules, pharmaceutical companies were to stop supplying medicine to them. Each of these measures contributed to the gradual consolidation of a formal medical community and a linked set of operational hierarchies.

The changes brought by socialism also had a direct impact on the architectural layout of clinics. For example, Chen Hongting's union clinic allocated a different room to each newly designated medical department. Chen's house is a large, traditional-style structure, with four rows of two rooms each. In the first row, the room on the left side housed the Chinese and Western pharmacies, while the one on the right was used as the waiting room for patients. In the second row, the left-hand room became the laboratory, while the right-hand room housed the obstetrics department. In the third row, the lobby was used as the consultation room, while the rooms on either side of it were the Chen family's bedrooms. The kitchen, storeroom, and bathroom comprised the fourth row. Chen's union clinic therefore adopted the institutional layout of a modern minihospital, with its architectural distribution reflecting the division of expertise and bureaucratic management. The restructuring of the clinic did not apply only to its physical layout—it also applied to the adoption of the organizational style of a hospital. Work was organized by rosters, and staff duties were laid out in detailed statements. The clinic had its own financial management and income distribution systems, and it provided training and development for staff members, as well as staff welfare programs. Union clinics also implemented a twenty-four-hour outpatient system, as established in a service vision statement of the time that declared that "outpatient services are available at any hour and house calls are accessible at any time."[17] In keeping with this new work structure, former private medical practitioners were also trained in new workplace behaviors. Sandun Union Hospital, in the district adjacent to Jiang Village, declared that all staff members should adhere to the hospital's timetable and should not be late for work in the morning or leave early. They were exhorted to be loyal and diligent in carrying out their duties during work hours.[18] In medical consultation, Chinese medicine doctors also started to learn how to write a new type of case record modeled on those of Western medicine.[19]

Another important step in the institutionalization of rural medicine was reformulating the coordination of medical service delivery both inside and outside of the clinics. From their establishment in the early 1950s onward, associations for medical practitioners and pharmaceutical shops were asked to "help each other."[20] Simultaneously, as the ideals of a new "socialist form of medical practice" emerged, the union clinics were required to create an environment in which practitioners would actively exchange their clinical experience—especially their knowledge about effective remedies—which they had previously guarded carefully from competitors in their private practices.[21] For example, Sandun Union Hospital required that "all medical staff of each department of this union clinic, each clinic branch, and each medical station should consult other colleagues if they encounter difficult, serious illnesses that are beyond their capacity to treat . . . [and that] staff members should work with solidarity and friendliness and offer assistance to each other in the workplace."[22] This type of cooperation was also required in epidemic prevention work, such as that undertaken by schistosomiasis prevention teams. Any cases that could not be treated effectively were then to be referred upward to ensure patient safety.[23] By late 1954, the Yuhang County Health Bureau claimed that solidarity among medical practitioners had greatly improved. Thus, the establishment of union clinics gradually changed the age-old tradition of "mutual elbowing out" between competing private medical practitioners.[24]

However, since this type of enhanced medical coordination was only initiated within township-based communities, it had little relevance outside of them. In fact, as late as the mid-1960s, coordination seldom occurred between clinics and hospitals at different levels, such as between district hospitals and commune clinics. This was partly because there was no ranking system to assess medical proficiency but also, and more importantly, because the way that the union clinics had been formed in the early 1950s inhibited such cooperation. As indicated in chapter 1, the union clinics below the county level were established according to population size and the geographic areas that needed to be covered, following the organizing principle of "one clinic per township." Rural union clinics were subdivided into state-owned central commune clinics and collectively owned commune clinics. Central commune clinics were generally later designated "district hospitals," although they were simply converted union clinics that just happened to be located in the district seats. In theory, district hospitals offered a better quality of assistance than the commune clinics within their districts, but in reality there was little difference between the medical proficiency of commune clinic staff and those at district hospitals. So while district hospitals were supposed to be more advanced medical service providers, they were frequently merely at a higher administrative level within the new organizational hierarchy.

The establishment of the union clinics as the first step in institutionalizing China's rural medical systems meant that the nature of villagers' medical encounters with doctors also gradually changed. In Jiang Village, Chen Zhicheng recalled that although union clinic doctors continued to operate in their home villages after 1952, they had to collect their medicine supplies from the union clinics because they no longer had them at home. Initially, doctors did not charge a specific fee for treating patients at home with the medicines they carried in their medical kits, which patients bought from them. At the end of the day, doctors would take the medicine fees back to the union clinic and replenish their medical kits. By 1956, this practice had gradually declined, and patients increasingly went to their union clinic for treatment, attracted partly by the clinics' specialist pharmacies and injection rooms. Moreover, as doctors found themselves dealing with a wider range of treatable diseases as the years went by, their medical kits were unable to hold a sufficient range and quantity of pharmaceuticals.[25] All the same, union clinics were not universally popular, in part because they were often dingy, poorly lighted, and generally unappealing. Many were in small buildings, so treatment, dressing changes, and filling of prescriptions all had to be done in the same room. Furthermore, union clinics' limited state subsidies and relatively low incomes compared to state medical units or hospitals meant that their level of service was limited.[26] Despite these factors, the union clinics gradually succeeded in relocating the practice of traditional medicine to an institutional setting. The earlier ambulatory practice of private medical practitioners who made house calls to their patients' homes shifted to a hospital-based bureaucratized collective medical practice.[27]

The residents of Jiang Village first started to access preliminary forms of hospitalization during the schistosomiasis prevention programs. Luo Zhengfu recalled that union clinic practitioners went out to the villages to provide treatment plans, which lasted for seven to ten days. Antimony treatment (*tiji liaofa*), which involved an intravenous injection, was the preferred treatment method, but the strong side effects it had on the heart led union clinic practitioners to bring patients together for monitoring over the week or ten-day period. The treatment group was usually composed of patients from three production brigades, who stayed at the village meeting hall for the duration of their treatment, together with the doctors attending them and a cook. Patients slept on the floor and supplied their own bedding and clothing. Luo described this setup as inpatient treatment in a temporary hospital ward.[28] According to a report in the *Hangzhou Daily*, "patients at treatment stations enjoy an orderly environment and have access to culture [books and newspapers]. Fifty-four patients are arranged into four wards according to their gender and their home villages. Every ward has a director and a vice director and a committee member in charge of food, in accordance with hospitalization regulations . . . patients' families make frequent visits to see their relatives."[29] This model also spread to other medical programs. For example, during the Great Leap Forward campaign, villages established delivery rooms for birthing mothers. One person was in charge of caring for the pregnant women in each village, who congregated at the delivery rooms to be treated by the designated caregiver and to be given their sugar and oil coupons.[30]

However, while an institutional medical structure came to the villages through these specific campaigns, the movement of villagers out into larger county or district hospital settings proceeded at relatively slow pace. Indeed, as for services beyond local communities, although hospitals in county seats had received state support for infrastructure since the mid-1950s, it was still difficult for villagers to seek treatment away from their homes. The factors inhibiting them included the strict service timetables, excessive bureaucracy and medical checkups, expensive medicine fees, overly complicated departmental structure, and complex process of transferring between departments.[31] The majority of villagers, who rarely went to the county seats, needed extensive guidance and assistance to seek hospital treatment. These procedures often seemed too complicated to villagers, who also feared the unfamiliar white-gowned doctors.[32] But the most important constraint of all was economic factors: patients and their families had to consider travel costs, living expenses while in the hospital, loss of work points, and medical fees.[33] As a result, until the advent of the barefoot doctors in 1969 and 1970, the scope of villagers' health-seeking practices was quite limited. As had long been the case, their medical encounters did not exceed the services provided by the commune—that is, their own local community.

Medical Stations, the Proficiency Hierarchy, and the Referral System

On January 11, 1970, when the Jiang Village Union Clinic was converted into a commune clinic, it established branches through the Luojiazhuang and Sanshen production brigades, with other brigades setting up their own medical stations, signifying a further downward extension of the two-tier (county- and commune-level) medical system.[34] The commune clinics and brigade medical stations were assigned different duties. As the medical units in charge of health administration and health work for the whole commune, commune clinics were required to provide medical treatment to the masses and deal seriously with the treatment of patients referred upward by brigade medical stations. Commune clinics were also asked to assist brigades in consolidating and developing the work of the whole cooperative medical service system by giving lessons and sharing information around the localities they served.[35] In turn, brigade medical stations and barefoot doctors were charged with "seriously conducting medical work, delivering medicine and services to villagers' doors, whole-heartedly serving the people, trying to improve the quality of medical services, and actively undertaking disease prevention work for common, frequent, and endemic diseases."[36] According to official media, poor and lower-middle peasants praised the barefoot doctors, saying, "there are doctors right there in front of us and a hospital right near our houses"(*yisheng jinzai yanmianqian, yiyuan banzai dui libian*).[37]

In this way, a medical community system based on the people's commune emerged in both policy and practice. The people's communes provided the final structural links between the different layers of medical service delivery that were available, and a noticeable hierarchy of medical personnel and facilities emerged as a result of the new three-tier medical system. The 1950s-era goal of coordinating medical services was realized in the 1970s, when patient referral became possible, and practical problems relating to patients moving beyond their villages and their local communities were solved. In fact, cooperative medical service listed "patient referral" as the key task of barefoot doctors and commune clinic doctors, and this institutional design guaranteed villagers access to a broader range of medical encounters.

Furthermore, the barefoot doctor program also overcame the financial impediments that villagers had previously encountered to hospitalization and treatment at higher-level hospitals. In the 1970s, cooperative medical services could be categorized into three main groups according to the origins of their funds: production brigades, the communes, or a combination

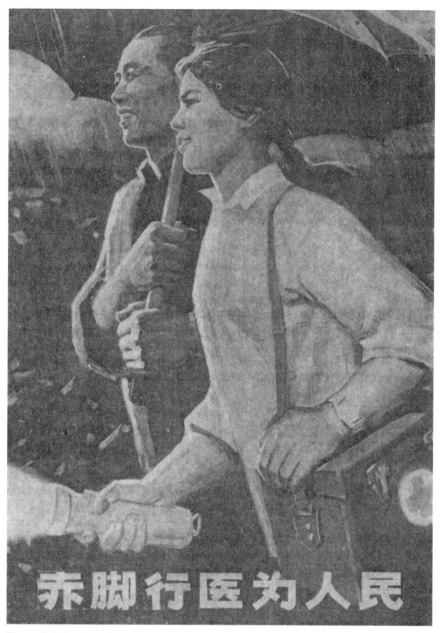

Figure 5.2. Serving the people barefoot. Chen Aikang, "Chijiao xingyi wei renmin" [Serving the people barefoot], *Gongnongbing huabao* [Pictorial of workers, peasants, and soldiers] 21 (1974). Reproduced with permission.

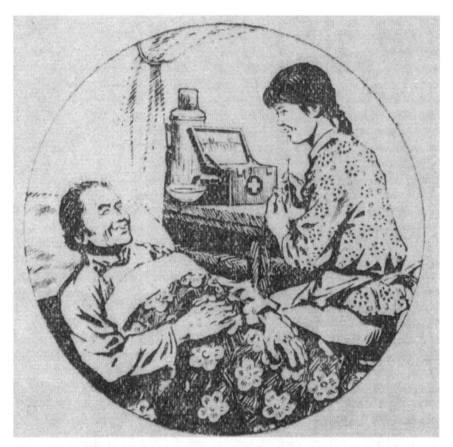

Figure 5.3. A barefoot doctor at a patient's bedside. *ZJRB*, October 23, 1974.
Reproduced with permission.

of the two. The first type was the most common in rural Hangzhou, while
the second and third types were less popular. Jiang Village Commune fell
into the third category. The commune clinic was in charge of the cooperative medical service, assisted by barefoot doctors in the production brigades.
Commune members paid RMB 2 per year to join the cooperative medical
service, which entitled them to RMB 0.05 consultations at the clinic and a
50 percent discount on pharmaceutical costs. Injections, outpatient visits,
operations, and acupuncture treatments were all free. This system also stipulated that when a commune member's illness could not be treated inside
the commune, the clinic had to refer the case to a higher-level hospital
and supply a referral letter by way of introduction. Once the patient was
being treated at this higher level, the commune clinic would reimburse 40
percent of the patient's medical fees. The referral letter was crucial to this

process: if a patient went to see a doctor in a neighboring commune clinic or hospital without one, his or her medical fees would not be reimbursed.[38] These regulations ensured that villagers sought treatment level by level up the three-tier system.[39] Therefore, the referral system and the reimbursement methods that were associated with it extended medical encounters by enhancing medical coordination and strengthening the proficiency hierarchy so that medical staff at the different levels could do what they were supposed to do. Another outcome of the referral system was that villagers' medical encounters shifted from home bedsides to hospital wards on a large scale. A new relationship emerged between patients, the family members taking care of or accompanying them (*peiban*), and doctors in an institutionalized medical context. This was different from the relationships within home-based medical encounters but reflected the same social, cultural, and psychological features of Chinese society.[40] Family members assumed much of the duty of taking care of patients in wards, even in critical care units. During the 1970s, family members stayed with hospitalized patients continually, taking care of them, cooking for them, sleeping on small beds alongside them or napping on the edge of patient beds at night. All these were considered family duties, helping patients to feel comfortable and relaxed in this strange environment. Although these practices were against hospital regulations, doctors had no problem with them.[41]

This shift of medical encounters from home to hospital was also significant for village women as, although they were accompanied by family members to the hospital, the family members no longer supervised the treatment itself. As patients, women encountered the new hierarchy of proficiency and division of expertise in hospitals and underwent physical examinations in a male-dominated institutionalized medical context. Another related consequence of the advent of modern medicine was the application of a series of new medical instruments for diagnosis and treatment. Each of these new technologies required greater physical intimacy between patients and doctors, as bodies were penetrated by needles and thermometers and heard and seen inside and outside by X-rays, blood pressure meters, and stethoscopes. Female patients were now required to expose more of their bodies to male physicians, and this exposure took place in hospitals rather than at their parental or marital homes. Under these circumstances, medical institutions and diagnostic instruments and methods changed the power relationship between doctors and women over women's bodies.

The Stratification of Medical Encounters across Villages

Despite the growing numbers of patients seeking treatment outside their homes at union clinics, as described above, in the late 1960s the family home remained an important venue for medical treatment. With the advent of the barefoot doctor program, the modes of medical encounters were diversified and greatly extended. The family home was still an important venue for the medical treatment of villagers at the beginning of the program, even after the establishment of the medical stations. As a commune clinic pharmacist recalled, "At that time, sick villagers sent their family members out to get the doctors—even those at the clinics—and bring them back to their homes. They usually preferred to ask the doctors to come to their homes."[42] However, this did not mean that the medical stations were not important hubs for treatment. One villager recalled how "later, the cooperative medical station was set up in the village. So when we had minor illnesses, we went to the medical station in the village meeting hall. I remember that the barefoot doctor gave me a few tablets of aspirin. They were wrapped in paper."[43] The short geographic distances within the villages made such medical encounters quick and convenient. In addition, the establishment of a communications system around 1969 through which each house had access to a loudspeaker hanging on the village wall meant that people could immediately summon barefoot doctors from any corner of the village in an emergency.[44] However, over time, medical consultations increasingly took place at clinics or medical stations, and by the late 1970s the home was no longer the main venue for medical encounters between barefoot doctors and villagers. According to WHO statistical data on villager consultation times drawn from four brigades in Ye County, Shandong Province, 81.5 percent of total medical consultations took place at brigade medical stations, while the remaining locations included homes and fields.[45]

The changes to medical encounters outside the communes were even more significant to villagers than those within. As mentioned above, partial reimbursement for medical fees reduced economic burdens on individual households and enabled villagers to seek treatment at hospitals, mainly county hospitals. Barefoot doctors played an important role in this process, becoming the necessary guides and administrative advisors and helping to solve villagers' difficulties with bureaucracy and to mitigate their fears about communication with hospital medical personnel. Jiang Village barefoot doctor Yan Shengyu recalled that when villagers could not be cured in the brigade medical stations or the commune clinics, they were usually referred to the Hangzhou City No. 2 Hospital. He said, "At that time, the Hangzhou City No. 2 Hospital was located in Gongchengqiao Bridge in the Hangzhou urban area. We rowed a boat along the canal to pick patients up and take them to the hospital."[46] Today, the villagers still have vivid impressions of the personal attention they received from the barefoot doctors on their way to county hospitals thanks to the referral system. As one villager explained, "In the old days, there was no bus service from here to the county town. So we had to go there by foot. A barefoot doctor from the village would carry the medical kit swaying on his hips and accompany patients when they walked to the county hospitals. In Chairman Mao's time, the barefoot doctors did very well in this regard. There were a lot of incidents like this in the village and in the neighboring villages."[47]

With the extension of medical encounters facilitated by the barefoot doctors, the stratification of medical service delivery and cooperation within it became increasingly consolidated. In 2006, I spoke to a seventy-year-old woman by the surname of Jiang who had suffered from chronic illnesses since middle age. Like the majority of elderly villagers, she could not recall what medication she took or how much money she paid for her medical expenses decades ago. However, she had a very clear recollection of her experience of being referred to a county hospital in 1978:

> That year, I had acute appendicitis. At first, the commune clinic doctor said it was acute appendicitis. The village barefoot doctor also said it was acute appendicitis. He said he could cure it. Anyway, there was a cooperative medical station in the village and it was convenient. The brigade cooperative medical station was located in a village meeting hall near my house. I received an intravenous medication for three days in the cooperative medical station, but it did not work. The appendix was getting worse and becoming rotten, and there was a pustule. The commune doctor criticized the village doctor, saying, "You shouldn't have tried to treat it if you knew that you couldn't do it." Since there was no other option, I was referred to the county hospital immediately. A lot of people accompanied me, including my eldest uncle, my third uncle, my fourth uncle, my youngest uncle, and my eldest daughter. The village barefoot doctor also came with me to the county hospital so he could give me intravenous medication on the road. After we arrived at the county hospital, we asked the doctor to wait for my second uncle before starting the operation, but the doctor got angry with us and started shouting, "What are you waiting for? Nonsense! You will die if the operation is not done immediately." So the operation began immediately. . . . I stayed in the hospital for a month. When I left, I also took some injections and medicines with me back to my home. The village doctor continued to give me injections.[48]

Jiang's vivid description indicates that operations and hospitalization in county hospitals were important events not only for the immediate family but also for the whole clan. More importantly, Jiang's case indicates that the barefoot doctor, the commune clinic, and the county hospital achieved the desired division of labor and cooperation in patient treatment stipulated by the new hierarchical medical system. In Jiang Village, the average medical fees per patient were as follows in 1971: brigade stations, RMB 0.13; Sanshen branch, RMB 0.24; Luojiazhuang branch, RMB 0.33; clinic headquarters, RMB 0.37, and hospital referrals, RMB 4.19 (see table 5.1). The spending at each level indicated the stratification of medical encounters that resulted from the different degrees of medical proficiency found at each level of

Table 5.1. Jiang Village Cooperative Medical Service outpatient visits and medical fees, 1971

Villages	Distance (km)	Headquarters			Sanshen branch			Luojiazhuang branch			Production brigade station			Patient referral		
		Visits	Fees (RMB)	Ave. (RMB)	Visits	Fees (RMB)	Ave. (RMB)	Visits	Fees (RMB)	Ave. (RMB)	Visits	Fees (RMB)	Ave. (RMB)	Visits	Fees (RMB)	Ave. (RMB)
Type I																
Jiang Village	0.0	4,518	1,254.30	0.28	32	5.87	0.18	8	2.47	0.31				122	262.65	2.15
Sanshen	1.5	712	286.36	0.40	7,393	1,612.00	0.22							124	419.30	3.38
Luojiazhuang	2.0	327	165.16	0.51	11	12.50	1.14	4,673	1,459.00	0.31				129	650.01	5.04
Dengyunwei	1.5	561	214.56	0.38	9	3.58	0.40	1,018	316.80	0.31				50	188.48	3.77
Subtotal		6,118	1,920.38	0.31	7,445	1,633.95	0.22	5,699	1,778.27	0.31				425	1,520.44	3.58
Type II																
Hejian	1.0	2,506	925.66	0.37	104	36.70	0.35	57	24.49	0.43	705	56.11	0.08	78	147.76	1.89
Shuanglong	1.5	1,452	551.22	0.38	7	1.25	0.18	51	24.00	0.47	1,171	132.30	0.11	60	151.10	2.52
Wulian	2.0	729	396.69	0.54	20	11.90	0.60	2,808	1,025.00	0.37	2,631	406.00	0.15	70	198.99	2.84
Subtotal		4,687	1,873.57	0.40	131	49.85	0.38	2,916	1,073.49	0.37	4,507	594.41	0.13	208	497.85	2.39
Type III																
Longzhang	1.0	1,470	636.93	0.43	60	25.20	0.42	1	0.06	0.06	6,849	1,026.00	0.15	99	538.08	5.44
Wangjiaqiao	1.8	271	131.59	0.49	302	109.00	0.36				1,340	201.90	0.15	13	83.97	6.46
Yangjiadai	2.0	929	358.42	0.39	4	1.41	0.35				1,740	127.70	0.07	24	194.70	8.11
Baojian	2.2	460	186.00	0.40	138	66.00	0.48	62	24.19	0.39	2,473	250.70	0.10	40	313.32	7.83
Zhoujiacun	3.0	430	253.21	0.59	433	181.00	0.42				2,541	343.30	0.14	36	395.19	10.98
Subtotal		3,560	1,566.15	0.44	937	382.61	0.41	63	24.25	0.38	14,943	1,949.60	0.13	212	1,525.26	7.19
Total		14365	5,360.10	0.37	8,513	2,066.41	0.24	8,678	2,876.01	0.33	19,450	2,544.01	0.13	845	3,543.55	4.19

Source: "Jiangcun hezuo yiliao kaizhi mingxibiao, 1971," supplied by barefoot doctor Hong Jinglin, Wulian Village.

the hierarchical medical system. In other words, medical units at each level treated illnesses with different levels of seriousness. Brigade medical stations treated minor illnesses, so medical expenses incurred there were the lowest, while expenses incurring from hospital referral were the highest, as they treated serious illness.

The Dual Role of Barefoot Doctors and the Embarrassment of the Commune Clinics

Barefoot doctors provided health care at the lowest end of the hierarchical medical system and were also responsible for the cooperative medical services and referral system. Their work ensured that the new medical hierarchy, the cooperative medical service's reimbursement methods, and the referral system all combined to extend the villagers' medical encounters from their home bedsides to hospital wards. During this process, the cooperative medical service's reimbursement scheme greatly relieved the villagers' medical expense burdens, while the barefoot doctors helped eliminate patients' difficulties in communicating with doctors and adjusting to institutionalized medical environments. Therefore, the economic, cultural, and bureaucratic factors that had inhibited the shift toward hospitalization in the past were generally resolved in rural China during the 1970s through the intervention of the barefoot doctors. However, there were a number of important deviations from this new pattern of institutionalized medical encounters, which emerged as a result of the dual roles played by barefoot doctors as health workers and physicians and the increasingly embarrassing conditions of the commune clinics.

Some works of scholarship, particularly those written in the People's Republic of China, have argued that barefoot doctors functioned in the same way as the health workers in C. C. Chen's experimental health program in Ding County in the 1930s.[49] In fact, the barefoot doctors were quite different from Chen's health workers. Nor were they the same as the peasants who became "health workers" in the 1950s and 1960s under the union clinic model, even though this group formed a core recruitment base for the barefoot doctor program. In these two earlier programs, the health workers basically undertook auxiliary public heath work at the village level, such as administering inoculations and collecting stool samples. According to Li Jinghan, the Ding County health-care workers of the 1930s received two weeks of training, which included courses on vaccination, water-well reconstruction, and the use of medical kits, and thus were not in any sense doctors or physicians.[50] Indeed, C. C. Chen repeated this basic point over and over again in his 1989 memoirs: "It was a cardinal principle in our system that the health worker should never act, or be called on to act, as physician."[51] In contrast, the barefoot doctors had their own medical stations and medical kits, and healing became an important part of their daily work, in addition to the epidemic prevention work associated with health workers. C. C. Chen also noticed a tendency among barefoot doctors in the 1970s and 1980s to overestimate their skills: "most [barefoot doctors] are trained to administer first aid or treat mild cases of common illnesses, [but] gradually [come] to regard themselves as fully trained physicians capable of practicing medicine."[52] In this sense, the barefoot doctors played a dual role throughout the 1970s, in that they were both health workers and physicians. In terms of public health, the advent of barefoot doctors greatly strengthened the three-tier medical system and enhanced its efficiency in large-scale health campaigns, such as inoculation and epidemic prevention.[53] However, the healing roles of barefoot doctors were more significant than their public health duties because they started to take over medical practice in the local community, which had previously been provided by commune clinics. Their healing roles therefore became a major influence on the structural evolution of the three-tier medical network.

Along with the dual roles of the barefoot doctors, the structural evolution of the three-tier medical network was also influenced by the nature of the prevailing medical facilities. In this regard, the commune clinics merit particularly detailed analysis as, in theory, they were the first resort for villagers seeking treatment outside of their home villages. The general condition of the union clinics was poor throughout the 1960s, right up to their conversion into commune clinics, which began in 1969. The Yuhang County Health Bureau admitted that "the majority of communes had union clinics, but they were old and fragile and could not serve the masses very well. County and district hospitals developed very slowly, and patients who needed appendectomies had to be transferred to the hospitals in the urban areas."[54] Some progress had been made beginning in the mid-1960s under Mao's "June 26 Directive" on health work, but conditions did not improve overnight. Chapter 1 pointed out that medical instruments were supplied to rural commune clinics in the early 1970s in order to improve the shortage of doctors and medicines in rural areas, following Mao's directive. However, commune clinics were only allocated vital medical equipment and instruments—such as instruments for obstetrics and minor and major surgery after 1975.[55] The general situation was not promising, as is illustrated in tables 5.2–5.4.

These tables show a total of 309 commune clinics and forty-six district hospitals in the seven counties of Hangzhou Prefecture in 1976, which was the peak year of the implementation of the cooperative medical service. However, 23.6 percent of the commune clinics (seventy-three clinics) had no clinic beds. As for medical instruments, only 8 percent (twenty-five clinics) of the commune clinics had the five basic types of medical instruments. There were only sixty-nine X-ray machines and a total of 210 microscopes in the

Table 5.2. Classification of commune clinics and district hospitals based on the numbers of clinic beds in Hangzhou Prefecture, 1974–76

Year	Clinic numbers	Clinic classification					
		0	1–6	7–10	11–20	21–30	31–50
Commune							
1974	309	110	118	44	25	7	3
1975	308	75	151	38	31	9	2
1976	309	73	138	46	38	8	5
District							
1974	41	8	4	9	7	4	2
1975	41	9	1	13	6	1	4
1976	46	16	4	9	6	2	5

Sources: Hangzhoushi weishengju [Hangzhou Prefecture Health Bureau], "Hangzhou diqu nongcun shengchan dadui he shengchandui weisheng zuzhi qingkuang" [Survey of health organizations in production teams and production brigades in rural areas of Hangzhou Prefecture], 1974, HZA, vol. 87-3-298; "Hangzhou diqu nongcun shengchan dadui shengchandui weisheng zuzhi qingkuang," 1975, HZA, vol. 87-3-302; "Nongcun chijiao yisheng weishengyuan jieshengyuan qingkuang" [Statistical data of rural barefoot doctors, health workers and midwives], 1976, HZA, vol. 87-3-307.

309 commune clinics. As for surgical skills, only 5.5 percent of the commune clinics (seventeen clinics) could handle both acute abdominal disease and difficult labor operations. For example, Jiang Village Commune Clinic had only two clinic beds for observing patients. Only in the late 1970s did the clinic spend RMB 1,000 to buy a refrigerator and a small X-ray machine.[56] Although the director of the Zhejiang Provincial Health Department, Li Lanyan, admitted Hangzhou Prefecture had poor medical facilities, it was not the worst in Zhejiang Province. About 31.7 percent of the district hospitals and commune clinics did not even have clinic beds.[57]

Even worse, a significant gap existed in the distribution of medical resources between the different counties of Hangzhou Prefecture. Tables 5.5 and 5.6 show that most of the prefecture's medical resources were controlled by three counties—Xiaoshan, Yuhang, and Lin'an—which are situated around Hangzhou city, the capital of both the prefecture and the province. The economic conditions in these counties were relatively better than those in the other four counties. They were also the favorite destinations of

Table 5.3. Key medical equipment and instruments owned by commune clinics and district hospitals in Hangzhou Prefecture, 1974–76

	Clinics		Medical equipment and instruments			
Year	Total	In possession of the "five types of equipment and instruments"*	Surgical scalpel set	Four family planning instruments (series)	X-ray machine	Microscope
Commune						
1974	309	11	140	287	34	171
1975	308	8	144	352	43	193
1976	309	25	166	404	69	208
District						
1974	41	8	33	95	28	53
1975	41	11	61	114	28	54
1976	46	25	83	148	39	62

Sources: Hangzhoushi weishengju [Hangzhou Prefecture Health Bureau], "Hangzhou diqu nongcun shengchan dadui he shengchandui weisheng zuzhi qingkuang" [Survey of health organizations in production teams and production brigades in rural areas of Hangzhou Prefecture], 1974, HZA, vol. 87-3-298; "Hangzhou diqu nongcun shengchan dadui shengchandui weisheng zuzhi qingkuang," 1975, HZA, vol. 87-3-302; "Nongcun chijiao yisheng weishengyuan jieshengyuan qingkuang" [Statistical data of rural barefoot doctors, health workers and midwives], 1976, HZA, vol. 87-3-307.

Hangzhou urban medical service teams in the 1960s and 1970s, whereas medical resources were quite scarce in Tonglu, Jiande, and Chun'an counties, which were located in relatively remote, poor areas.

Commune clinics were also highly understaffed: in Yuhang County, which had a population of 820,000, there were only five secondary medical school students working in fifty commune clinics, and there were no medical university graduates in any of the commune clinics even as late as 1986. The remaining medical staff consisted of educated youth or barefoot doctors recruited after 1970.[58] In neighboring Fuyang County, the majority of commune clinic leaders were recruited from the available pool of young villagers, and they knew nothing of professional management.[59] In Jiang Village, a few medical school students were assigned to the clinic at one point. However, the roads of Jiang Village were quite poor, and this made access to the

Table 5.4. Surgical skills at commune clinics and district hospitals in Hangzhou Prefecture, 1974–76

Year	Clinic	Treatment of acute abdominal pain and difficult labor	Emergency abdominal surgery only	Treatment of difficult labor only	Four types of family-planning operations	Insertion of IUDs and performing abortions and female sterilization
Commune						
1974	309	4	9	43	56	82
1975	308	16	11	56	48	100
1976	309	17	11	51	66	102
District						
1974	41	22	4	3	25	3
1975	41	16	2	7	29	2
1976	46	15	6	7	29	4

* The "five types of equipment and instruments" referred to the X-ray machine, microscope, high pressure sterilizer, four family planning instruments, and any one of three types of surgical scalpel bags.

Sources: Hangzhoushi weishengju [Hangzhou Prefecture Health Bureau], "Hangzhou diqu nongcun shengchan dadui he shengchandui weisheng zuzhi qingkuang" [Survey of health organizations in production teams and production brigades in rural areas of Hangzhou Prefecture], 1974, HZA, vol. 87-3-298; "Hangzhou diqu nongcun shengchan dadui shengchandui weisheng zuzhi qingkuang," 1975, HZA, vol. 87-3-302; "Nongcun chijiao yisheng weishengyuan jieshengyuan qingkuang" [Statistical data of rural barefoot doctors, health workers and midwives], 1976, HZA, vol. 87-3-307.

village difficult, even on foot. There was no canteen or accommodation for the students, so they all left shortly after starting work.[60] Not until 1996 did the Jiang Village Commune Clinic receive its first ever university medical graduate.

The poor medical facilities in the commune clinics and district hospitals during the 1970s prompted one barefoot doctor to claim that "the commune clinic was basically not different from our services. There were only a few doctors, and we had the same instruments that they had."[61] Because of this situation, patients with relatively serious illnesses who could not be treated by the brigade medical stations could not be treated by the commune clinics, either. Instead, they had to be referred to higher-level hospitals, thus

Table 5.5. Distribution of medical equipment and instruments owned by commune clinics in Hangzhou Prefecture, 1976

County	Clinic	X-ray machines	Microscopes	"Five types of medical equipment and instruments"	Operation bags	Family planning resources
1. Xiaoshan	56	33	55	17	48	177
2. Yuhang	49	13	44	3	33	83
3. Lin'an	45	8	20	4	30	20
4. Tonglu	29	1	10	1	8	18
5. Fuyang	40	3	25	0	14	15
6. Jiande	37	7	34	0	15	51
7. Chun'an	53	4	20	0	18	40
Total	309	79	208	25	166	404
Counties 1–3	150 (48.5%)	54 (78.3%)	119 (57.2%)	24 (96%)	111 (66.9%)	280 (69.3%)

Source: "Nongcun chijiao yisheng, weishengyuan, jieshengyuan qingkuang" [Statistical data of rural barefoot doctors, health workers and midwives], 1976, HZA, vol. 87-3-307.

skipping the commune clinics. Even today, villagers still have vivid memories of this situation:

> I remember clearly how my wife and I were laboring in the fields on the mountain one day in 1973. My father came to the field and told us that our second daughter had suddenly developed a serious illness. The village barefoot doctor made a diagnosis and told us to go to the district clinic immediately. We carried our daughter in our arms and went to the district clinic with the barefoot doctor. He knew that if he could not cure this disease, the doctors in the commune clinic would not be able to cure it either. They did the same work, and they [the barefoot doctors] were very familiar with the details of the commune clinics.[62]

The Formation of the Dumbbell-Shaped Structure of the Three-Tier Medical System

As the discussion in the previous section indicated, the three-tier medical network in rural China went through a series of major changes and challenges

Table 5.6. Surgical skills in commune clinics in Hangzhou Prefecture, 1976

County	Clinic	Treatment of acute abdominal pain and difficult labor	Emergency abdominal operations only	Treatment of difficult labor only	Four types of family-planning operation	Insertion of IUDs, performing of abortions and female sterilization only
1. Xiaoshan	56	6	6	29	19	31
2. Yuhang	49	2	0	0	13	25
3. Lin'an	45	8	1	19	9	15
4. Tonglu	29	0	2	1	15	7
5. Fuyang	40	0	0	0	2	0
6. Jiande	37	1	2	2	8	24
7. Chun'an	53	0	0	0	0	0
Total	309	17	11	51	66	102
Counties 1–3	150 (48.5%)	16 (94.1%)	7 (63.6%)	48 (94.1)	41 (62.1%)	71 (69.6%)

Source: "Nongcun chijiao yisheng, weishengyuan, jieshengyuan qingkuang" [Statistical data of rural barefoot doctors, health workers and midwives], 1976, HZA, vol. 87-3-307.

during the 1970s. First, the barefoot doctors emerged not only as health workers but also as physicians providing treatment. Because they fulfilled healing roles, the barefoot doctors therefore had similar medical expertise to commune clinic doctors. Second, the conditions of the commune clinics were embarrassing, as they lacked the necessary equipment, supplies, and personnel to provide the medical services delegated to them by the system. Third, the popularization of brigade medical stations, which had the authority to refer patients to the top of the medical hierarchy, made villagers bypass the commune clinics altogether. These factors contributed to the reshaping of the three-tier medical network, with the second (or middle) tier—the commune clinics—becoming largely redundant. The decline of the commune clinics made the rural medical network take on a dumbbell shape: the middle part (the commune clinics) shrank, while the top and bottom (the county hospitals and the brigade medical stations) became increasingly important.

In Jiang Village Commune, patient attendance at commune clinics, branch clinics, and brigade medical stations during 1971 reflected this change (see table 5.1). At that time, the villages that made up Jiang Village

Commune could be grouped into three categories (which I will refer to as types 1, 2, and 3) according to their geographic distance from the commune seat of Jiang Village and patient attendance. Type 1 villages were the four production brigades that lacked medical stations: Jiang Village Brigade, which was the commune clinic headquarters; Luojiazhuang and Sanshen brigades, which each had branch clinics; and a small brigade in the central commune. Type 2 villages were those surrounding the headquarters and its branch clinics, which had three production brigades one to two kilometers from Jiang Village. In these three brigades, the patients' visits to the brigade medical stations were 43 percent lower than visits to the clinic headquarters and the two branch clinics. In the type 3 villages, there were five production brigades, one to three kilometers from the Jiang Village Commune Clinic headquarters. The total patient visits to these brigade stations were 3.3 times greater than those to the headquarters and the branch clinics. In this type 3 area, the commune clinic had already lost its advantages in attracting patients. Because the Jiang Village Cooperative Medical Service was jointly run by the commune clinic and the brigade medical stations, the commune clinic and its two branches attracted quite a few patients from each brigade. However, in the communes where the cooperative medical service was implemented by the brigade medical stations, the commune clinics lost their advantages in attracting patients altogether because of the cooperative medical service's reimbursement policy and the convenience of the services provided by medical stations. As mentioned above, cooperative medical services run by production brigades were the most common type in rural Hangzhou. Furthermore, as the previous chapter has already pointed out, even when the cooperative medical service ceased to function, the majority of medical stations continued to provide medical services. The structure of the medical community therefore began to change following the creation of the cooperative medical services and brigade medical stations.

The discussion above has already shown that the medical resources available in the commune clinics of Xiaoshan County were the best of the seven counties within Hangzhou Prefecture. According to statistical data for the ten cooperative medical stations of Ningwei Commune in July 1972, the total number of patient visits to the brigade cooperative medical stations was 12,845, while the number of patient visits to commune clinics was 2,496, or 16.27 percent of the total for the whole commune. Of the 1,289 patients who were referred by the brigade barefoot doctors for treatment at a higher level, 630 (48.8 percent) went to a commune clinic, while the remainder went to district or county hospitals.[63] The decline of commune clinics in less developed counties such as Chun'an was even more marked: when asked what percentages of villagers were treated by barefoot doctors after 1970, the barefoot doctor Xu Peichun immediately replied that it was about 90 percent,[64] and the villagers in the same commune recalled that it was at least 80 percent.[65]

Official reports also admitted that the commune clinics were experiencing a decline in patient numbers and highlighted their dilemma: "When the cooperative medical services are implemented effectively, commune clinic profits decrease correspondingly."[66] C. C. Chen, who strongly disapproved of the fact that barefoot doctors regarded themselves as physicians, also noticed the decline of the commune clinics in Shaifang County, Sichuan Province: "Some *xiang* (township) health centers received fewer patients than in the past and, accordingly, were experiencing some financial difficulties. . . . People now have bicycles, and many villages even have tractors. Thus it has become quite easy in recent years to transport people to the county hospitals."[67] Financial matters were made worse by the health work assigned by the County Health Bureau and higher levels, which put further pressure on the commune clinics. As one commune clinic complained in September 1974, "health clinics have to do a great deal of epidemic prevention work, and medical staff members have a heavy workload. Thus, the expenditure of the health clinic has increased correspondingly."[68] In Fuyang, the County Health Bureau reported that some commune clinic directors and medical staff did not welcome the cooperative medical service, and some even refused to accept the barefoot doctor program in their communes: "Each commune clinic physician received a monthly salary of only 30 to 40 yuan. If cooperative medical services were set up, fewer patients would come to the commune clinic, and the salaries would not be paid anymore." The County Party Committee warned that it would not subsidize the commune clinics unless they helped production brigades build the cooperative medical services and assist the barefoot doctors.[69]

However, this action did not reverse the decline of the commune clinics. According to the statistical data on patient visits to the county hospitals and from the district and commune clinics in Jiande County from 1973 to 1983, the number of patient visits to the county hospitals increased by 23.7 percent, from 321,786 visits to 398,117, while the number of patient visits to the commune and district clinics increased by only 0.22 percent, from 718,410 visits to 720,021. During the same period, the total population of Jiande County increased by 9.4 percent, from 404,800 to 442,700.[70] Thus, the number of patient visits to the county hospitals in Jiande County from 1973 to 1983 increased at two and a half times the rate of population increase during that period, while the number of patient visits to the district and commune clinics increased by a statistically insignificant amount, which actually represented a substantial decline of 8 percent per capita.

In an attempt to shore up the system, the roles of rural commune clinics were redefined and reemphasized in late 1977, under the reign of Hua Guofeng. According to the new regulations, commune clinics were the key level of the rural medical network and were required to provide technical guidance for the medical and health work within their communes.[71] After the 1978 economic reforms, the commune clinics adopted a bonus system to reward personnel for hard work in order to improve the quality of medical service delivery and enhance work efficiency, but even this still did not reverse the decline. At the same time, commune clinics were experiencing even more intense competition from barefoot doctors, who had accumulated even more medical expertise and had grown yet more familiar with their patients in the villages than the commune clinic doctors had. The relationship between the two groups evolved into an all-out competition. As the 1978 economic reforms brought an end to the cooperative medical service, reimbursement regulations ceased to be the central pillar of the referral system. Villagers were now more familiar with hospitals and had higher incomes because of economic reforms. As villagers now paid for medical services by themselves, they had much greater flexibility when choosing doctors, and improved transportation also facilitated these choices.[72] In the meantime, government subsidies to the commune clinics (now called township clinics) also declined, so much so that some township clinics could not even afford to pay their employees full salaries. In some areas of rural Hangzhou, the township clinics were auctioned or rented out to their own medical staff by the middle of the 1990s, and the number of medical staff shrank tremendously. Furthermore, there was still very little difference between the medical proficiency of township clinics and village clinics run by former barefoot doctors (now called village doctors).[73] As a result, former commune clinics were soon so marginalized that their duties became purely administrative— for example, they reported on public health data, such as vaccination rates and incidence of disease.

This dumbbell-shaped structure has continued to characterize the rural medical network. In 2003, one Chinese research team on rural medicine and health described the township clinics in the three-tier medical system as "quite embarrassing." They argued that the present rural medical service system is composed of "village clinics (former brigade medical stations), township clinics (former commune clinics), and county hospitals." The basic aim of this structure is to divide patients among the three service points. That is, patients who could not be treated in village clinics were to be referred to township clinics, while those seeking treatment at township clinics could be referred to county hospitals. However, the actual operation of the three-tier medical system did not follow the institutional design. There were no noticeable medical advantages to township clinics in comparison to the barefoot doctors' medical stations. According to a survey of one thousand peasants, 58 percent of "serious illnesses" were treated at county hospitals and hospitals above the county level, while only 12 percent were treated at the township clinics. Village clinics treated about 47 percent of minor illnesses, while township clinics only treated about 18 percent.[74] Therefore, township clinics could not compete against county hospitals in treating serious illnesses and could not compete with village clinics in treating minor illnesses, either. They lost their medical authority and dominance over village clinics in the township communities.

Ironically, some union clinic doctors had foreseen the effects that training a third tier of medical personnel would have on the future of clinics when they had been required to train half-peasant, half-doctors in 1965. Official reports from the time criticized medical staff at some clinics for being reluctant to teach these health workers. The doctors in question compared the initiative to "putting porridge stalls in front of restaurants . . . committing suicide . . . [and putting the] hospital above, the health workers below, and killing [the clinics] in the middle."[75] More than forty years later, the township clinics that had replaced the union clinics and the commune clinics ended their roles in the local communities and faded out of the medical life of villagers completely. The barefoot doctors, the "newly emerged things" of the Cultural Revolution, obtained medical dominance within their local communities.

The process that started in the early 1950s of institutionalizing medical services in China's villages included the construction of new medical institutions, the formalization of modes of medical encounters, the implementation of a scheme for coordinating medical delivery, and the creation of a medical community in which knowledge could be shared. The birth of the union clinics in the 1950s was the first step in the process of drawing villagers into a formal medical service, in which treatment was delivered outside of their homes. The subsequent advent of barefoot doctors enabled the provision of a linked system of medical proficiency that moved from brigade medical stations, up to the commune clinics, and finally to the county hospitals. This structure completed and enhanced a medical coordination program that revolved around the proficiency hierarchy of the three-tier medical system. At the same time, the implementation of the cooperative medical service's reimbursement policy removed the economic restrictions that had previously prevented villagers from accessing medical services outside their local communities. Barefoot doctors played significant roles as participants, promoters, and guides during the process of institutionalizing villagers' medical encounters with doctors into the hierarchical medical system. As a result, villagers started to move beyond their home villages to access new medical services in modern medical settings, mainly county hospitals.[76] In this sense, the barefoot doctors helped speed up the shift of medical encounters from bedsides to hospitals.

During this process, the barefoot doctors inadvertently caused the hollowing out of the three-tier medical network, resulting in its eventual dumbbell-shaped structure. By the early 1980s, the barefoot doctors and their village clinics (the former brigade medical stations) had replaced township clinics (the former commune and union clinics), thus achieving medical dominance in local communities. Meanwhile, the township clinics largely degenerated into administrative medical units. The rise of this dumbbell-shaped structure contributed, in turn, to the medical institutionalization of barefoot doctors and their clinics: in the late 1980s, the government required that each barefoot doctor's village clinic have a pharmacy, a consultation room, and an infusion room for the intravenous administration of medication. These increasingly formal medical settings made the barefoot doctors look more and more professional. Moreover, the shift from bedside medicine to hospital medicine meant that the venues of significant life events for Chinese villagers—such as birth, illness, ageing, and death—were completely relocated.[77] This change in the social medical institution occurred in tandem with the increasingly Westernized medical knowledge structure that resulted from the introduction of Western medicine into rural China.[78] The fates of commune clinics were similar to those of Chinese medicine doctors. The clinics declined as traditional establishments evolved into modern medical institutions, while Chinese medicine doctors either gradually faded out of the village medical world or transformed themselves by adopting Western medical knowledge and techniques.

Chapter Six

Group Identity, Power Relationships, and Medical Legitimacy

In his *Profession of Medicine*, Eliot Freidson showed that in all societies people diagnose sickness and devise methods for its management. Some individuals are thought to be especially knowledgeable about sickness and are regularly sought out by patients or their families. In many cases, these individuals have other trades or professions and simply perform healing tasks on the side to supplement their income, while others develop a sufficient practice to make a living solely from healing and so develop a specialist vocation. He notes that not all healers are called doctors or physicians, nor are they necessarily considered professionals.[1] Freidson's general observations apply to the traditional medical world of rural China. In his investigation of rural doctors in Ding County, northern China, Li Jinghan said, "Naturally, the medical expertise of these doctors is mediocre. Anyone willing to treat illnesses could be counted as a doctor." He also pointed out that most rural doctors practiced medicine as a secondary occupation, rather than depending solely on it to make a living.[2] In the eyes of the peasants of Ding County, old age and experience signified reliable medical expertise and an increased likelihood of effective treatment. Patients were not required to make monetary payments to doctors—instead, they gave "acknowledgments" (*daxie*) of gratitude, often in the form of a few gifts during a community festival.[3]

This general pattern continued in China's villages into the late 1950s, in part because of the absence of an alternative. Most people continued to seek medical care from their local folk healers, fellow villagers who were deemed to have special healing talents. Both patients and healers depended on agricultural labor to make a living—very few professional doctors supported themselves entirely from their medical practice. By the early 1960s, the situation had not changed much in this respect: the newly designated health workers also labored alongside their fellow villagers and still received payment in the same way as the village healers of earlier decades. The difference was that they carried medical kits into the fields to perform basic first aid on the spot, such as daubing cuts and grazes with mercurochrome solution or gentian violet and bandaging open wounds to minimize infection. At this point, there were only a few union clinic doctors based at each commune seat, and the average villager still did not have a clear concept of "doctors" as a group of professionals with a discrete identity in their own villages. However, this situation would change in the late 1960s with the advent of the barefoot doctor program and its penetration into the countryside. Although the very name "barefoot doctor" implies that it was their duty to participate in agricultural work in the paddy fields, and thus that medical practice was not their only work, villagers soon formed new perceptions of medical professionals as a result of their interactions with the barefoot doctors.

Doctors Wearing Shoes

During the 1970s, official Chinese discourse repeatedly claimed that participation in agricultural labor was one of the main duties of the barefoot doctors: "To be a good barefoot doctor, one should first be a good commune member. If one does not participate in labor, one is not a barefoot doctor. . . . Whether or not the barefoot doctors continue to participate in agricultural labor depends on the crucial question of which road they are taking and whether or not they have deviated from the correct path."[4] In 1974, Deng Xiaoping, who was then the vice premier of the State Council, told foreign guests that "having barefoot doctors is better than being without doctors. Being barefoot means that they participate in labor, on the one hand, and yet they treat patients, on the other hand. In the beginning, the barefoot doctors' knowledge was limited, and they could only cure common diseases. In a few years, they will wear grass shoes, to indicate that their knowledge has increased. After a few more years, they will progress from grass shoes to cloth shoes, and then from cloth shoes to rubber shoes."[5] Deng's speech inspired a series of heated debates in the official media, which criticized him for insulting the medical abilities of the "newly emerged things" of the Cultural Revolution with "a speech about the barefoot doctors wearing shoes" (*chijiao yisheng chuanxielun*). This was part of the campaign attacking Deng which ran from 1975 to 1977 and was known as "criticize Deng and repulse the right-deviationist wind to reverse the verdicts" (*pideng fanji youqing fan'anfeng*).[6]

However, revolutionary discourse was always far removed from actual practice in socialist China. Not long after the nationwide promotion of the barefoot doctor program in 1969 and 1970, the barefoot doctors had already donned shoes and separated themselves from agricultural labor. There were two barefoot doctors on Jiang Village Commune's Longzhang Brigade prior to 1978, but neither worked in the fields. The first, Yan Shiwei, was already in his seventies and had worked in Chen Hongting's union clinic for a number of years but had had to stop when he contracted tuberculosis and so returned to his home brigade. The second was Niu Shuiying, a woman barefoot doctor in charge of the pharmacy, giving injections, and delivering babies. Niu said that both she and Yan Shiwei usually remained at the medical station and did not go out to treat patients.[7] The former barefoot doctors and their fellow villagers explain this deviation from the propagandized norm in quite practical ways. Barefoot doctor Xu Peichun argued that the number of diseases among villagers during the 1970s meant that he and his colleagues simply did not have time to participate in agricultural labor in addition to their medical tasks.[8] A villager who was asked about this had a slightly different interpretation, but it still reflects the magnitude of the barefoot doctor's duties: "Calls for treatment came at uncertain times; sometimes [people would need a doctor] at midnight. Anyway, there were around 500 commune members in a village so it was okay to support him [the barefoot doctor] even though he did not take part in [agricultural] labor."[9] Moreover, even if barefoot doctors participated in agricultural labor, it was often just for symbolic purposes. For example, 163 barefoot doctors in Tangxi District of Yuhang County participated in agricultural labor for a total of 143 days in one month. This was less than one day per person per month.[10]

The barefoot doctors' removal from agricultural labor meant that they gradually became a special category of commune member, distinguished by their professional knowledge and specialist work, which became the prime feature of their new group identity. Interestingly, when barefoot doctor Xu Peichun described his activity and that of the agricultural laborers, he used two different Chinese terms for work: "When the commune members went out to work (*chugong*) in the field, we went to work (*shangban*) in the medical stations."[11] The use of these two different expressions is an important linguistic distinction—each had precise meanings within the villagers' vocabulary, and they were never used interchangeably. In general terms, the two words relate to the household registration system: *shangban* was used only for workers who held urban household registration status, while *chugong* was associated exclusively with those with rural household registration status. Furthermore, *shangban* denotes the performance of skilled work, while *chugong* refers to "unskilled" manual labor in the fields. In this sense, the difference between *chugong* and *shangban* is comparable to the difference in English between blue-collar workers and white-collar professionals. This word choice reveals that, in the villagers' eyes, barefoot doctors were already effectively "doctors with shoes," even before Deng's declaration. Unlike ordinary commune members who earned work points through participating directly in agricultural labor, the barefoot doctors had a discrete identity and a different relationship to the brigade's "work."

Harmonizing with Colleagues and Peers

The formation of peer relationships is another important aspect of group identity. There is an old Chinese saying that goes, "Colleagues in the same trade are enemies" (*tonghang shi yuanjia*), and this was certainly applicable to the daily practice of medical work in China's past.[12] Important insights into the negative impact of this phenomenon can be found in the writings of Chen Cunren, a prominent Chinese medicine doctor in Shanghai during the 1920s and 1930s. He became famous for being one of five delegates who traveled to Nanjing to protest the Nationalist government's resolution abolishing Chinese medicine in 1929. According to Chen, medical practitioners usually despised their peers and made negative comments about each other in their efforts to attract patients. They dismissed their opponents' skills and bragged about their own medical excellence. He described the situation shortly after he had become a physician: "Old physicians used to shake their heads when they looked at the prescriptions I wrote. It seemed that my prescriptions were always wrong. Some never even glanced at my prescriptions. Actually it was the habit of patients in old Shanghai to invite two to three doctors to write prescriptions, which they then checked with other doctors. However, among doctors, usually doctor A said doctor B was wrong, while doctor B said doctor A was wrong."[13] Chen's description continued to hold true for a few years into the new regime. According to an investigative report on the union clinics that was published in 1957, "Some union clinic doctors who were trained in the old society still maintain remnants of old thoughts and strong clan inclinations. They do not recognize the medical proficiency of other doctors. They attack other doctors, brag about themselves, and try to elbow others out."[14]

Fractious peer relationships and open displays of jealousy were mainly manifested in competition over patients, sparked by the desire for profit, fame, and publicly recognized medical authority. These habits were exacerbated by the absence of state regulations and self-regulation within the medical profession. The establishment of the union clinics and the founding of the state medical system marked the start of the state's disciplining of the "old society" healers. The state's goals in regulating and standardizing daily medical practices were twofold: it sought to promote new ethical and ideological principles, such as "serving people," and also to organize interactions between patients and doctors into state-controlled medical units. For the doctors, the union clinics solved the earlier problem of needing to solicit patients to secure an income. Under the new system, they had guaranteed salaries that were determined according to a complex formula based on the gross income of the clinic as well as each doctor's medical proficiency and medical qualifications, their fame among the masses, and their family's particular needs, as chapter 1 described. The implementation of these dramatic measures led rural medical practitioners to gradually develop a collective professional identity within an over arching socialist rubric. This trend toward a socialist professional medical identity continued when the barefoot doctor system was introduced between 1969 and 1970.

In the 1970s, barefoot doctors were mainly responsible for the medical and public health work of their own production brigades, and they did not intervene in each other's geographical domains. Meanwhile, the reimbursement policy of the cooperative medical services and the subsidized pharmaceuticals the barefoot doctors prescribed confined their patients to their own brigade's medical stations, which minimized competition between colleagues in neighboring villages. The relatively standardized training of the barefoot doctor program brought an end to the variation in medical proficiency—be it perceived or real—that underpinned the vying for patients typical of the old system. As Jiang Village barefoot doctor Zhou Yonggan said, "We did not have too much to do with the barefoot doctors of other villages. Patients would not go to other villages to seek treatment. In general . . . all barefoot doctors' proficiencies were at almost the same level."[15] In rare situations, barefoot doctors went to other villages to treat patients outside of their official jurisdiction. But for the most part, there was little conflict and competition. The barefoot doctors' salaries or work points depended on their production brigade's economic conditions, not the number of patients they treated. As such, an individual doctor would not be affected financially by another barefoot doctor operating in his home village.[16]

Inside the medical stations, the nonprofit orientation of the cooperative medical services and salary calculation methods also minimized internal competition. Like their fellow villagers, each barefoot doctor was paid according to the work points system, in which an individual's daily work points depended on his or her physical capability for performing agricultural labor. This system also applied to the barefoot doctors, meaning that neither their individual medical qualifications and proficiency nor the numbers of patients that each treated affected their income. As ordinary female commune members generally received fewer work points than their male counterparts, female barefoot doctors were paid fewer work points than their male counterparts.[17] Zhang Ahhua, a barefoot doctor on Jiang Village Commune's Hejian Brigade, described the methods of payment and income: "The production team registered our work points for us, referring to us as ordinary commune members. Usually, there were 3,500 work points for each normal laborer per year, ten points for each day, and RMB 1.2 per ten work points. We barefoot doctors received the same work points as normal male laborers."[18]

This method was also applied to medical stations with more than one barefoot doctor. In Jiang Village, when Yan Shengyu joined the Longzhang Brigade medical station in 1978, he became the station's third barefoot doctor. According to Yan, all three were given work points for thirty days per month, but the number of points varied. Yan Shiwei had started practicing medicine in 1958, but he was only given 8.5 points in 1976 because of his old age.[19] Yan Shengyu received ten work points, like a normal male laborer.

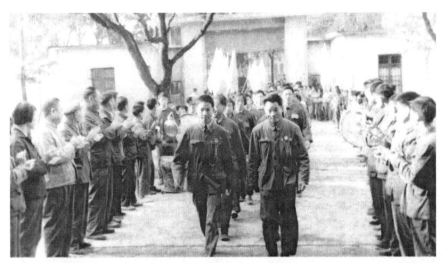

Figure 6.1. Barefoot doctors walking into a meeting hall, October 18, 1976. Reproduced with permission from the Fuyang City Archives, Zhejiang Province, China.

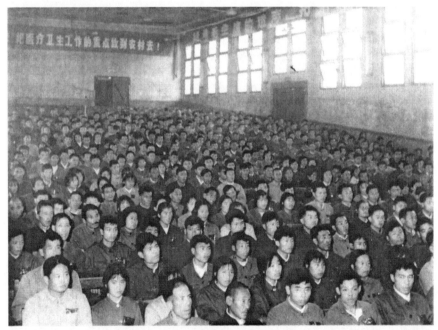

Figure 6.2. Fuyang County barefoot doctor and cooperative medical services meeting, October 18, 1976. The banner on the rear wall says "Stress rural areas in medical and health work!" The banner on the right wall says "Inherit Chairman Mao's unfulfilled wishes and carry on the proletariat revolution to the end!" Reproduced with permission from the Fuyang City Archives, Zhejiang Province, China.

Niu Shuiying, the female barefoot doctor in charge of the pharmacy, giving injections and delivering babies, got six work points and was paid an additional RMB 1.35 by the family if a baby was born at night. She reported that she submitted these extra payments to the brigade.[20] Medical station colleagues happily accepted this method of allocating wages, and discrepancies in earnings did not affect the working relationship between the barefoot doctors. Notably, both female villagers and female barefoot doctors seem to have accepted the fact that they earned less than their male counterparts as a fact of life, because they assumed that men's labor ought to be more valuable than women's.

The factors explored above all minimized conflicts among the barefoot doctors in terms of personal incomes and professional prestige during the 1970s.[21] They contributed to the formation of their sense of a group identity, which was particularly important for their development in the early years of the program. Alongside this new, noncompetitive medical structure, a new system of politicized medical ethics was promoted.[22] As indicated earlier, medical ethics assumed a new political meaning under the socialist government, which demanded that doctors conform to the image of an ideal doctor who was both "red and expert," meaning socialist in spirit and medically proficient.[23] After 1970, the government further promoted medical ethics and introduced a series of awards that gave public recognition to outstanding doctors and promoted a sense of group identity. "Model barefoot doctors" were celebrated at representative meetings, which also involved group political training of the barefoot doctors to further encourage the formation of an *esprit de corps* and a unified idea of medical ethics. The ideologically charged atmosphere of these meetings exerted a subtle influence on the daily behavior of the barefoot doctors. At the same time, villagers also formed their own expectations of the barefoot doctors based on the political indoctrination that they received about the doctors' role. One barefoot doctor said that she chose not to carry a medicine box: "I thought that if I carried a medical kit, the villagers would regard me as a doctor rather than a villager. I am a very sensitive person. Sometimes the villagers joked with me: 'Hey, you are a barefoot doctor. Why aren't you barefoot?' I immediately reflected [on my behavior] and whether I was keeping myself too aloof from the masses."[24]

A Steep Career Ladder and Blocked Social Mobility

The formation of a sense of group identity was also closely associated with the barefoot doctors' career and mobility prospects. Like other professionals in other social settings, the barefoot doctors pursued their careers and strove for upward social mobility within their particular social contexts, although this was significantly affected by their twin identities as doctors and villagers. While they were considered doctors at the village level of the state's three-tier medical system, they were not considered to be formal staff of this same system. As a result of this ambiguity, the barefoot doctors were denied institutional opportunities for advancement. Instead, they were regular commune members who were affiliated with particular production brigades. Just like their fellow villagers, they had limited scope for progress beyond the village because the urban and rural household system that had been in place since 1958 created a rigid barrier to social mobility for China's rural residents.[25] Sulamith and Jack Potter outlined the paths for social mobility among villagers under the people's commune system in the 1970s as follows: serving in the armed forces, rising within the organization of the Communist Party, or making a great academic achievement.[26] According to their fieldwork in Zengbu Brigade, Guangdong Province, the rate of villagers who changed their household status from rural to urban was 3.6 per 1,000 per year over the whole fourteen-year period from 1965 to 1978.[27] As villagers described themselves, "The production brigade was a big jar. We look like crabs in the jar. We kept trying to climb out of the jar again and again, but we failed every time."[28] In this sense, the production brigades isolated the villages from wider society during the 1970s, and the barefoot doctors experienced the same limitations on social mobility as their fellow brigade members.

Nonetheless, advancement within the system was sometimes possible for the barefoot doctors. During the 1970s, when the commune clinics needed additional staff as a result of the shortage of medical personnel, the barefoot doctors were seen as ideal candidates for recruitment. This represented a promotion for the barefoot doctors and was the most important path to upward social mobility.[29] This was the case for Jiang Jingting, Mr. Cat-Dog, of Sanshen Village, who retired from the Jiang Village Township Clinic in 1996 after twenty-seven years of medical service in the commune clinic, during which time he experienced shifting models of health-care delivery. In 1965, the young Mr. Cat-Dog was selected to be among the first batch of health-care workers, who were then renamed "barefoot doctors" in 1968, when his main responsibility was to help the commune clinic conduct schistosomiasis prevention work, as the disease was rampant in Sanshen Brigade. In 1970, Jiang Village Commune Clinic set up a branch in Sanshen, and Mr. Cat-Dog was assigned to take charge of the schistosomiasis prevention work for the commune.[30] Similarly, Zhou Yonggan and two of his classmates, who had been selected to study at Yuhang County People's Hospital, were recruited by the commune clinic in 1973 because of the shortage of medical personnel. Zhou is still working at Western City Hospital (as the clinic is now called).[31] However, this kind of upward social mobility was rare among the Jiang Village barefoot doctors, and only Mr. Cat-Dog, Zhou, and Zhou's classmates moved upward throughout the 1970s. To a great extent, this kind of upward social mobility depended on the individual's performance, hard work, and popularity among both commune clinic doctors and other villagers, but there was also an element of luck.[32] The promotion to clinic doctor changed the employee's household registration from rural to urban, and this single shift meant they could enjoy a series of welfare benefits unavailable to ordinary villagers in the commune era. Working in the commune clinics also enabled those who had been promoted to enhance their medical skills, which in turn further advanced their careers.

Besides advancement within the state medical system, barefoot doctors had the same, albeit limited, opportunities as their fellow villagers to achieve upward social mobility in the 1970s. In 1971, one Jiang Village barefoot doctor by the surname of Lu had the good fortune to join the People's Liberation Army, which not only changed his fate but also brought great honor to him, his family, and even his fellow production brigade members.[33] Xu Shuilin, who became a barefoot doctor in 1968, was another unusual case.[34] He enrolled in the Hangzhou Health Professional Secondary School following the waiver of the entrance examination in 1975. This meant that his household status was converted from rural to urban, and after his graduation he was assigned a job by the state in the Hangzhou Medicine Experimental Workshop, where he has been working ever since. Today, he is famous for his expertise in snake bite antidotes in the suburban areas of western Hangzhou.[35] Of the total twenty-four barefoot doctors in Jiang Village Commune, Xu and Lu were the only ones who managed to achieve upward social mobility by going to school or joining the army.

Not everyone was as fortunate in achieving upward social mobility as the barefoot doctors mentioned above, because such opportunities were very scarce in Chinese village societies during the 1970s. Therefore, both upward and downward social mobility mainly occurred inside the production brigades, such as barefoot doctors resigning from their medical and health-related duties to do other kinds of work. One barefoot doctor returned to agricultural labor in 1970, while another became the brigade party secretary in 1972. The resignations of these barefoot doctors created vacancies, which led to another opportunity for upward social mobility: the selection of replacements. For example, Zhang Ahhua was selected to fill the barefoot doctor post vacated by Xu Shuilin. Zhang recalled, "I served as a health worker under Xu's supervision. There were eleven production teams, and each of them had one health worker like me. We health workers were all working part-time. When the brigade barefoot doctor came to our team to do epidemic prevention vaccinations or other things, we assisted him. In 1975, when Xu Shuilin was sent to study at the secondary technical school, I was selected to be a barefoot doctor in our brigade."[36]

The limited opportunities for social advancement are clearly reflected in the systematic survey of 818 barefoot doctors in Jiande County conducted in

1974. According to this survey, only 3 barefoot doctors went to study at universities, while 44 went to commune clinics, 8 worked in district hospitals. In total, only 55 (less than 7 percent) left their home villages.[37] Paths to promotion and upward social mobility were haphazard, uncertain, and noninstitutionalized and obviously differed from those of the formal medical profession or the staff of the Chinese state medical system.[38] Nonetheless, the fact that the barefoot doctors were part of the three-tiered system, however marginal their role within that structure, facilitated their stability as a group and contributed to the formation of a sense of group identity. This helped increase the speed of the decline of their medical "competitors" in the villages.

Demarcating and Marginalizing "Competitors"

Historically, the group identity of medical practitioners develops from limiting the competitive power of other social groups that show an interest in health and illness.[39] In China, this process was based on dominant medical practitioners setting themselves apart from other healers and clearly demarcating their activity through regulation—either their own or that of the state. Over the centuries, China's Confucian scholars repeatedly denounced shamans and local healers for their supernatural leanings and declared that such practices were inconsistent with Confucian values. Nonetheless, it was not their goal to eradicate these medical traditions.[40] But after 1949, the state took a firmer view and explicitly excluded folk healers who contradicted state ideology from the state system. Therefore political campaigns against "illegal healers" who might still be practicing medicine in the villages regularly enhanced the barefoot doctors' group identity.[41] As the description in chapter 1 indicated, healers in religious orders and supernatural sects were criticized and then eventually prohibited from operating at the beginning of the Cultural Revolution.[42] From the late 1960s onward, the new regulations declared that "vagrant healers and witch doctors should be strictly controlled. Each level of government should take serious measures to control them. Health departments at each level should also enforce the management and supervision [of medical work] in order to protect the health of the masses."[43] Barefoot doctors were asked to fight against feudal superstition as part of their daily work, while the advantages of the cooperative medical service were actively publicized.[44] Although "superstitious healers" and their practices did not disappear entirely from the villages upon the announcement of these policies, the villagers dared not seek treatment from these traditional sources openly. In Jiang Village, although the blind and crippled fortune-teller was severely criticized at the start of the Cultural Revolution, he was still popular among his fellow villagers, who would often carry him to a private corner and ask him to tell them their fortunes.[45]

Moreover, with the establishment of a rural health-care network and the campaign against superstition, modern medical knowledge was disseminated through public broadcasts, blackboards, and health posters. Old villager Luo, who was in charge of the Jiang Village Commune Cooperative Medical Service Committee in the early 1970s, said, "At meetings, we were told repeatedly, 'don't listen to superstition and talk about ghosts.'"[46] Commune members were advised to see doctors when they were ill because, according to the officials, Buddha did not exist.[47] Medical anthropological studies based on Yunnan Province also found that, although the campaign against superstition was not entirely successful in the areas where the Yi ethnic minority lived, it was impressive enough for Yi villagers to know that holding healing rituals was considered bad and dangerous.[48] As one foreign scholar observed, the traditional religious methods of treating disease seem to have been replaced by secular ones on the Chinese mainland by 1978.[49] This shift provided barefoot doctors with a much bigger space in which to practice medicine and build their sense of group identity.

Meanwhile, the criticism and prohibition policies were also extended to healers or physicians who attacked the "newly emerged things." Shen Yutian was an eighty-seven-year-old independent medical practitioner in Yuhang County who specialized in Chinese internal medicine. An official report criticized him for delaying the treatment of a child's measles, which led to the child's death. He was also denounced for using Chinese medicine to perform an illegal abortion on an unmarried girl that almost caused her death. In addition, he concealed an epidemic when he performed 116 treatments on 71 measles patients. Because of his malpractice and his illegal medical practice, he was severely criticized in official instructions which were circulated county-wide by the Yuhang County Health Bureau in 1974. The official instructions pointed out:

> It was not exceptional in our county for the illegal practice of medicine to lead to serious [negative] consequences, such as in the case of Shen Yutian. Some people, like the "bragging doctors" (*shuozui langzhong*), were dismissed from their medical units because they didn't have any medical skills. Some of them were witches who murdered and cheated patients for money; some of them were class enemies evading participation in agricultural work under the surveillance of the masses. Some of them have even infiltrated the brigade medical stations. They have cheated and bragged, told lies, sold fake medicine and cheated for money. They fiercely persecute the masses, attack the barefoot doctors, undermine the foundation of the cooperative medical service, and destroy the rural health revolution.[50]

Soon, Shen Yutian was ordered to make a self-criticism, and his medical license was cancelled. The new order demanded a dogged struggle against such quacks. "We must whole-heartedly support the 'newly emerged things'—the barefoot doctors and the cooperative medical service." The state further urged local officials to pay "revolutionary attention" to the matter and educate the masses not to believe in superstition or be cheated by quacks. Finally, it exclaimed "Trust our own barefoot doctors."[51] The official marginalization of these other healers and the new medical education given to the villagers expanded the rural medical world and further benefited the gradual development of a sense of group identity among barefoot doctors.

Changes in the Doctor-Patient Power Relationship

Group identity is closely associated with the doctor-patient power relationship. However, this power relationship is characterized by two diametrically opposed dynamics in elite classical Chinese medicine—in which doctors were subordinate to patients—and modern Western medicine—in which patients are subordinated to doctors. In pre-twentieth-century China, patients controlled their medical interactions with their doctors and enjoyed greater autonomy than did their Western counterparts, particularly in the upper levels of society.[52] In the absence of an external accreditation body, both doctors and patients depended heavily on a tight personal trust network. Given that a doctor's credibility was based on a patient's public praise of his work or a celebrity's recommendation of his skills, patients enjoyed extraordinary power over their physicians.[53] In contrast, in Western medical settings, including those in China, doctors had absolute power while their patients had little or none. As Kleinman noticed, Western-style practitioners in Taiwan's Chinese society gave instructions regarding treatment without much margin for interpretation and had noticeably more authority than their counterparts among the Chinese-style practitioners, who offered explanations and even negotiated diagnoses and treatment.[54] This situation was heightened by the increasing complexity of modern medical sciences and the rise of medical institutions and technologies. Practitioners of Western medicine claim exclusive accuracy: there is only one correct view, and it derives from the scientific basis of the medicine they practice. This medicine is the domain of experts; therefore, the patient has to take on a submissive role in the treatment process.[55] There is no room for social negotiation of roles: doctors and patients do not come to a consensus about the nature of an illness or its treatment, nor do the patient's friends and relatives usually participate in the discussion of the disease, its origin, or its prognosis.[56] In Chinese hospitals, the expression *tinghua* ("do as you are told," or "listen to what is said") is a common patient instruction.[57]

However, the dramatic difference in doctor-patient power relationships between elite Chinese medicine and Western medicine is not observed in rural Chinese medicine. On the one hand, before the advent of the barefoot doctors, the village medical world was dominated by folk healers, while ordinary villagers were not able to choose professional doctors as the wealthy elite did. More importantly, doctors and patients were both villagers from the same enclosed communities and were familiar with each other, in stark contrast to the relationships within Chinese medicine among the urban elites. On the other hand, village patients, their families, and relatives could all participate in the healing process, which adhered to the pattern found in the Chinese medicine setting. The barefoot doctors' relationship with their fellow villagers emerged in this social context.

As mentioned earlier, the notion of barefoot doctors can be traced back to the village health workers of the experimental health program in Ding County in the 1930s. Its director, C. C. Chen, once explained that the decision to select village health workers from among local youths rested on more than just economic considerations. In his opinion, it was also because these young villagers were honest, hardworking, and familiar with their fellow villagers.[58] Chen's predecessor, Hsun-yuan Yao, who is paid less attention by current scholarship, once emphasized the importance of village health workers "who speak the local dialect, who are acquainted with local conditions and are 'unspoiled.'"[59] Similarly, Lisowski also pointed out the advantages of selecting barefoot doctors from their home villages: "Being part of it [the village], they understand the everyday problems of the people they serve. They stay in the countryside, for that is their home. Their patients are their neighbors, co-workers, and relatives, and their work gives them immense satisfaction."[60] In discussing the social relations between barefoot doctors and villagers, recent scholarship argues that the state used the kinship affection network to mobilize villagers to be barefoot doctors, giving rise to an equal power relationship between barefoot doctors and villagers.[61] For example, Yang Nianqun argues that barefoot doctors were under the dual control of a kinship affection network and institutionalized political atmosphere, which contributed to the success of the epidemic prevention system during the 1970s.[62]

Indeed, the proximity of the personal relationships in these tightly knit communities made a positive impact on doctor-patient power relations. The villagers felt quite relaxed about communicating with "one of their own" about their diseases. If they went outside the locality to a more formal setting, such as a district clinic or a county hospital, they would encounter doctors who wore white gowns and masks and who might speak Mandarin instead of their own dialect. These doctors made the villagers feel shy and vulnerable, a reaction described as "white gown syndrome." The barefoot doctors overcame this problem for the villagers because they emerged from within the villages themselves in a fashion that was similar to the earlier folk healers or medical practitioners. However, the power relationship between barefoot doctors and villager patients was dynamic rather than static, even in the specific social and medical contexts of an enclosed village society during the 1970s, and barefoot doctors gradually obtained more power over time.

Understandably, the villagers initially had limited faith in the barefoot doctors. After all, these doctors often had only a few months of training. An educated youth from Fuyang County called Liu described the villagers' distrust of the barefoot doctors:

> When I had just become a barefoot doctor in the village, the son of a peasant developed a high fever. When I heard this news, I went to his home without being asked. But his father insisted that the fever was due to mischief caused by ghosts and gods. He set up a shrine and burned spirit paper, and then he mixed the ashes with water and asked his son to drink this mixture. However, his child's fever became more and more serious.[63]

Because of the increasingly serious nature of the illness and the absence of any alternative course of action, the child's father finally agreed to let Liu treat the fever using his medicine. The child was suffering from pneumonia that had developed from a common cold, so after just a few doses of herbal medicine the child's temperature dropped. Liu said, "After this event, the people living in nearby villages were willing to ask me to treat them."[64]

However, growing acceptance and trust meant that the power relationships between the barefoot doctors and the villagers gradually became unbalanced and asymmetric. Because barefoot doctors primarily treated commune members in their own production brigades under the policy of "medical regionalization," they basically treated their fellow villagers. The doctors became more and more familiar with the health problems of their fellow villagers as they gained experience. Although the barefoot doctors did not usually write prescriptions or keep written case records, as well-educated physicians did, their memories effectively served this purpose.[65] Under the dumbbell-shaped structure of the three-tier medical network, the barefoot doctors' medical territories and their patients gradually stabilized, enabling them to eventually gain the villagers' trust and take on the dominant role in the doctor-patient relationship. Compared to their predecessors in the village health context, the barefoot doctors had several advantages. As the Porters pointed out in *Patient's Progress*, the premodern practitioner did not have miracle cures to command the unqualified submission and lasting gratitude of his patients. Medical treatments often resulted in failure or only partial success, and patients often died or did not respond to treatment.[66] Modern pharmaceuticals and medical instruments—such as antibiotic tablets, injections, and infusions—have enhanced modern medical practitioners' power in their interactions with their patients. As a result of these factors, doctors started to assume control over treatment regimes. For example, even the presence of a stethoscope reshaped the relationship between doctors and patients, in that it took the mantle of illness out of the hands of their patients.[67] Villagers were amazed by the ability of the physician to learn about the inner structure of the human body through the use of a stethoscope, based on sounds that were inaudible to the patients themselves.[68] Liu recalled his experience of using a stethoscope on an old village man for the first time. When Liu put the stethoscope under his clothes, the old man was very nervous, and a lot of villagers crowded around and watched with great curiosity.[69]

The increasing power of the doctors over their patients is also reflected in their responsibility for malpractice. Another barefoot doctor, Shang, recalled her medical practice in an anthology of the experiences of educated youth in villages:

> When I was a barefoot doctor, I did not actually have too much medical knowledge. Administering injections and prescribing medicines were sufficient for minor illnesses. . . . The procedure was also quite simple. I just put the needles and syringes in boiling water, and pushed and pulled a few times before the instruments were sterilized. During the several years that I worked as a barefoot doctor, no infections ever occurred. I don't know whether it was due to my luck or to the kindness of the masses.[70]

However, not everyone was as lucky as Shang. Barefoot doctors made mistakes that in today's terms would be considered malpractice. The problem was that the health bureaus did not criticize this kind of malpractice because they wanted to protect and promote the development of these "newly emerged things." A poisoning accident that occurred in Fuyang County illustrates this point well. In July 1972, Nan'an Commune Clinic surveyed the malaria patients in the commune according to the instructions issued by the County Health Bureau. The commune clinic determined that commune members in Longshan Brigade should take a malaria medicine called ethylamine pyridine, and the district hospital issued the clinic with instructions regarding formal treatment methods for malaria and the medicine dosage chart. The medicine began to be distributed on July 20. At the start, Dr. Fang from the commune clinic, who was in charge of this work, directed the barefoot doctor of Longshan Brigade to give a dosage of sixteen pills at a time, although the actual recommended dosage was only eight. This mistake caused serious poisoning in the village, including ten cases of stomach cramps, twenty headaches, one case of diarrhea, and one case of serious poisoning. The commune clinic was severely criticized, and Dr. Fang was dismissed. The brigade's own barefoot doctor was absolved of any responsibility for the incident, though he should have been suspicious about the high dosage that the doctor had prescribed.[71] Incidents of medical malpractice committed by barefoot doctors were not included in the health bureau's official documents, while those committed by doctors at other medical units were included. After the rural economic reforms, however, when some bare-foot doctors moved from villages to urban areas, reports of their medical malpractices emerged in large numbers. These doctors were referred to by disparaging titles, such as "itinerant charlatans" (*jianghu youyi*), just as some folk healers of the 1950s and 1960s had been ridiculed before them. Nonetheless, the state's denial of medical malpractice among barefoot doctors throughout the 1970s greatly contributed to the ascending authority of doctors in the doctor-patient power relationship in the early years of the barefoot doctor program. These points indicate that the power relationship between barefoot doctors and villagers was not equal, despite the minimal geographical and psychological distance between them.

Reinterpreting Legitimacy: Disintegration as a New Beginning

The state's played a crucial role in the formation of a group identity for the barefoot doctors and their ascendance in the doctor-patient power relation-ship in the 1970s. But the villagers' positive experience of the rapid effects of Western medicine administered by the barefoot doctors during these years was also fundamental to improving the barefoot doctors' authority.[72] In a political climate where "both redness and expertise" were emphasized rather than professional medical expertise alone, the barefoot doctors did not need to invoke the authority of a medical registration board or a university degree. As Chen Zhicheng said, there was no medical qualification requirement for doctors at the union clinics, nor was there a ranking system for doctors in rural areas.[73] However, this situation would change dramatically with Deng Xiaoping's reforms, which were initiated in the late 1970s, when the emphasis on barefoot doctors' qualities shifted from "redness" to "expertise."[74] In the health sector, this socialist modernization reform program was evident in the new attention paid to medical professionalization, improving the quality of hospital services, and increasing the use of technology.[75]

To motivate the barefoot doctors to improve their medical proficiency and to enhance the quality of the cooperative medical service, in October 1979 the State Council proposed holding examinations to certify the barefoot doctors,[76] a quarter of whom were to attain a medical proficiency level akin to that of secondary technical school graduates within a five-year period.[77] In Hangzhou Prefecture, the content of the examinations included political performance, medical theories, and practical skills. The doctor's political performances were assessed by the Communist Party branches of their pro-duction brigades and then checked by their commune party branches. The district and commune clinics assessed their technical expertise, including basic medical skills such as giving injections, changing medicines, cleaning and suturing wounds, and treating common diseases, as well as their abilities regarding artificial respiration, vaccinations, antisepsis, quarantine, water purification, epidemic reporting, and acupuncture. A medical theory examination was central to the accreditation process and was designed by each county according to the practical needs of each locale. Those demonstrated good political performances and practical skills, and who passed the medical theory exam, were certified as barefoot doctors by Zhejiang Province.[78] The new accreditation and testing system started in 1981 when examinations and assessments of village doctors were held in Hangzhou Prefecture.[79] Barefoot doctors who passed the medical theory and basic medical technique examinations and who were also regarded as having above-average political track records were certified as village doctors by the authorities in Zhejiang Province.[80] However, neither process prohibited those who failed to succeed from practicing medicine in the villages, so, in this regard, these accreditation programs were not formal medical qualifications.

Concurrently, rural economic reforms started to occur around Hangzhou Prefecture that would lead eventually to decollectivization and the fragmentation of the commune system. As one villager recalled, "In 1978, we ordinary masses just knew that there was an experiment taking place in Anhui Province. At that time, some villagers began to work less than before. In 1979 and 1980, there was chaos in the production teams. It was different than before."[81] A few production brigades and teams began changing the existing collective labor and distribution methods. Some implemented a contract-bonus system that reallocated responsibility for labor and output to individuals. In this system, commune members signed contracts with the production teams that specified a certain output and the work points and production costs of achieving that output. If the actual output exceeded that contracted, the individuals received a bonus. If the output was less than that specified in the contract, they were required to compensate the production team.[82] This system therefore gave commune members huge incentives to work and greatly increased their incomes. However, barefoot doctors, who still depended on the fixed work point system, were not able to sign similar contracts with production brigade. As a result, the income balance between the commune members and the barefoot doctors was gradually severed. There were immediate negative consequences for the doctors.[83]

In December 1980, Xixing Commune, in the north of Jiang Village Commune, reported that some barefoot doctors were reluctant to continue their work and wanted to change their profession because of their dissatisfaction with their wages since the implementation of the rural reform policy.[84] In February 1981, Health Minister Qian Xinzhong admitted that some barefoot doctors had given up practicing medicine and reverted to farming or primary school teaching. Even some who had been barefoot doctors for more than ten years and who had received considerable training were changing their jobs.[85] In the early years of the reforms, the results of barefoot doctors departing because of changes in wages were not all that serious, because the people's commune system was still largely intact. But, by 1983, the rural household contract responsibility system was fully implemented in the villages, and this posed a major threat to the continuation of the barefoot doctor program.[86] Under the contract responsibility system, all the land in each brigade was divided up and allocated to individual households on a per capita basis, so that each commune member—barefoot doctors included—received an equal share of the land. Each household managed their own landholdings and grew whatever crops they wanted, and they submitted a certain amount of grain and tax to the state.[87] Meanwhile, collective properties were also sold off or allocated to individual households, so barefoot doctors and cooperative medical stations lost the support of the collective economy.[88] As collective property, the medical stations were contracted to the barefoot doctors within the production brigades, and were then, in most cases, operated as private village clinics.[89]

The barefoot doctor program disintegrated in the context of this dual process of new medical certification and the implementation of the household responsibility system. The state effectively changed the definition of medical legitimacy by prioritizing medical proficiency over other factors. Simultaneously, the core institutional context that had supported the barefoot doctors, the cooperative medical service, ceased to exist with the end of the people's communes (now known as townships). The barefoot doctors had to make a living out of medicine on their own initiative rather than from work points allocated by the commune's production brigades (now known as administrative villages). Villagers were no longer confined to the medical jurisdictions of their own villages (the former production brigades) and were now free to seek medical attention elsewhere.

In 1980, Jiang Village Commune had a total of fourteen brigades. All the villages except Jiang Village, the commune seat, had medical stations and barefoot doctors, who totaled eighteen in the commune. Only two of them did not receive their barefoot doctor certification on May 25, 1980,[90] but they were still practicing medicine in 1983 when the household responsibility system was implemented. From then on, new certification programs and medical proficiency standards started to differentiate the more highly skilled members of the barefoot doctor groups from the less skilled ones. In villages that had two barefoot doctors, one of them usually stopped and switched to another line of work. The only exception was Wulian Village, where two barefoot doctors, Shen Guanrong and Hong Jinglin, continued to practice medicine at the same medical station, one in the morning and the other in the afternoon. For others, as Yan Shengyu explained, "the low income was the main reason [they stopped practicing medicine]. The majority of them had low skill levels, which affected their incomes."[91] They moved to more lucrative work, such as carpentry or raising pigs. In Longzhang Village, Niu Shuiying and Yan Shengyu

Table 6.1. Barefoot doctors in Jiang Village Commune after 1980

Village	Name of barefoot doctor	Attained barefoot doctor certification (1980)?	Attained village doctor certification (1988)?	Year he/she stopped working	Reason he/she stopped working	New job
Jiang village						
Yangjiadai	Yang Zhihua	√		1985	Low income	Carpenter
	Qian Xuechang	√		1983	Low income	Carpenter
Shuanglong	Zhou Honggen	√		1983	Heavy financial burdens	
	Yang Lingjuan	√		1990	Low income	
Luojiazhuang	Yang Aifa	√		1983	Better job offer	Village secretary
	Luo Xuejuan	√	√	1994	Better job offer	Factory doctor
Longzhang	Yan Shengyu	√	√			
	Niu Shuiying			1983	New regulations around 1987 requiring that women should only give birth in hospitals.	Shop assistant at the power station
Hejian	Zhang Ahhua	√	√			
Dengyunwei	Xu Jinfeng	√		1983		Raising pigs

(continued)

Table 6.1. Barefoot doctors in Jiang Village Commune after 1980—(concluded)

Village	Name of barefoot doctor	Attained barefoot doctor certification (1980)?	Attained village doctor certification (1988)?	Year he/she stopped working	Reason he/she stopped working	New job
Wulian	Shen Guanrong	√	√	2004	Stopped in 2004 because of new regulations, continued to practice at home, and stopped in 2008 because of cancer.	
	Hong Jinglin	√	√	2004	Stopped in 1997, resumed in 2002, stopped in 2004, then practiced at home until 2006, stopped because of new regulations.	
Shentankou	Shen Jinrong			1999	Old age	
Sanshen	Wu Miaorong	√	√	1994	Low income	Raising pigs
Baojian	Bao Ahyu	√		1987	Low income	
Zhoujiacun	Fei Baofa	√	√	2002	Better job offer	Full-time village cadre
Wangjiaqiao	Jiang Huamao	√	√	1996	Illness	
	Zhong Xingfa	√		1983	Low proficiency	

Sources: Chen Zhicheng, interview, January 9–10, 2005; November 6, 2009; Yan Shengyu, interviews, November 3 and 23, 2009.

divided their medicine supply and shelving between them, and each carried their shares home on shoulder poles. Niu stopped working as a barefoot doctor, but she continued to work as a midwife in the village until 1987, when the government ruled that women should give birth only in hospitals, so there was no longer a need for her services. Meanwhile, the medical station was contracted to Yan, who continued to practice medicine.

After 1983, there were still 12 barefoot doctors practicing medicine in the villages of Jiang Village Township (see table 6.1). By 1988, when the village doctor certificates were issued in Yuhang County, two more barefoot doctors quit their jobs because of their low incomes. The remaining ten barefoot doctors were spread across nine villages.[92] Eight of them obtained both the barefoot doctor certificates issued in 1980 and the village doctor certificates in 1988. The other two were Shen Jinrong and one woman barefoot doctor surnamed Yang. Shen Jinrong had neither the barefoot doctor certificate nor the village doctor certificate because of his old age and illiteracy. However, he had decades of experience because he had started to practice medicine following his grandfather at the age of fourteen. Although barefoot doctor Yang did secure her barefoot doctor certificate, she gave up this work two years later because her income was too low. By 1990, the remaining nine barefoot doctors generally had higher levels of medical proficiency than those leaving the profession, and they remained a relatively stable group between 1990 and 2004. Departures from the group during this time were due to natural processes, such as aging and illness.[93] According to Luo Zhengfu, the director of Jiang Village Township Hospital after 1978, there was no new impact on rural health and medicine after the initial reshuffling associated with the end of collectivization. Those who continued practicing medicine did so largely because they felt more confident about their levels of medical proficiency.[94]

The reduction in barefoot doctor numbers that resulted from the inability of individual doctors to meet new medical proficiency standards during the 1980s was highly significant for both the state and the barefoot doctors themselves. The state's implementation of professional qualifications caused some individuals to leave the sector, even though failing medical examinations did not mean they had to stop practicing medicine. This process thereby raised the barefoot doctors' expertise as a group, because those remaining had necessarily attained these qualifications. This increase in expertise simultaneously contributed to the consolidation of their authority among their fellow villagers. In the meantime, barefoot doctor certificates or village doctor certificates also enhanced their authority because, in villagers' eyes, these barefoot doctors now were accredited by the state. As a result of this process, the barefoot doctors increased their legitimacy in the eyes of both the government and their fellow villagers. Their rise in social and economic status further separated the barefoot doctors from their fellow villagers and positioned them as a professional group in possession of specialist knowledge to which they had privileged access. In April 2004, one barefoot doctor with whom I developed a close relationship told me that he earned RMB 80,000 per year, which was three times as much as local primary school teachers in this relatively less-developed county in a mountainous area. According to Gail Henderson's studies in the late 1980s, in some very wealthy rural areas, village doctors earned two to three times as much as their urban counterparts.[95]

Current scholarship argues that the disintegration of the barefoot doctor program indicated the beginning of the decline of health services in China's villages due to the decline in the number of barefoot doctors and the dismantling of the cooperative medical service.[96] However, this argument does not hold true for Hangzhou Prefecture nor for many other parts of China.[97] During the 1970s, the average number of barefoot doctors per brigade was above 1.5, and the maximum average reached 2.5 at one point. From 1983 to 1988, each village (or former production brigade) in Hangzhou, and in China as a whole, had one or more barefoot doctor (see fig. 6.3). Although this indeed represented a decline in doctor numbers since the 1970s, it does not necessarily indicate a decline in the quantity and quality of the medical services provided in the villages. One barefoot doctor operating alone could manage all aspects of treatment, pharmacy, and accounting duties in his or her medical station.

Another factor suggesting that rural health care did not necessarily decline was that the majority of the medical stations and clinics continued to operate despite the diminution in barefoot doctor numbers. According to data from Hangzhou Prefecture, Zhejiang Province, and China as a whole, the percentage of brigades implementing the cooperative medical service dropped to its lowest level in 1983, but the number of village clinics (the former brigade medical service stations) still remained high. In the nation as a whole, 90 percent of villages had clinics, while the figure for Zhejiang Province was around 70 percent (see fig. 6.4).[98] From 1983 to 1988, these figures basically remained stable, and in some areas the percentage of villages with clinics increased even after the implementation of the rural reforms. Residents of villages without clinics could access the medical services provided by barefoot doctors in neighboring villages more easily because the improved economic conditions had also made transportation more convenient for the rural population.[99]

The public health network in the villages was also maintained and improved during the reform years, despite recent scholarship claiming that this network was disrupted by the administrative changes that resulted from the reforms.[100] In the meantime, epidemic prevention was further institutionalized by the standardization of vaccine supply, inoculation periods, and management and assessment processes.[101] According to the *Yuhang County*

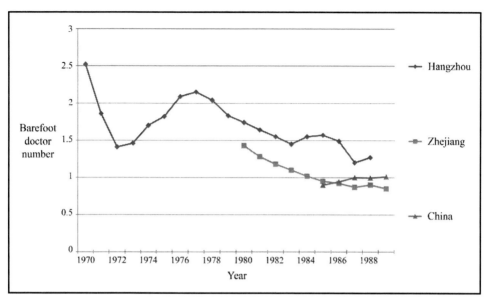

Figure 6.3. Average numbers of barefoot doctors in each production brigade (village) in Hangzhou, in Zhejiang Province, and in China as a whole, 1970–89 (unit: person). Data from (1) Hangzhou: Hangzhoushi weishengju Hangzhoushi weishengzhi bianji weiyuanhui, *Hangzhoushi weishengzhi*, 84–87; Hangzhoushi weishengju [Hangzhou Prefecture Health Bureau], "Hangzhou diqu nongcun shengchan dadui ji shengchandui weisheng zuzhi qingkuang" [Survey of Health Organizations in Production Brigades and Production Teams in Rural Areas of Hangzhou Prefecture], 1973, HZA, vol. 87-3-29; (2) Zhejiang: Zhejiangsheng tongjiju [Zhejiang Province Bureau of Statistics], ed., *Zhejiang tongji nianjian 1984* [Zhejiang Statistical Year Book, 1984] (Hangzhou: Zhejiangsheng tongjiju, 1984), 248; Zhejiangsheng tongjiju, *Zhejiang tongji nianjian 1985* [Zhejiang Statistical Year Book, 1985] (Hangzhou: Zhejiangsheng tongjiju, 1985), 192; Zhejiangsheng tongjiju, *Zhejiang tongji nianjian 1988* [Zhejiang Statistical Year Book, 1988] (Hangzhou: Zhejiangsheng tongjiju, 1988), 347; Zhejiangsheng tongjiju, *Zhejiang tongji nianjian 1989* [Zhejiang Statistical Year Book, 1989] (Hangzhou: Zhejiangsheng tongjiju, 1989), 372; Zhejiangsheng tongjiju, *Zhejiang tongji nianjian 1990* [Zhejiang Statistical Year Book, 1990] (Hangzhou: Zhejiangsheng tongjiju, 1990), 410; (3) China: Zhongguo weisheng nianjian bianzhuan weiyuanhui [Editorial Board of China Health Yearbook], ed., *Zhongguo weisheng nianjian 1990* [China Health Yearbook 1990] (Beijing: Renmin weisheng chubanshe, 1991), 459.

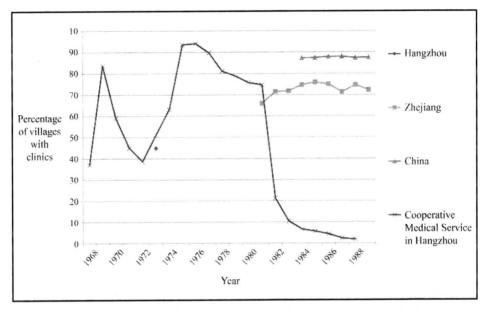

Figure 6.4. Percentages of villages with clinics, 1970–89 (unit: percentage). Data from (1) Hangzhou: Hangzhoushi weishengju Hangzhoushi weishengzhi bianji weiyuanhui, *Hangzhoushi weishengzhi*, 84–87; Hangzhoushi weishengju [Hangzhou Prefecture Health Bureau], "Hangzhou diqu nongcun shengchan dadui ji shengchandui weisheng zuzhi qingkuang" [Survey of Health Organizations in Production Brigades and Production Teams in Rural Areas of Hangzhou Prefecture], 1973, HZA, vol. 87-3-29; (2) Zhejiang: Zhejiangsheng tongjiju, *Zhejiang tongji nianjian 1984*, 248; Zhejiangsheng tongjiju, *Zhejiang tongji nianjian 1985*, 192; Zhejiangsheng tongjiju, *Zhejiang tongji nianjian 1988*, 347; Zhejiangsheng tongjiju, *Zhejiang tongji nianjian 1989*, 372; Zhejiangsheng tongjiju, *Zhejiang tongji nianjian 1990*, 410; (3) China: Zhongguo weisheng nianjian bianzhuan weiyuanhui, *Zhongguo weisheng nianjian 1990*, 459.

Health Gazetteer, there were two stages of vaccination work. In the period from 1949 to 1970, vaccinations were conducted according to the number of vaccines supplied by the higher authorities. Then, between 1971 and 1982, vaccines were allocated according to the number of people who were supposed to be vaccinated. After 1983, the planned vaccination program (*jihua mianyi*) was implemented,[102] which institutionalized the supply and delivery of vaccines. Barefoot doctors were in charge of administering vaccinations and distributing vaccination notices to the villagers.[103] In villages that had no clinics, barefoot doctors still attended local meetings where people would line up to be vaccinated. In the township government bureaucracies, a medical staff member was specially delegated to oversee this work.[104] In the words of a Jiang Village barefoot doctor, this was "voluntary work" (*yiwugong*). The village usually paid a subsidy of RMB 60 per month to the village doctors.[105] At the end of each year, the township hospital would invite them to a dinner in recognition of their voluntary service.[106]

In general, the provision of basic medical services and public health-care standards in China's countryside have greatly improved since the rural reforms because the barefoot doctor group has remained largely intact and has indeed been strengthened in many ways through the reforms. A survey of patient satisfaction with medical services and their physician's abilities in two townships in Yuhang County indicated that health-care facilities and services had improved since the beginning of the economic reforms. Many informants said that they were dissatisfied with what they described as the "poorer conditions" of the past and that they regarded the present economic development as beneficial to their health-care services.[107] But, while they were happy with the services and their doctors' skills, they were dissatisfied with the high price of medical services in the new market economy.[108]

On January 24, 1985, the health minister Chen Minzhang announced during the concluding session of the National Health Bureau Directors' Meeting that the term "barefoot doctor" would no longer be used in China:

> The term "barefoot doctor" was put forward by Zhang Chunqiao in an article published in the early stages of the Cultural Revolution. Soon afterward, it was used everywhere on a large scale. The implications of this term are not clear. We have now decided that we will not use it anymore. From now on, those barefoot doctors who reach the proficiency level of secondary technical school (*yishi*) shall be called "village doctors"(*xiangcun yisheng*), while those who cannot reach the *yishi* level shall be called "health workers"(*weishengyuan*).[109]

The term "barefoot doctor" thus disappeared from official documents, though it was still popular among the villagers in their daily lives.

The story of the barefoot doctors, from their emergence in 1968 to the demise of their name in 1985, is unique in medical history. Barefoot doctors were effectively government-recognized "healers" who were inserted by means of a political campaign into the rural medical world, where they quickly ascended to a position of dominance. In the socialist period under Mao, the state played a key role in the formation of the barefoot doctors' group identity in an enclosed village society. It did so by minimizing group conflicts, consolidating group consciousness, inhibiting social mobility, and marginalizing competitors. Moreover, the expansion of Western medicine facilitated by the barefoot doctors and the state's continued support for their practice contributed to the barefoot doctors' ascending authority within the doctor-patient relationship. After the start of the rural reforms in the late 1970s, the state reinterpreted the barefoot doctors' medical legitimacy by implementing a medical examination system, in which medial expertise was the main criterion. While this new requirement for achieving minimum standards of medical expertise led to a fragmentation of the barefoot doctors' sense of group identity, it also brought significant positive results. In this sense, the rural reforms and the rise of the market economy can be said to have actually contributed to the barefoot doctors' professionalization. More specifically, the group identity, credibility, and authority that the barefoot doctors gained in the villages during the 1970s remained intact in spite of the rural reform process. Moreover, as the rural reforms progressed, the remaining barefoot doctors (now called village doctors) became village elites in terms of their increased incomes, professional expertise, and social status.

Chapter Seven

Conclusion

In 1952, when Chen Hongting and his father welcomed the doctors from neighboring villages to their family clinic in order to establish the Jiang Village Union Clinic, they could never have imagined the radical changes that would take place in the following decades. Chen Hongting could not have foreseen the dramatic ups and downs he would experience in both his life and career—from being a founding director of the clinic to being demoted, criticized, and even forcibly paraded through the street wearing a dunce cap, until finally retiring as an ordinary staff member. Nor could he have anticipated that the conversion of his home clinic into a union clinic marked the beginning of the transformation of the medical world of Jiang Village. The far-reaching consequences of that day in 1952 include the triumph of Western medicine over Chinese medicine (including the widespread use of Western pharmaceuticals), the establishment of the three-tier rural medical system, and the rise of barefoot doctor group. Chen Hongting himself studied Western medical knowledge and techniques, led his staff in undertaking public health work, and regularly received ideological indoctrination in socialist medical ethics. As a Chinese medicine doctor who practiced medicine under both the Nationalist and Communist regimes, his personal fate was tied up with the social changes brought about by the continuous political campaigns instigated after 1949. However, one theme dominated both the social transformation of rural Chinese medicine and Chen Hongting's medical career above all others: the introduction of Western medicine into China's villages.

The Village Medical World and Barefoot Doctors in the Postsocialist Era

In 2003, when I first visited Jiang Village, more than two decades had passed since the implementation of Deng Xiaoping's rural reforms, during which time Jiang Village—and Chen Hongting—had undergone a further series of tremendous changes. After stepping down from his position as clinic director during the Cultural Revolution, Chen Hongting worked as an ordinary staff member in the clinic until his retirement in 1979. His salary, which had been cut during the Cultural Revolution as a result of his demotion, was eventually repaid. His nephew, Chen Zhicheng, led the clinic rebellion against Chen Hongting in the early days of the Cultural Revolution and became the new director in 1968. Zhicheng left the clinic in 1976 but was rehired in 1981 and two years later was given an honorary title by the Yuhang County Health Bureau for his performance at work. The two Chens lived in separate houses but shared a common dividing wall. Despite this proximity, they never visited each other—indeed, whenever Chen Hongting was ill, he would ask the barefoot doctor Zhang Ahhua to give him intravenous drips. Chen Hongting died in 2007 without having reconciled with his nephew.

In 1996, Jiang Village was incorporated into Xihu District of urban Hangzhou as a township (*xiang*) and was no longer part of Yuhang County. As Hangzhou's suburbs expanded, Jiang Village became increasingly urbanized. By 2004, Wulian Village and Luojiazhuang Village, in the eastern part of the township, had been completely urbanized and the streets had become bustling roads lined with tall buildings. The other villages in Jiang Village Township were still designated as rural. The headquarters of Jiang Village Township Clinic were moved to the site of a former branch clinic in Luojiazhuang Village and was renamed Western City Hospital. The building that had originally been the headquarters was relegated to branch status, while another former branch was totally dismantled. Four barefoot doctors were still practicing medicine in their own village clinics: Yan Shengyu in Longzhang Village, Zhang Ahhua in Hejian Village, and two other barefoot doctors in Wulian Village. Their normal work routine was to open their clinics for treatment sessions in the mornings and then close for the afternoons. Their patients included not only their fellow villagers but also more and more rural migrant workers who were pouring into the region to make a living. At certain times of the year they distributed notices about organized vaccination drives for children and infants to parents in their areas. Every month, they attended a meeting convened by Western City Hospital to learn about the latest programs and policies. For example, when SARS broke out in 2003, they donned chemical-proof suits and carried out disinfection and quarantine work in their jurisdictions.

The postsocialist era brought other changes as the deep penetration and firm control of political power during the socialist period receded from the villages. Despite having been dominated by Western medicine at the height of the commune era, the medical world of Jiang Village—which had been constantly differentiated by political campaigns since 1949 and finally reconstructed at the height of the Cultural Revolution—has returned to its pluralistic pre-1949 form. The blind, crippled fortune teller known as the "Living Buddha," who had been criticized during the Cultural Revolution and paraded down the river in a boat, regained his popularity. Demand for his services meant that he made a lot of money, and envious villagers reported that he had already built many multistory houses. The temples around Jiang Village have also regained their prosperity since the early

1980s and have again become sites of healing rituals. The most prosperous temple in the Hangzhou urban area, Lingyin Temple, serves as a model for this religious resurgence. On the ninth and nineteenth days of each month, old women from Jiang Village and other neighboring villages pray to the Buddha and chant scriptures in a renovated Yuanjue Temple, which had been destroyed during the Cultural Revolution but was reconstructed in the late 1990s. The return of a plurality of health beliefs is indicated by the behavior of the former "revolutionary" union clinic director, Chen Zhicheng. Chen reads pulses and treats patients using both Chinese and Western medicine at his unauthorized private clinic in the morning and then reads and copies Buddhist sutras in the afternoon, and he visits the temple each month. Despite the resurgence of healing rituals, folk medicine practices such as bone setting and bloodletting are gradually fading out as old folk healers pass away, though their family members claim that they still know a few techniques.

The wheels of history never stop turning. Jiang Village is located in the Xixi wetland, and the Hangzhou city government launched a huge project to construct the Xixi National Wetland Park in 2004, the year after I started my fieldwork in Jiang Village. The residents of eleven villages dismantled their homes and were relocated into two residential communities in stages, as the new apartments constructed for them became ready. They were given compensation for this based on the condition of their houses, and their household registration status was changed as part of the so-called Rural-to-Urban Conversion Project (*nongzhuanju*). This was completed by 2008, by which time all villagers had been assigned to their new residential communities, and Jiang Village no longer belonged to a rural region. The Western City Hospital set up the Jiang Village Community Health Service Center and satellite health service stations in each residential community.

Accompanying the changes in administrative jurisdictions brought by urban development and the Rural-to-Urban Project, the qualifications for practicing medicine correspondingly changed. In 2006, Wulian Village Clinic was the first to be shut down. The two barefoot doctors who had worked there for more than 30 years were deemed ineligible to practice medicine in urban areas because their village doctor certificates were insufficient qualifications—urban areas require medical personnel to hold the assistant medical practitioner license (*zhiye zhuli yishi zigezheng*). After health service stations were established in each residential community in 2008, Zhang Ahhua and Yan Shengyu's village clinics were also abolished for license-related reasons. Only Yan was successful in upgrading to become an assistant medical practitioner (*zhiye zhuli yishi*), and he was incorporated into one of the health service stations. He is paid a fixed salary by the center and no longer has to worry about making a living based on patient demand. Though Zhang Ahhua is no longer eligible to practice medicine, he is still providing treatment to his fellow villagers at his underground (i.e., illegal) clinic, which is located just next to another health service station. Thus, of the entire cohort of barefoot doctors who worked in the former Jiang Village Commune from 1968 onward, Yan Shengyu is the only one who is still legally eligible to practice medicine. Interestingly, he was also the last to join the Jiang Village barefoot doctor group, which he did in 1978.

When Jiang Village was undergoing the changes to its medical system resulting from becoming an urban area, in other counties of Hangzhou Prefecture a similar readjustment called the "integrated management of rural health" (*nongcun weisheng yitihua guanli*) was implemented in 2008–10. According to the regulations, each former township clinic or hospital was converted into a community health service center. Extant village clinics were abolished, while county governments established new health service stations or converted extant village clinics into health service stations. Each station has an outpatient room, treatment room, pharmacy, and transfusion room (for intravenous drips). Health service stations were located according to the "twenty-minute service circle," a distribution principle that ensured nobody would be more than twenty minutes away from a health service station by foot. Village doctors were incorporated into these health service stations, because unlike their "urban" counterparts in Jiang Village, they were not required to hold the assistant medical practitioner license. However, the majority had to leave the home-based clinics they had been operating from since the early 1980s because they were assigned to neighboring villages or even other townships. Instead of the twenty-four-hour service village doctors previously provided, they now work according to a strict timetable at the new community health service centers and stations. The regulations specify that these centers and stations must provide "six-in-one" services to villagers (now called rural residents), which encompass prevention, treatment, promotion of health and well-being, rehabilitation, health education, and family planning advice.

At the same time as this major restructuring of the rural medical system was going on, the National Basic Pharmaceutical Catalog (*guojia jiben yaowu mulu*) was put into effect. It regulated that rural community health services could prescribe 307 pharmaceuticals (205 types of Western medicines and 102 types of Chinese patent medicines). As economic conditions vary nationwide, local governments are authorized to complement the national catalog with extra pharmaceuticals. For example, Zhejiang Province added 150 types, while Hangzhou Prefecture added 50, bringing total of basic pharmaceuticals for some counties within Hangzhou Prefecture up to 507 types. These pharmaceuticals are supplied to health service centers through the collective bidding system, while health service centers implement zero-profit sales, in which there is no difference between the wholesale and retail prices.

Meanwhile, since the majority of current village doctors (*nongcun shequ yisheng*) will be retiring soon, each county government started training rural community doctors to fill these forthcoming vacancies in 2009. Senior middle school students who sat for the national college entrance examination were selected and sent to study clinical medicine for three years at Zhejiang Medical College and will be assigned to health service stations after graduation. Without any doubt, the barefoot doctors of the Cultural Revolution era will completely disappear from the medical world of China's villages in the near future.

Barefoot Doctors and Western Medicine

The social transformation of rural medicine in Jiang Village was a microcosm of the long-term historical development of Chinese and Western medicine in rural China since the early twentieth century, including a series of landmark events—the initiation of the experimental rural health programs in the 1930s, the founding of the Communist regime in 1949, the popularization of the barefoot doctor program in 1968, the disintegration of the barefoot doctor group around 1983, and the recent rural medical reform. This book has shown how Western medicine, as modern medicine, marginalized the Chinese medicine that had dominated the medical world of Chinese villages. It has argued that the barefoot doctor program, which lasted from 1968 to 1983, was a pivotal stage in the displacement of Chinese medicine by Western medicine in rural China.

When the debates between Chinese and Western medicine occurred in the late 1920s and early 1930s, Chinese medicine still enjoyed widespread practical legitimacy, although the state was reluctant to offer official support. Chinese medicine even had some therapeutic advantages over Western medicine, especially prior to the introduction of antibiotics. However, from the 1950s onward, Western medicine marched briskly into Chinese villages because of changes in knowledge transmission modes, the extension of pharmaceutical sales networks, and the decline in pharmaceutical prices. This process fundamentally changed villagers' medical beliefs and rural pharmaceutical consumption structures. Although Chinese medicine—that is, herbal medicine, acupuncture, and Chinese *materia medica*—was legitimized by the state, it lost practical acceptance among the villagers. This completely contrasts with its status in the first half of the twentieth century. The integration of Chinese and Western medicine widely promoted by the state after the mid-1950s and enhanced by the barefoot doctor program after 1968 was an asymmetrical process that was ultimately dominated by Western medicine. Simultaneously, with the decline of Chinese medicine in rural China, Chinese medicine underwent processes of standardization and urbanization. On the one hand, the state's support for Chinese medicine as a legitimate set of healing practices promoted the development of Chinese patent medicine through standardized production and consumption convenience, which was influenced by Western medicine. On the other hand, as Chinese medicine use was dwindling in the villages, it was gaining popularity among the cosmopolitan, urban middle class as a *Chinese* health-care method.[1] In contrast to this decline and transformation of Chinese medicine, Western medicine has reached new heights of market dominance. As this book has thoroughly analyzed, Western pharmaceuticals have been seriously overused since the advent of barefoot doctors in the early 1970s. Today, the overuse of Western medicine also includes that of medical technology. The most noticeable example of this is the high caesarean section rates that are becoming more and more obvious in rural China.

Medical institutionalization was the second key aspect of Western medicine's expansion into Chinese villages. As this book has demonstrated, after 1949, the Communist government established the state medical system by differentiating and reorganizing the extant plural medical systems, according to the Communist Party's political ideologies. These processes had dramatic impacts on the transformation of Chinese medicine in terms of notions of a medical community, hierarchical structures, and coordinated service delivery within formal institutional settings. This book has argued that the birth of the union clinics in the early 1950s was the first step toward medical institutionalization, cooperation, and stratification within the two-tier medical system. Later, through the barefoot doctor program and the associated cooperative medical service, a hierarchical and coordinated medical system was established, while a medical community of professionals with similar interests based in each commune was strengthened under the three-tier medical system. Correspondingly, medical encounters between villagers and doctors shifted from home bedsides to hospital wards. However, the institutionalization of rural medicine in China led to the three-tier medical system taking on the dumbbell-shaped structure identified throughout this volume. This transformation revealed that the barefoot doctors had certain advantages over the commune clinics in expanding Western medicine's reach through the medical community in the 1970s. More importantly, the process also indicated the embarrassment of Chinese medicine as represented by commune clinics. The dumbbell-shaped structure this book proposes also provided a new explanation for the so-called crisis of China's rural medical system in the postsocialist era. This book argues that the decline of township clinics started with the advent of the barefoot doctors in the early 1970s and continued into the 1980s because of more fierce competition from the latter. Meanwhile, there was a gradual implantation of modern hospitals and clinics in villages, from union clinics in the 1950s, cooperative medical stations in the 1970s, to health service stations in around 2008. Though very preliminary, these rural clinics and stations had the basic features of modern medical institutions, including division of expertise, internal layout, and institutional management.

Since the early twentieth century, the impact of Western medicine on Chinese medicine and its ensuing legitimacy crisis not only awakened the consciousness of Chinese medical practitioners but also initiated the state's attempts at professional management of Chinese medicine in the early twentieth century. This book has shown that this contestation of Chinese medicine by Western medicine continued at a more rapid pace after the formation of the People's Republic of China. From 1949 to the mid-1960s, the new government reeducated the medical practitioners of the "old society" in order to form a socialist medical profession, mainly through indoctrinating them with a new concept of medical ethics revolving around socialist ideological principles. The barefoot doctor group emerged as a political creation in this context. By the early 1980s, the state had secured the group identity of the barefoot doctors and enhanced their authority as medical providers. Their power relative to their patients was enhanced through a series of institutional arrangements, such as "inclusion" and "exclusion," demarcation from competitors, and the intentional waiver of responsibilities for medical malpractice. These were all largely positive developments for the barefoot doctor group in an enclosed village society, particularly in the early stages of the program. Paradoxically, while the barefoot doctors were drawn from among the villagers themselves, their experience of state-sponsored training and certification also paved the way for the subsequent redefinition of medical legitimacy in which medical proficiency was emphasized. This credential-based health world led to some barefoot doctors evolving into village doctors or assistant professional medical practitioners over the course of the 1980s and beyond. This process represented a special path toward the formation of a medical profession, initiated by a political campaign, developed in an enclosed village society, and strengthened through the professionals in question having survived profound social changes. The rise of barefoot doctor group was also a process of marginalization of Chinese medicine in Chinese villages.

Barefoot Doctors, the Socialist State, and Villagers

As this book has revealed, state power penetrated every aspect of rural medicine since 1949, including the mobilization of private medical practitioners into establishing union clinics, the implementation of the barefoot doctor program, the large-scale decrease in pharmaceutical prices, the establishment of a hierarchical and coordinated medical system, and the definitions of medical legitimacy. Within this context, Western medicine was introduced into Chinese villages under socialism in just three decades. The significance of the barefoot doctors lies in their role in the contestation between Chinese and Western medicine in the village arena, the evolution of the three-tier medical system, and the formation of a new professional group. In the meantime, as this book has shown, the development of rural medicine and health occurred in the context of the wide gap in medical resource distribution between rural and urban areas, even though political discourse insisted on "emphasizing rural areas." Therefore, the violation of political ideology and the use of state power occurred simultaneously. However, such contradictions were not unusual in the socialist state.

Entering the twenty-first century, the state still plays the leading role in the transformation of rural medicine. The recent medical reforms have made the dumbbell-shaped structure of the three-tier medical system disappear overnight, simply by ceasing the annual renewal of business licenses for village clinics and thus rendering any medical practice there illegal. As this book has argued, the barefoot doctor group evolved the whole medical system toward this dumbbell-shaped structure in the 1970s, a process which then continued throughout the 1980s, 1990s, and the first decade of the new millennium. Therefore, the recent medical reform represented a significant restructuring of the rural medical system. In the meantime, through the newly implemented National Pharmaceutical Catalog, the state aimed to control the practice of overprescribing to increase earnings (known as "supporting doctors by selling medicines") through policy design, though the outcomes of this are uncertain at the moment. Furthermore, just as the barefoot doctor program was initially promoted nationwide because of a single investigative report including Mao's comments in *The People's Daily*, the medical legitimacy of the barefoot doctors was equally rapidly and dramatically reversed in the medical reforms of 2008–10.

Though the recent rural medical reform radically changed the structure and operational features of the rural medical system that barefoot doctors had dominated since the early 1970s, the essence of this reform was still the same—the introduction of Western medicine (i.e., modern medicine) in terms of scientificization, institutionalization, and professionalization. The differences between the two eras lie in specific policies. The barefoot doctors who played pivotal roles in the introduction of Western medicine into villages since the early 1970s were not able to escape the general trend which led to their exclusion as a result of similar processes promoted by the state in the new century. To varying degrees, their roles and fates were similar to those of rural Chinese medicine doctors during the 1950s and 1960s, in that both declined because of a new system that required the study, dissemination, and practice of Western medicine.

However, the introduction of Western medicine into the villages was not only a top-down process dependent on the power of the state but also a bottom-up process of acceptance and adaptation. As Scheid argues, while political processes have been an important factor in these changes, they are by no means the only factor that shaped contemporary Chinese medicine. He argues that "grassroots pressure for a more modern Chinese medicine expressed locally by patients through such mechanisms as practitioner selection, demand for certain kinds of diagnosis or treatment, or simply through bringing to the clinical encounter certain kinds of problems cannot be ignored."[2] This book is a micro study of the barefoot doctors and the medical world of the Chinese villages that they dominated under socialism—as such, it is a history written from below. The choice of this methodology is significant at least in three aspects. First, this book places barefoot doctors within a very broad context of the social history of medicine in the twentieth century. The analysis of the medical world of Chinese villages before and after 1949 presented a picture that differed from those indicated in extant studies of history of Chinese medicine in late imperial China, which are basically examinations of elite society. Second, as a broad description based on local archives and personal interviews, it challenges the prevalent arguments that dominate current scholarship on medicine and health care in rural China in both the socialist and postsocialist eras. Third, the medical world of Chinese villages after 1949 began a thorough and radical social transformation that would bring Western medicine—as modern medicine—to even the most remote areas of the country with the gradual establishment of state medical system. The impact of Western medicine on village society was comprehensive, reflecting the features of socialist politics and Western medicine. Therefore, the village-centered study of the introduction of Western medicine into China indicates that this process followed a path different from those in other social settings, such as those spread via colonial medicine.

As the villagers experienced their health-care providers transforming from "old things" to "newly emerged things," they necessarily experienced a dramatic shift in their health worlds and underwent significant changes as citizens and patients. Their participation in public health campaigns fully reflected the features of body politics in socialist contexts, such as submitting stool samples in the morning and allowing doctors to take blood samples from their ears in the evening. The villagers quickly formed their own comparative medical beliefs about Chinese and Western pharmaceuticals, as a result of which Chinese medicine was soon relegated to a secondary position. Thanks to medical institutionalization, the scope of the villagers' medical encounters was greatly expanded and extended beyond their home village boundaries. The establishment of the state medical system and the formation of a socialist medical profession also diversified their relationship with doctors. The traditional practice of "doctors never knocking at the patients' doors" was first discarded when doctors were asked to deliver pills to the villagers' homes to oversee their consumption during various public health campaigns. With the advent of barefoot doctors, villagers enjoyed a relatively equal relationship with their medical service providers in the enclosed societies of their home villages. However, the advent of medical commercialization under the market economy not only brought more plentiful medical resources, it also worsened the doctor-patient relationship, leading to mutually negative images of each other.

In general, barefoot doctors, the socialist state, and villagers each played their own roles in the social transformation of rural medicine under socialism. Without any doubt, as the performers of state policies and medical service providers to villagers, the barefoot doctors played the most important roles in this transformation. They increased the speed of the irreversible global trend toward Western medicine and ensured that it reached down to even the most isolated villages in China. The foundations laid by the barefoot doctors in rural medical health—scientificization, medical institutionalization, and professionalization—are still the key themes of rural medicine in present-day China. Meanwhile, the recent radical medical reform has intended to tackle a few thorny challenges, including ending the abuse of pharmaceuticals, demolishing the dumbbell-shaped structure of medical system, and improving the proficiency of rural medical personnel. These main challenges are similar to those faced by modern medicine today throughout the world. Therefore, even the challenges that now face medicine in rural China—and will continue to confront it for the foreseeable future—are further evidence of the great transformation in rural health that was brought about in large part by the barefoot doctor program.

Appendix One

The Organization of the
Three-Tiered Medical System in
Rural China, 1968–83

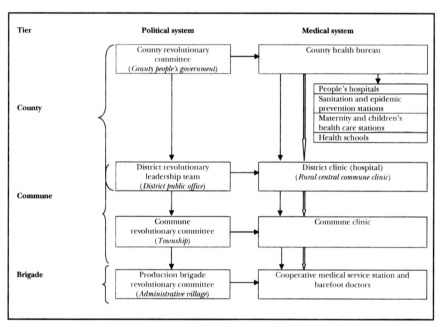

Notes: Terms in parentheses are those used after the political reforms of the early 1980s. Black arrows indicate a relationship of administrative authority (*xingzheng lingdao*), which affected policy, personnel, and budget. As each medical unit was under the dual leadership of the horizontal government systems and vertical medical systems, the administrative authority therefore included both political and medical administrative bodies and processes. The hollow arrows indicate a relationship of technical supervision (*yewu zhidao*) with the vertical medical system. Women barefoot doctors also undertook maternity and children's health care work.

Source: Yuhangxian weishengju weishengzhi bianzhuanzu, *Yuhangxian weishengzhi*, 79; Xu, *Fuyangxian weishengzhi*, 27–39; Lin'anxian weishengzhi bianzhuan weiyuanhui, *Lin'anxian weishengzhi*, 44; Chen, *Medicine in Rural China*, 152–53; Yip, *Health and National Reconstruction in Nationalist China*, 199.

Appendix Two

Common Medicines in Chinese Villages during the 1960s–70s

Part 1: Western Medicines

Name	Chinese name	Ingredients	Presentation/ doses	Clinical usage	Notes
1. Antibiotics					
Penicillin	青霉素		1. Penicillin G sodium injection: 0.2 million units, 0.4 million units, and 0.8 million units; 2. Penicillin G procaine injection: 0.4 million units and 0.8 million units.	Pyogenic streptococcal infections (such as scarlet fever, tonsillitis, erysipelas, and endocarditis), sensitive *Staphylococcus aureus* infections, pneumococcus infections, furuncles, and carbuncles.	Side effects include allergic reactions and shock.
Chloromycetin	氯霉素		50 mg, 0.25 g tablets, 0.125 g and 0.25 g injections	Typhoid, paratyphoid, urinary tract infections, bacillary dysentery, typhus, whooping cough, epidemic cerebrospinal meningitis, and other bacterial infections.	Side effects include nausea, vomiting, loss of appetite, and stomatitis; in some cases can cause skin rash; a large dosage could poison a newborn baby.
Syntomycin	合霉素		50 mg, 0.25 g tablets, and 0.25 g injection	Similar to Chloromycetin (see above).	Side effects are similar to those of Chloromycetin (see above).

(continued)

Name	Chinese name	Ingredients	Presentation/ doses	Clinical usage	Notes
Tetracycline	四环素		50 mg, 0.125 g, and 0.25 g tablets, 0.125 g, and 0.25 g injections	Urinary tract infections, hematosepsis, biliary tract infections, and bacillary dysentery caused by typhus fever, atypical pneumonia, and sensitive bacteria	Side effects include nausea, vomiting, discomfort in the upper abdomen, diarrhea, stomatitis, liver damage due to prolonged oral administration or large intravenous dosages; in children, delayed bone growth, limited tooth enamel growth, and yellow or decaying teeth.
Terramycin	土霉素		50 mg, 0.125 g, 0.25 g tablets, 0.1 g injections, 0.1 g and 0.25 g powder injections	Similar to tetracycline (see above), particularly good for enteric infection and amebic dysentery.	Side effects are similar to those of tetracycline (see above).

(continued)

Name	Chinese name	Ingredients	Presentation/ doses	Clinical usage	Notes
Streptomycin	链霉素		1.Streptomycin sulfate, 0.1 g tablet, 0.25 g and 0.5 g injections, 1 g and 2 g powder injections (to be diluted in saline or glucose solution) 2.Dihydrostreptomycin: 0.5 g, 1.0 g, and 2.0 g powder injections	Tuberculosis, urinary tract infections, enteric infections, bacillary meningitis, and whooping cough caused by Gram-negative bacilli. As above, for patients who are allergic to streptomycin sulfate.	Side effects include numbness, dizziness, aching around mouth and face, and tinnitus and deafness due to long-term use.
2. Sulfonamide drugs					
Sulfapyridine	磺胺嘧啶		0.5 g tablets, 0.4 g and 1g injections.	Infections caused by hemolytic Streptococcus, Staphylococcus, Neisseria meningitides, Streptococcus pneumonia, gonococcus, Escherichia coli, bacillus dysenteriae, and trachoma virus.	Side effects include headache, dizziness, loss of appetite, nausea, vomiting, and decline of white blood cells, etc.
Children's Sulfadimidine powder	小儿安	0.15 g Sulfadimidine, 0.1 g sulfaguanidine, and 0.1 g sodium bicarbonate	Powder	Upper respiratory tract infection, enteritis, otitis, and conjunctivitis.	
Sulphaguanidine	磺胺脒		0.5 g tablets	Bacillary dysentery and enteritis.	

(continued)

Name	Chinese name	Ingredients	Presentation/ doses	Clinical usage	Notes
Antidysentery tablets	止痢片	sulfaguanidine	0.5 g tablets	Bacillary dysentery and enteritis.	
Anti-inflammatory tablets	消炎片	sulfonamide antibacterial drug	Tablets		
3. Antipyretic and analgesic drugs					
Fever-reducing painkillers	解热止痛片		Tablets	Antipyretic and analgesic drug	
Fever-reducing and pain-relieving powder	解热止痛散		Powder	Antipyretic and analgesic drug	
Analgin	安乃近片		0.5 g tablets	High fever, headaches, influenza, muscle pain, toothache, joint pain, menstrual pain, and rheumatic arthritis.	Side effects include drug rash, allergic purpura, exfoliative dermatitis, and decline of white blood cells.
Antondin	安痛定		Tablets	Nonsteroidal anti-inflammatory, analgesic, and antipyretic. For headaches, fever, joint pain, menstrual pain, and neuropathic pain.	

(continued)

Name	Chinese name	Ingredients	Presentation/ doses	Clinical usage	Notes
Painkiller tablets	去痛片	0.15 g amidopyrine and 0.15 g phenacetin per tablet	Tablets	Antipyretic and analgesic drug.	Large dosages cause exhaustion, sweating, and facial pallor; sometimes causes nausea, vomiting, and the decline of white blood cell count.
Children's fever-reducing tablets	小儿退热片	0.0567 g aspirin and 0.041 g phenacetin per tablet	Tablets		
4. Stomach drugs					
Gastropin tablets	胃舒平片		Tablets	Hyperchlorhydria, gastric ulcers, and gastric diseases.	
Sodium bicarbonate tablets	小苏打片		Tablets	Stomachache caused by hyperchlorhydria.	
5. Antiparasitic drugs					
Antimalarial tablets	止疟片	Chloroquine	Tablets	Treatment or prevention of malaria.	
Ascarid-repelling tablets	驱蛔灵片	Piperazine citrate	0.5g tablets	Ascariasis	Sometimes causes nausea, vomiting, dizziness, and abdominal pain.

(continued)

Name	Chinese name	Ingredients	Presentation/ doses	Clinical usage	Notes
Precious Pagoda Lozenges	宝塔糖	Purified from Santonica wormseed.	tablets	To expel or destroy parasitic intestinal worms.	Listed as Western medicine; the most popular over-the-counter anthelmintic in the 1950s–1970s. Originally sold in tablet form, sugar was added to help children take it. The tablets' pale yellow and pink conical shape gave rise to the name "Precious Pagoda Lozenges" or "Pagoda Candy." After the early 1980s, this type of lozenge gradually disappeared and was replaced by one containing trochisci piperazini phosphatis.

(continued)

Name	Chinese name	Ingredients	Presentation/ doses	Clinical usage	Notes
6. Drugs for surgical and topical uses					
Gentian violet	紫药水			Common mucocutaneous disinfectant.	
Iodine	碘酒			Antiseptic disinfectant for surgery and topical applications.	
Mercurochrome solution	红药水			Sterilization, disinfection, and antisepsis, etc.	
Paste for chilblains	冻疮膏			Chilblains	
Paste for sores	疮药膏			Various skin ulcers	
Beriberi-clearing liquid	脚气水			To treat beriberi, the disease caused by vitamin B1 deficiency, which is endemic in eastern and southern Asian countries.	
Anti-itch lotion	癣药水	6 g salicylic acid, 12 g benzoic acid and 100 ml alcohol		To diminish inflammation, disinfect and relieve itching; for tinea corporis and tinea manus and pedis.	Dermatological medicine
Toothache drops	牙痛水	Camphor, clove oil, and chloral hydrate.		Toothache	

(continued)

Name	Chinese name	Ingredients	Presentation/doses	Clinical usage	Notes
7. Respiratory drugs					
Children's cough syrup	小儿止咳糖浆	ephedrine, ammonium chloride, phenobarbital, licorice, platycodon root, fritillary, and almond	Bottles of syrup	Coughing in children	
Cough relief tablets	止咳片		Tablets	Coughing	Listed as Western medicine, several brands
Ephedrine tablets	麻黄素片		Tablets	Bronchial asthma, anaphylactoid reactions, and hypotension.	Listed as Western medicine
8. Ophthalmologic drugs					
Chlortetracycline eye ointment	金霉素眼膏		2 g tins	Bacterial conjunctivitis, viral conjunctivitis, and trachoma.	
Eye drops	眼药水	Chloromycetin		Bacterial conjunctivitis, viral conjunctivitis, and trachoma.	Many brands available.
		Cortisone acetate		Allergic conjunctivitis and nonulcer keratitis.	

Part 2: Chinese Herbal Medicines

Latin name	English name	Chinese name	Clinical use
Andrographis paniculata	Herba Andrographitis	穿心莲 *chuanxinlian*	Infections of the respiratory, digestive, and urinary tracts, and purulent infections.
Herba Senecionis Scandentis	Climbing groundsel herb	千里光 *qianliguang*	Various inflammations, such as bacillary dysentery, enteritis, acute appendicitis, acute conjunctivitis, and sore throats.
Codonopsis pilosula	Radix Codonopsis Pilosulae	党参 *dangshen*	To reinforce and invigorate the function of the spleen and lungs.
Rhizoma Coptidis	Coptis Root	黄连 *huanglian*	To drain dampness and relieve toxicity, such as high fever, irritability, disorientation, delirium, sore throats, boils, carbuncles, and abscesses.
Semen Crotonis Pulveratum	Croton Seed Powder	巴豆霜 *badoushuang*	Highly toxic; for abdominal pain and constipation, convulsions, profuse sputum, and edema.
Solidago Virgaaurea Linn	Goldenrod	一枝黄花 *yizhihuanghua*	Sore throats, tonsillitis, snake bites, influenza, and bleeding from knife wounds.
Radix Glycyrrhizae	Liquorice root	甘草 *gancao*	Spleen and stomach deficiency, sores and boils, coughs caused by bronchitis and inflammation of the upper respiratory tract, and spasmodic abdominal pain.
Flos Lonicerae	Honeysuckle flowers	金银花 *jinyinhua*	Carbuncles, erysipelas, pharyngitis, acute dysentery, infection of the upper respiratory tract, and epidemic febrile diseases.
Herba Menthae	Mint	薄荷 *bohe*	To dispel heat and toxins, such as influenza, fever, headache, sore throat, and aphtha.
Paris polyphylla smith	Rhizoma paridis	七叶一枝花 *qiyeyizhihua*	To clear away heat and toxic matter and soothe swelling.
Plantago asiatica	Chinese plantain	车前草 *cheqiancao*	For nephritis, edema, and acute urinary tract infections, etc.

Part 3: Chinese Patent Medicines

Name	Chinese name	Ingredients	Clinical use
Berberine tablets	黄连素片 *huangliansu pian*	Purified from the Chinese herb *Rhizoma coptidis* (coptis root, *huanglian*).	Acute gastroenteritis, dysentery, and eye infection.
Cooling ointments (or Tiger Balm)	清凉油 *qingliangyou*	Menthol, peppermint oil, camphorated oil, camphor, and eucalyptus oil.	Insect bites and stings, headaches caused by heatstroke and for colds, dizziness, and carsickness, etc.
Human Elixir	人丹 *rendan*	Menthol, borneol, cloves, catechu, and fennel.	Sunstroke and heatstroke, dizziness and vomiting, travel sickness.
Shidishui tincture	十滴水 *shidishui*	Camphor, dried ginger, and *Rheum officinale.*	Dizziness, nausea, and stomachaches caused by heatstroke.
Cow bezoar antidotal tablets	牛黄解毒片 *niuhuang jiedupian*	Cow bezoar, Rabiagar, gypsum fibrosum, *Rheum officinale, Scutellaria baicalensis,* and platycodon root.	To dispel heat and toxins, such as flu, sore throats, and pulmonary infections.
Fructus forsythiae antidotal tablets	银翘解毒片 *yinqiao jiedupian*	Honeysuckle flower, *Fructus Forsythiae, Radix Isatidis,* platycodon root, liquorice root, and menthol.	Colds, fevers, and sore throats.

Source: Hangzhou yiyao shangyezhi bianzhuan weiyuanhui, *Hangzhou yiyao shangyezhi,* 126–27; Fuyangxian weishengju, fuyangxian shangyeju, fuyangxian gongxiaohezuoshe [Fuyang County Health Bureau, Fuyang County Commerce Bureau, Fuyang County Supply and Marketing Cooperative], "Nongcun gongxiao hezuoshe hezuo shangdian hezuo xiaozu jianying chengyao cankao mulu" [Reference List of Pharmaceuticals Sold at Rural Supply and Marketing Cooperatives, Cooperative Stores, and Cooperative Teams], February 27, 1963, FYA, vol. 74-1-13; Zhejiangsheng geweihui shengchan zhihuizu weishengju, *Zhejiang minjian changyong caoyao,* vol.1; Chuanshaxian jiangzhen gongshe chijiao yisheng, *Chijiao yisheng changyong yaowu;* Beijing yixueyuan yingu jiaoyanshi hanying changyong yixue cihui bianxiezu [Editorial team of Chinese-English common medical vocabularies of Beijing Medical College English teaching and research], ed., *Hanying changyong yixue cihui* [Chinese-English common medical vocabularies] (Beijing: Renmin weisheng chubanshe, 1982); Cochran, *Chinese Medicine Men,* 44–51; *Cihai (xiudinggao)/ yiyao weisheng fence* [Unabridged comprehensive dictionary (revised edition): Medicine, pharmaceutical and health] (Shanghai: Shanghai cishu chubanshe, 1978).

Abbreviations

Archives:

CAA	Chun'an County Archives, Zhejiang Province
FYA	Fuyang City Archives, Zhejiang Province
HZA	Hangzhou Prefecture Archives, Zhejiang Province
JDA	Jiande City Archives, Zhejiang Province
JSA	Jiangsu Province Archives, Jiangsu Province
LAA	Lin'an City Archives, Zhejiang Province
PDA	Pudong New District Archives, Shanghai Municipality
RAC	Rockefeller Archival Centre, USA
SDA	Sandun Township Integrated Chinese and Western Medicine Hospital, Hangzhou City, Zhejiang Province
SHA	Shanghai Municipal Archives, Shanghai Municipality
SXA	Shaoxing Prefecture Archives, Zhejiang Province
XSA	Xiaoshan District Archives, Hangzhou City, Zhejiang Province
YHA	Yuhang District Archives, Hangzhou City, Zhejiang Province
ZJA	Zhejiang Province Archives, Zhejiang Province

Newspapers:

HZRB	*Hangzhou ribao*	[Hangzhou Daily]
RMRB	*Renmin ribao*	[People's Daily]
ZJRB	*Zhejiang ribao*	[Zhejiang Daily]

Measurements:

1 *mu* = 666.66 square meters
1 *jin* = 500 grams

Glossary

Ah Bao xiansheng	阿宝先生
Autumn-Snow Temple	秋雪庵
Baicaoyuan	百草园
Bannong banyi	半农半医
Baojian Village	包建村
Beizhan, beihuang, weirenmin	备战、备荒、为人民
Biwendan	避瘟丹
Buwei liangxiang, bianwei liangyi	不为良相，便为良医
Caocao bangbang	草草棒棒
Changxing County	长兴县
Chanpo	产婆
Chaxu yiliao wangluo geju	差序医疗网络格局
Chi dashitang	吃大食堂
Chijiao	赤脚
Chijiao yisheng	赤脚医生
Chijiao yisheng chuanxielun	赤脚医生穿鞋论
Chuansha County	川沙县
Chugong	出工
Chun'an County	淳安县
Chunmiao	《春苗》
Dan'ganfeng	单干风
Dashu	大暑
Dengyunwei Village	登云圩村
Diaoping senlin	吊瓶森林
Duangen	断根
Duilai duiqu	队来队去
Fenpian baogan	分片包干
Fuyang County	富阳县
Gongfei yiliao	公费医疗
Gongfen	工分
Gongsi heying	公私合营
Guojia jiben yaowu mulu	国家基本药物目录
Guolu langzhong	过路郎中
Guoyaodian	国药店
Guoyi	国医
Hang County	杭县

Hangzhou Prefecture	杭州市
Hejian Village	合建村
Hezuo yiliao	合作医疗
Hongbao	红暴
Hongyu	《红雨》
Hongyu	红雨
Hujizhi	户籍制
Huopusa	活菩萨
Jiande County	建德县
Jiang Village	蒋村
Jianghu youyi	江湖游医
Jiao	角
Jieshengpo	接生婆
Jihua mianyi	计划免疫
Jin	斤
Jingzhe	经折
Jinpingmei	金瓶梅
Jiushiwu	旧事物
Jiuyi	旧医
Langzhong	郎中
Lao sanjian	老三件
Laobao yiliao	劳保医疗
Laozhongyi	老中医
Liangguan wugai	两管五改
Liangtiaotui zoulu	两条腿走路
Lianhe zhensuo	联合诊所
Lianzong	联总
Lin'an County	临安县
Lingling yi dabao, jianjian yi daguo, hehe yi dawan	拎拎一大包，煎煎一大锅，喝喝一大碗
Lingyin Temple	灵隐寺
Liqiu	立秋
Longzhang Village	龙章村
Luojiazhuang Village	骆家庄村
Maijue	脉诀
Miaoshou huichun	妙手回春
Minglaozhongyi	名老中医
Miwan	蜜丸
Nongcun shequ yisheng	农村社区医生
Nongcun weisheng yitihua guanli	农村卫生一体化管理
Nongzhuanju	农转居
Peiban	陪伴
Pideng fanji youqing fan'anfeng	批邓反击右倾翻案风

Pidou	批斗
Sanshen Village	三深村
Santu sizi	三土四自
Shangban	上班
Shayao	痧药
Shehui kaiyeyi	社会开业医
Shehui yiwu gongzuozhe	社会医务工作者
Shejue	舌诀
Shentankou Village	深潭口村
Shuanglong Village	双龙村
Shuangqiang	双抢
Shuiwan	水丸
Shuozui langzhong	说嘴郎中
Sibing	四病
Sifen huozhi	死分活值
Songyao shangmen, kanyao luodu	送药上门，看药落肚
Tangtouge	汤头歌
Temple of Lord Jiang	蒋公庙
Tian Chunmiao	田春苗
Tianjia Temple	田家庵
Tiji liaofa	剃剂疗法
Tinghua	听话
Tonghang shi yuanjia	同行是冤家
Tonglu County	桐庐县
Toutong xun lieque, yatong hegushou, dufu sanli liu, yaobei weizhong qiu	头痛寻列缺，牙痛合谷收，肚腹三里留，腰背委中求
Tuanjie zhongxiyi	团结中西医
Wang, chu, kou, ting	望、触、扣、听
Wang, wen, wen, qie	望、闻、问、切
Wangjiaqiao Village	王家桥村
Weishengyuan	卫生员
Western City Hospital	城西医院
Wugong	误工
Wulian Village	五联村
Wupo	巫婆
Xiafang	下放
Xiang	乡
Xiangcun yisheng	乡村医生
Xianyan houtang, xiankuai houman, jianniao bujia, ningqian wuguo	先盐后糖、先快后慢、见尿补钾、宁欠勿过
Xiaoshan County	萧山县
Xihu District	西湖区
Xingjunsan	行军散

Xingzheng lingdao	行政领导
Xinsheng shiwu	新生事物
Xinyi	新医
Xinzhen liaofa	新针疗法
Xiucai xueyi, longzhong zhuoji	秀才学医，笼中捉鸡
Xixi National Wetland Park	西溪国家湿地公园
Xiyao lai de kuai, zhongyao lai de man	西药来得快，中药来得慢
Xiyao zhibiao, zhongyao zhiben	西药治标，中药治本
Xiyi xiyao	西医西药
Yangjiadai Village	杨家埭村
Yangyao	洋药
Yanmin hupan	《雁鸣湖畔》
Yaoxingfu	药性赋
Yewu zhidao	业务指导
Yi	医
Yibu sanshi, bufu qiyao	医不三世，不服其药
Yigen yinzhen, yiba caoyao	一根银针、一把草药
Yiliao wangluo chaxu geju	医疗网络差序格局
Yinchen	茵陈
Yinhetang	殷和堂
Yinpian	饮片
Yisheng jinzai yanmianqian, yiyuan banzai dui libian	医生近在眼面前，医院办在队里边
Yisheng jiti suoyouzhi	医生集体所有制
Yishi	医士
Yiwugong	义务工
Yiyao heyi	医药合一
Yiyao yangyi	以药养医
Yuanjue Temple	圆觉庙
Yuhang County	余杭县
Zhiye zhuli yishi	执业助理医师
Zhiye zhuli yishi zigezheng	执业助理医师资格证
Zhongcaoyao yundong	中草药运动
Zhongyang qingtu	重洋轻土
Zhongyao	中药
Zhongyi	中医
Zhoujia Village	周家村
Zhulinsi	竹林寺
Zibenzhuyi weiba	资本主义尾巴
Zuotangyi	坐堂医

Notes

Introduction

1. Ralph Croizier, *Traditional Medicine in Modern China: Science, Nationalism, and the Tensions of Cultural Change* (Cambridge, MA: Harvard University Press, 1968), 2.

2. Ibid., 229.

3. "Cong 'chijiao yisheng' de chengzhang kan yixue jiaoyu geming de fangxiang: Shanghaishi de diaocha baogao" [Fostering a revolution in medical education through the growth of the barefoot doctors: An investigative report from Shanghai municipality], *RMRB*, September 14, 1968. This article first appeared in *Hongqi* [Red Flag] on September 10, 1968.

4. "Shenshou pinxia zhongnong huanying de hezuo yiliao" [Cooperative medical service warmly welcomed by poor and lower-middle peasants], *RMRB*, December 5, 1968.

5. Victor W. Sidel, "The Barefoot Doctors of the People's Republic of China," *New England Journal of Medicine* 286, no. 24 (1972): 1292–1300; World Bank, *China: Long-Term Issues and Options in the Health Transition* (Washington, DC: The World Bank, 1992), 18.

6. In this vein, Judith Farquhar writes of the "apple-cheeked" images of women barefoot doctors. See Judith Farquhar, "Market Magic: Getting Rich and Getting Personal in Medicine after Mao," *American Ethnologist* 23, no. 2 (May 1996): 252.

7. There have been numerous studies and accounts of barefoot doctor programs. In her ethnographically based case study of Tiger Springs Village, Sydney D. White assessed the merits of these works, which she grouped into three waves: 1969 to 1978, the early 1980s to mid-1980s, and the late 1980s to late 1990s. See Sydney D. White, "From Barefoot Doctors to Village Doctor in Tiger Springs Village: A Case Study of Rural Health Care Transformations in Socialist China," *Human Organization* 57, no. 4 (Winter 1998): 480–90.

8. Peter Worsley points out that the World Health Assembly passed a resolution in 1976 requesting that member states take steps to develop primary health-care programs. He argues that the major stimuli for this change in orientation included the enormous publicity given in the West to Chinese acupuncture, the traditional pharmacopoeia used by the barefoot doctors, and the system of primary health care that centered on them. See Peter Worsley, "Non-Western Medical Systems," *Annual Review of Anthropology* 11, no. 1 (1982): 340; and World Health Organization and the United Nations Children's Fund, "Primary Health Care: A Joint Report by the Director-General of the World Health Organization and the Executive Director of the United Nations Children's Fund," International Conference on Primary Health Care, Alma-Ata, USSR, September 1978.

9. For the latest research, see Yang Nianqun, "The Memory of Barefoot Doctor System," in *Governance of Life in Chinese Moral Experience: The Quest for an Adequate Life,*

ed. Everett Zhang, Arthur Kleinman, and Tu Weiming (London: Routledge, 2011), 131–45; Jane Duckett, *The Chinese State's Retreat from Health: Policy and the Politics of Retrenchment* (Abingdon, UK: Routledge, 2010), 6–7; Arthur Kleinman and James L. Watson, "SARS in Social and Historical Context," in *SARS in China: Prelude to Pandemic?* ed. Arthur Kleinman and James L. Watson (Stanford, CA: Stanford University Press, 2006), 1–16; David Blumenthal and William Hsiao, "Privatization and Its Discontents—The Evolving Chinese Health Care System," *New England Journal of Medicine* 353, no. 11 (September 2005): 1165–69; Liu Yuanli, "China's Public Health-Care System: Facing the Challenges," *Bulletin of the World Health Organization* 82, no. 7 (July 2004): 532–38; and Wang Shaoguang, "Zhongguo gonggong weisheng de weiji yu zhuanji" [China's public health: Crisis and opportunity], *Bijiao* [Comparative Studies] 7 (2003): 52–88.

10. Since 2002 Chinese scholars have been making pioneering studies of the rise, development, and decline of the barefoot doctor program. For a summary of recent literature, see Li Decheng, "Chijiao yisheng yanjiu shuping" [Comments on the studies of barefoot doctors], *Zhongguo weisheng chuji baojian* [Chinese Primary Health Care] 21, no. 1 (January 2007): 6–8. The initiation of the experimental New Rural Cooperative Medical Service in 2003 has given rise to economic and policy studies of the new scheme in both Chinese and English literatures, which usually included accounts of the barefoot doctor program during the 1970s as historical background. Similar descriptions also appeared in media discussions on current rural health. For the latest and most representative research, see "Missing the Barefoot Doctors," *Economist* 385, no. 8550 (October 13, 2007): 27–30; Sascha Klotzbucher, Peter Lässig, Qin Jiangmei, and Susanne Weigelin-Schwiedrzik, "What's New in the 'New Rural Co-Operative Medical System'? An Assessment in One Kazak County of the Xinjiang Uyghur Autonomous Region," *China Quarterly* 201 (March 2010): 38–57; and Wang Shaoguang, "Xuexi jizhi yu shiying nengli: Zhongguo nongcun hezuo yiliao tizhi bianqian de qishi" [Learning and adapting: The case of rural health-care financing in China], *Zhongguo shehui kexue* [Social Sciences in China] 6 (2008): 111–33.

11. Henry E. Sigerist, "The Social History of Medicine," paper presented to the California Academy of Medicine in San Francisco, March 11, 1940, in *Henry E. Sigerist on the History of Medicine*, ed. Felix Marti-Ibanez (New York: MD Publications, 1960), 25–33.

12. Nathan Sivin, "Science and Medicine in Chinese History," in *Heritage of China: Contemporary Perspectives on Chinese Civilization*, ed. Paul S. Ropp (Berkeley: University of California Press, 1990), 182. See also Francesca Bray, "Chinese Medicine," in *Companion Encyclopedia of the History of Medicine*, ed. W. F. Bynum and Roy Porter, vol. 1 (London: Routledge, 1993), 730.

13. Bray, "Chinese Medicine," 744; Bridie Andrews, "The Making of Modern Chinese Medicine, 1895–1937" (PhD diss., University of Cambridge, 1996), 258.

14. Yi-li Wu, "The Bamboo Grove Monastery and Popular Gynecology in Qing China," *Late Imperial China* 21, no. 1 (June 2000): 41.

15. Volker Scheid, *Currents of Tradition in Chinese Medicine, 1626–2006* (Seattle, WA: Eastland Press, 2007), 56, 101, 258.

16. Yi-li Wu, *Reproducing Women: Medicine, Metaphor, and Childbirth in Late Imperial China* (Berkeley: University of California Press, 2010), 16; Bray, "Chinese Medicine," 744; and Andrews, "Making of Modern Chinese Medicine," 258.

17. Charlotte Furth, *A Flourishing Yin: Gender in China's Medical History, 960–1665* (Berkeley: University of California Press, 1999), 266–300.

18. Bray, "Chinese Medicine," 744; Francesca Bray, *Technology and Gender: Fabrics of Power in Late Imperial China* (Berkeley: University of California Press, 1997), 310; Paul Unschuld, *Medical Ethics in Imperial China* (Berkeley: University of California Press, 1979), 73; Linda L. Barnes, *Needles, Herbs, Gods and Ghost: China, Healing and the West to 1848* (Cambridge, MA: Harvard University Press, 2005), 244; and Wu Lien-Teh, *Plague Fighter: The Autobiography of a Modern Chinese Physician* (Cambridge, UK: W. Heffer & Sons, 1959), 578.

19. Joanna Grant, *A Chinese Physician: Wang Ji and the "Stone Mountain Medical Histories"* (New York: Routledge Curzon, 2003), 91.

20. Sean Hsiang-lin Lei, "Fu zeren de yisheng yu you xinyang de bingren: Zhongxiyi lunzheng yu yibing guanxi zai minguo shiqi de zhuanbian" [Accountable doctor and loyal patient: Transformation of doctor-patient relationships in the Republican Period], *Xinshixue* [New History] 14, no. 1 (March 2003): 45–96.

21. Furth, *Flourishing Yin*, 224–65.

22. Grant, *Chinese Physician*, 87.

23. Sean Hsiang-lin Lei, "When Chinese Medicine Encountered the State, 1928–1937," accessed June 30, 2009, http://www.ihp.sinica.edu.tw/~medicine/active/years/hl.PDF, 14.

24. Warwick Anderson argued that "delimited historical and anthropological studies of traditional Chinese medicine, in elite and vernacular forms, abound." See Warwick Anderson, "Biomedicine in Chinese East Asia: From Semicolonial to Postcolonial?" in Leung and Furth, *Health and Hygiene in Chinese East Asia*, 274.

25. Kim Taylor argues that acupuncture and herbal medicine fitted well with the growing perception of the limitations and harmfulness of Western science (and medicine) in the West in postwar and postmodern society. See Kim Taylor, "Divergent Interests and Cultivated Misunderstanding: The Influence of the West on Modern Chinese Medicine," *Social History of Medicine* 17, no. 1 (2004): 95. For Chinese medicine in developing countries during the 1970s, particularly Africa, see Stacy Langwick, "From Non-Aligned Medicines to Market-Based Herbals: China's Relationship to the Shifting Politics of Traditional Medicine in Tanzania," *Medical Anthropology* 29, no. 3 (2010): 20–21.

26. Arthur Kleinman, *Patients and Healers in the Context of Culture: An Exploration of the Borderland between Anthropology, Medicine, and Psychiatry* (Berkeley: University of California Press, 1980), 24.

27. Ibid., 26.

28. However, Wu Lien-Teh argued that the precise origins of the Chinese terms meaning "Chinese medicine" (*zhongyi*) and "Western medicine" (*xiyi*) are rather obscure. He attributed them to the early nineteenth-century introduction of vaccination into south China. See Wu Lien-Teh, "A Hundred Years of Modern Medicine in China," *Chinese Medical Journal* 50, no. 2 (February 1936): 152.

29. Kim Taylor, *Chinese Medicine in Early Communist China, 1945–1963: A Medicine of Revolution* (New York: Routledge Curzon, 2005), 79.

30. Ibid.

31. Ibid., 84.

32. Volker Scheid, *Chinese Medicine in Contemporary China: Plurality and Synthesis* (Durham, NC: Duke University Press, 2002), 3.

33. Paul Unschuld, *Medicine in China: A History of Ideas* (Berkeley: University of California Press, 1985), 5.

34. Andrew Cunningham and Bridie Andrews, *Western Medicine as Contested Knowledge* (Manchester: Manchester University Press, 1997), 14.

35. Croizier, *Traditional Medicine in Modern China*, 234.

36. Unschuld, *Medicine in China: A History of Ideas*, 247.

37. Taylor, *Chinese Medicine in Early Communist China*, 30–31.

38. Ibid., 12.

39. Ibid., 147. See also Scheid, *Chinese Medicine in Contemporary China*, 65.

40. C. C. Chen, *Medicine in Rural China: A Personal Account* (Berkeley: University of California Press, 1989), 147.

41. Sydney D. White, "Deciphering 'Integrated Chinese and Western Medicine' in the Rural Lijiang Basin: State Policy and Local Practice(s) in Socialist China," *Social Science & Medicine* 49, no. 10 (1999): 1333–47.

42. Stella R. Quah and Li Jingwei, "Marriage of Convenience: Traditional and Modern Medicine in the People's Republic of China," in *The Triumph of Practicality: Tradition and Modernity in Health Care Utilization in Selected Asian Counters*, ed. Stella R. Quah (Singapore: Social Issues in Southeast Asia, Institute of Southeast Asia, 1989), 19–42.

43. Ibid., 5–6.

44. World Health Organization, *The Promotion and Development of Traditional Medicine: Report* (Geneva: World Health Organization, 1978), 18.

45. Unschuld, *Medical Ethics in Imperial China*, 4.

46. Asaf Goldschmidt, *The Evolution of Chinese Medicine: Song Dynasty, 960–1200* (Abingdon, UK: Routledge, 2008), 5–6; Scheid, *Currents of Tradition in Chinese Medicine*, 37; and Benjamin Elman, *A Cultural History of Modern Science in China* (Cambridge, MA: Harvard University Press, 2006), 209.

47. Ralph Croizier, "Medicine and Modernization in China: An Historical Overview," in *Medicine in Chinese Culture: Comparative Studies of Health Care in Chinese and Other Societies*, ed. Arthur Kleinman, Peter Kunstadter, E. Russell Alexander, and James L. Gale (Bethesda, MD: National Institutes of Health, 1975), 25.

48. Milton J. Lewis and Kerrie L. MacPherson, *Public Health in Asia and the Practice: Historical and Comparative Perspectives* (London, New York: Routledge, 2008), 5; and Carol Benedict, "Policing the Sick: Plague and the Origin of State Medicine in Late Imperial China," *Late Imperial China* 14, no. 2 (December 1993): 73.

49. Andrews, "Making of Modern Chinese Medicine," 50.

50. An Elissa Lucas, "Changing Medical Models in China: Organizational Options or Obstacles?" *China Quarterly* 83 (September 1980): 479; C. C. Chen, *Medicine in Rural China*, 423; and Yip Ka-Che, *Health and National Reconstruction in Nationalist China: The Development of Modern Health Services, 1928–1937* (Ann Arbor, MI: Association for Asian Studies, 1995), 76–77.

51. An Elissa Lucas, *Chinese Medical Modernization: Comparative Policy Continuities, 1930s–1980s* (New York, NY: Praeger, 1982). See also Yip, *Health and National Reconstruction in Nationalist China*, 6.

52. Lucas, "Changing Medical Models in China," 471–72.

53. Ibid., 461–89.

54. David Lampton, "Performance and the Chinese Political System: A Preliminary Assessment of Education and Health Policies," *China Quarterly* 75 (September 1978): 509–39; Mark G. Field, "Health and the Polity: Communist China and Soviet Russia," *Studies in Comparative Communism* 7, no. 4 (Winter 1974): 420–25; and Michel Oksenberg, "The Chinese Policy Process and the Public Health Issue: An Arena Approach," *Studies in Comparative Communism* 7, no. 4 (Winter 1974): 375–408.

55. David Lampton, *The Politics of Medicine in China: The Policy Process, 1949–1977* (Boulder, CO: Westview, 1977).

56. Kleinman, *Patients and Healers in the Context of Culture*, 49–50. Other scholars classify healers differently. For example, Stella Quah offers the following categories: Western biomedicine, traditional medicine, and popular medicine. See Stella Quah, "Health and Culture," in *The Blackwell Companion to Medical Sociology*, ed. William C. Cockerham (Oxford: Blackwell, 2001), 35.

57. Kleinman, *Patients and Healers in the Context of Culture*, 53.

58. Ibid., 59.

59. Ibid., 50.

60. For the state of the field of scholarship on medical pluralism in the history of Chinese medicine, see T. J. Hinrichs, "New Geographies of Chinese Medicine," in *Osiris*, 2nd ser., vol. 13, *Beyond Joseph Needham: Science, Technology, and Medicine in East and Southeast Asia*, ed. Morris F. Low (Chicago: University of Chicago Press, 1998), 287–325.

61. Christopher Cullen, "Patients and Healers in Late Imperial China: Evidence from the *Jinpingmei*," *History of Science* 31, no. 2 (June 1993): 99–150.

62. Elisabeth Hsu, *The Transmission of Chinese Medicine* (Cambridge: Cambridge University Press, 1999), 8–13.

63. Sydney D. White, "Medicines and Modernities in Socialist China: Medical Pluralism, the State, and Naxi Identities in the Lijiang Basin," in *Healing Powers and Modernity: Traditional Medicine, Shamanism, and Science in Asian Societies*, ed. Linda H. Connor and Geoffrey Samuel (Westport, CT: Bergin & Garvey, 2000), 172.

64. Yüan-ling Chao, *Medicine and Society in Late Imperial China: A Study of Physicians in Suzhou, 1600–1850* (New York: Peter Lang, 2009), 170.

65. Marta Hanson, "Inventing a Tradition in Chinese Medicine: From Universal Canon to Local Medical Knowledge in South China, the Seventeenth to the Nineteenth Century" (PhD diss., University of Pennsylvania, 1997), 1.

66. Yuet-Wah Cheung, *Missionary Medicine in China: A Study of Two Canadian Protestant Missions in China before 1937* (Lanham, ND: University of America Press, 1988), 73.

67. Zhao Hongjun, "Chinese versus Western Medicine: A History of Their Relations in the Twentieth Century," *Chinese Science* 10 (December 1991): 22.

68. Croizier, *Traditional Medicine in Modern China*, 40.

69. Zhao, "Chinese versus Western Medicine," 22.

70. Cheung, *Missionary Medicine in China*, 77; and M. Cristina Zaccarini, "Modern Medicine in Twentieth-Century Jiangxi, Anhui, Fujian and Sichuan: Competition, Negotiation and Cooperation," *Social History of Medicine* 23, no. 2 (2010): 343.

71. Kerrie L. MacPherson, *A Wilderness of Marshes: The Origins of Public Health in Shanghai, 1843–1893* (Hong Kong: Oxford University Press, 1987), 11; and Benjamin Elman, *On Their Own Terms: Science in China, 1550–1900* (Cambridge, MA: Harvard University Press, 2005), 406.

72. Edward Shorter, "The History of the Doctor-Patient Relationship," in *Companion Encyclopedia of the History of Medicine*, ed. W. F. Bynum and Roy Porter, vol. 2 (London, New York: Routledge, 1993), 789; and Paul Unschuld, *Medicine in China: Historical Artifacts and Images* (Munich: Prestel Verlag, 2000), 16.

73. Charles Rosenberg, *The Care of Strangers: the Rise of America's Hospital System* (New York: Basic Books, 1987), 342.

74. Andrews, "Making of Modern Chinese Medicine," 281.

75. Michelle Renshaw, *Accommodating the Chinese: The American Hospital in China, 1880–1920* (New York: Routledge, 2005), 140.

76. Unschuld, *Medicine in China: A History of Ideas*, 241.

77. Chen, *Medicine in Rural China*, 20.

78. Thomas Lewis, *The Youngest Science: Notes of a Medicine-Watcher* (New York: Viking Press, 1983).

79. See Liu Xiaoxing, "Change and Continuity of Yi Medical Culture in Southwest China" (PhD diss., University of Illinois at Urbana-Champaign, 1998), 17.

80. There were many such reports on Chinese medicines in villages during the 1970s. See Sidel, "Barefoot Doctors," 1292–300; Victor W. Sidel and Ruth Sidel, *Serve the People: Observations on Medicine in the People's Republic of China* (Boston: Beacon Press, 1973); and H. Jack Geiger, "Health Care in the People's Republic of China: Implications for the United States," in *Culture and Healing in Asian Societies: Anthropological, Psychiatric and Public Health Studies*, ed. Arthur Kleinman, Peter Kunstadter, E. Russell Alexander, and James L. Gate (Boston: G. K. Hall, 1978), 386.

81. Henry E. Sigerist, *A History of Medicine*, vol. 2, *Early Greek, Hindu, and Persian Medicine* (New York: Oxford University Press, 1961), 69.

82. Renshaw, *Accommodating the Chinese*, 24.

83. Ibid., 18.

84. Goldschmidt, *Evolution of Chinese Medicine*, 63–65.

85. K. C. Wong and Wu Lien-Teh, *History of Chinese Medicine: Being a Chronicle of Medical Happenings in China from Ancient Times to the Present Period*, 2nd ed. (Shanghai: National Quarantine Service, 1936), 137.

86. Renshaw, *Accommodating the Chinese*, 140.

87. Croizier, *Traditional Medicine in Modern China*, 43.

88. Other medical institutions also emerged in China, such as psychiatric hospitals. Peter Paul Szto argues that the establishment of the Western-style psychiatric hospital in China was a transfer of institutions, or "social technology": the psychiatric hospital is a social technology that centralized care of severe mental illnesses (SMI) outside the domain of the household. See Peter Paul Szto, "The Accommodation of Insanity in Canton, China, 1857–1935" (PhD diss., University of Pennsylvania, 2002), 33.

89. Scheid, *Currents of Tradition in Chinese Medicine*, 194.

90. Ray H. Elling, "Medical Systems as Changing Social Systems," *Social Science & Medicine* 12 (April 1978): 107–15.

91. Li Peiliang and Xu Huiying, "Yiliao weishengwang" [Medical and health network], in *Renmin gongshe yu nongcun fazhan: Taishanxian doushan gongshe de jingyan* [People's commune and rural development: Experiences of Doushan Commune, Taishan County], ed. Li Peiliang and Liu Zhaojia (Hong Kong: Chinese University of Hong Kong Press, 1981), 89.

92. Pi-Chao Chen, "The Chinese Model of Rural Health Service," in *Population and Health Policy in the People's Republic of China*, Occasional Monograph Series, No. 9 (Washington: Interdisciplinary Communications Program, Smithsonian Institution, 1976), 65.

93. Ding Xueliang, "Yingdui SARS weiji de sanzhong tizhi: Qiangzhi, fazhi, ruozhi" [Three systems responding to the SARS Crisis: Mandatory, legal, and weak methods], accessed March 20, 2011, http://www.aisixiang.com/data/7243.html; and Yang Nianqun, "Disease Prevention, Social Mobilization and Spatial Politics: The Anti-Germ Warfare Incident of 1952 and the Patriotic Health Campaign," *Chinese Historical Review* 11, no. 2 (Fall 2004): 156–57.

94. Patricia M. Thornton, "Crisis and Governance: SARS and the Resilience of the Chinese Body Politic," *China Journal*, 61 (January 2009): 39; and Jonathan Schwartz, R. Gregory Evans, and Sarah Greenberg, "Evolution of Health Provision in Pre-SARS China: The Changing Nature of Disease Prevention," *China Review* 7, no. 1 (Spring 2007): 82–87.

95. Eliot Freidson, "The Profession of Medicine," in *The Sociology and Politics of Health: A Reader*, ed. Michael Purdy and David Banks (New York: Routledge, 2001), 130–34; Eliot Freidson, *Profession of Medicine: A Study of the Sociology of Applied Knowledge* (Chicago: University of Chicago Press, 1988); and Eliot Freidson, "The Sociology of Medicine," *Current Sociology* 10, no. 11 (1962): 123–92.

96. John Burnham, *How the Idea of Profession Changed the Writing of Medical History* (London: Wellcome Institute for the History of Medicine, 1998).

97. Nathan Sivin, *Traditional Medicine in Contemporary China: A Partial Translation of Revised Outline of Chinese Medicine* (Ann Arbor, MI: Center for Chinese Studies, University of Michigan, 1987), 21–23.

98. Nathan Sivin, "The History of Chinese Medicine: Now and Anon," *Positions* 6, no. 3 (Winter 1998): 750.

99. Bray, "Chinese Medicine," 743.

100. Bray, *Technology and Gender*, 306.

101. For a more detailed discussion, see Chao, *Medicine and Society in Late Imperial China*, 8–14; and Yüan-ling Chao, "The Ideal Physician in Late Imperial China: The Question of Sanshi 三世," *East Asian Science, Technology, and Medicine* 17 (2000): 68. See also Angela Ki Che Leung, "Medical Instruction and Popularization in Ming-Qing China," *Late Imperial China* 24, 1 (June 2003): 148; Scheid, *Currents of Tradition in Chinese Medicine*, 105; Unschuld, *Medical Ethics in Imperial China*, 23.

102. Grant, *Chinese Physician*, 38–39.

103. For the systemic discussions on medical administrations in each dynasty, see Chen Bangxian, *Zhongguo yixueshi* [Chinese medical history] (Beijing: Shangwu yinshuguan, 1998), 1–142. See also Joseph Needham and Lu Gwei-Djen, "China and the Origins of Qualifying Examinations in Medicine," in *Clerks and Craftsmen in China and the West: Lectures and Addresses on the History of Science and Technology*, ed. Joseph Needham (Cambridge: Cambridge University Press, 1970), 379–95.

104. Goldschmidt, *Evolution of Chinese Medicine*, 42–68.

105. Sivin, "History of Chinese Medicine," 750. See also Leung, "Medical Instruction and Popularization in Ming-Qing China," 148–49.

106. Elman, *Cultural History of Modern Science in China*, 209.

107. Ye Xiaoqing, "Regulating the Medical Profession in China: Health Policies of the Nationalist Government," in *Historical Perspectives on East Asian Science, Technology and Medicine*, ed. Alan K. L. Chan, Gregory K. Clancey, and Hui-Chieh Loy (Singapore: Singapore University Press, World Scientific, 2001), 198–213; Karen Minden, *Bamboo Stone: The Evolution of a Chinese Medical Elite* (Toronto: University of Toronto Press, 1994); and John Z. Bowers, *Western Medicine in a Chinese Palace: Peking Union College, 1917–1951* (New York: Josiah Macy Jr. Foundation, 1974).

108. Angela Ki Che Leung, "Yiliaoshi yu Zhongguo xiandaixing wenti" [The medical history and modernity], *Zhongguo shehui lishi pinglun* [China Social History Review] 8 (2007): 4.

109. Xu Xiaoqun, *Chinese Professionals and the Republican State: The Rise of Professional Associations in Shanghai, 1912–1937* (Cambridge, New York: Cambridge University Press, 2001), 190–214; Yang Nianqun, *Zaizao "bingren": Zhongxiyi chongtuxia de zhengzhi kongjian, 1832–1985* [Remaking "patients": Spatial politics in the conflicts between Chinese and Western medicine, 1832–1985] (Beijing: Zhongguo renmin daxue chubanshe, 2006), 243–99; Scheid, *Currents of Tradition in Chinese Medicine*, 186–87, 125–26; Sean Hsiang-lin Lei, "When Chinese Medicine Encountered the State: 1910–1949" (PhD diss., University of Chicago, 1999), 67–120; Taylor, *Chinese Medicine in Early Communist China*, 7; Croizier, "Medicine and Modernization," 27; and Andrews, "Making of Modern Chinese Medicine," 193–205.

110. Daniel M. Fox, "Medical Institutions and the State," in Bynum and Porter, *Companion of the Encyclopedia of the History of Medicine*, 1223.

111. Gail Henderson, "Physicians in China: Assessing the Impact of Ideology and Organization," in Hafferty and McKinlay, *Changing Medical Profession*, 185; and Julio Frenk and Luis Duran-Arenas, "The Medical Profession and the State," in Hafferty and McKinlay, *Changing Medical Profession*, 29.

112. Judith Farquhar, *Knowing Practice: The Clinical Encounter of Chinese Medicine* (Boulder, CO: Westview Press, 1994), 12.

113. Yuhangxian diming weiyuanhui [Yuhang County Geographic Name Committee], ed., *Yuhangxian dimingzhi* [Yuhang County Geographic Name Gazetteer] (Yuhang: Yuhangxian diming weiyuanhui, 1987), 3.

114. Ibid., 256.

115. Qin Xiangguan in Hubei Province and Wang Guizhen in Shanghai Municipality were the protagonists of reports on cooperative medical services and barefoot doctors in the *People's Daily* in September and December 1968, which initiated the popularization of barefoot doctors nationwide. Qin was described as the founder of the cooperative medical service in China. I spent one week interviewing Qin at his home in March 2004, which was quite productive. Wang was described as the first Chinese barefoot doctor. She was promoted to the rank of vice minister of the Ministry of Health of the People's Republic of China during the Cultural Revolution. However, her family resolutely declined my interview request in June 2004 on the grounds that she did "not (wish) to recall the tragic memory." The only positive outcome of the day I spent finding her house and the half day I spent waiting outside it was that I managed to obtain access to important documents in the archives of her hometown. These included a text of a draft of her speech to a mass rally promoting

the barefoot doctor program in 1969 and her later self-criticism, which showed how the Gang of Four controlled the health front in 1978.

Chapter One

1. Chen Hongting, interview, April 16–20, 2004; January 24, 2005; March 25, 2007; and Zhu Shouhua, interview, January 5, 2005.

2. Zhou Lingen, ed., *Yuhang zhenzhi* [Yuhang Township Gazetteer] (Hangzhou: Zhejiang renmin chubanshe, 1992), 255.

3. Shao Jungen, interview, November 20, 2009. See also Paul Unschuld, *What is Medicine? Western and Eastern Approaches to Healing* (Berkeley: University of California Press, 2009), 118–19.

4. Yang Lixing and Shi Guanzhen, eds., *Xinchangxian weishengzhi* [Xinchang County Health Gazetteer] (Shanghai: Tongji daxue chubanshe, 1992), 161.

5. Zheng Jinzhu, interview, November 19, 2009. See also Scheid, *Currents of Tradition in Chinese Medicine*, 183.

6. Zhejiangsheng weishengchu [Zhejiang Province Health Department], "Guanyu yiwu renyuan guanli banfa ji xingyi zhizhaodengji" [Management regulations for medical practitioners and medical license registration], 1947, YHA, vol. 517 (Hang County, Republic of China).

7. Hangxian zhongyishi gonghui [Hang County Chinese Medicine Doctors Guild], "Zhongyishi gonghui ji shenqingshu" [Chinese Medicine Doctors Guild and application documents], 1946, YHA, vol. 91-3-499 (Hang County, Republic of China).

8. Yuhangxian weishengju weishengzhi bianzhuanzu [Editorial board of Yuhang County Health Gazetteer], ed., *Yuhangxian weishengzhi* [Yuhang County Health Gazetteer] (Hangzhou: Yuhangshi renmin yinshuachang, 1988), 84–85.

9. Chen Hongting, interview, April 20, 2004.

10. Yan Youxiang, ed., *Jiandexian yiyao weishengzhi* [Jiande County Pharmaceutical and Health Gazetteer] (Jiande: Jiandexian weishengju, 1985), 78.

11. Jiang Sheng'e, interview, November 11, 2009.

12. Liping Wang, "Paradise for Sale: Urban Space and Tourism in the Social Transformation of Hangzhou, 1589–1937" (PhD diss., University of California, San Diego, 1997), 89–137.

13. Chen Zhicheng, interview, January 6, 2005.

14. Shen Qinyang, interview, January 19, 2005; and Chen Zhicheng, interview, January 6, 2005.

15. Wu, *Reproducing Women*, 54.

16. Hong Jinglin, interview, January 11, 2005.

17. Jiandexian renmin weiyuanhui weishengke [Health Bureau of the Jiande County People's Committee], "Jiandexian shehui yiyao qingkuang diaocha zongjie baogao" [Investigative Summary Report of Social Medicine and Pharmaceuticals in Jiande County], October 1957, JDA, vol. 31-1-22.

18. Hangzhoushi renmin zhengfu weishengju [Health Bureau of the Hangzhou City People's Government], "1950 nian gongzuo zongjie" [Work Summary for 1950], 1950, HZA, vol. 87-3-3.

19. Lucas, *Chinese Medical Modernization*, 99; and Croizier, *Traditional Medicine in Modern China*, 163.

20. Regarding terms for Chinese medicine doctors, see Scheid, *Currents of Tradition in Chinese Medicine*, 295; and Taylor, *Chinese Medicine in Early Communist China*,79, 84.

21. Hangxian weisheng gongzuozhe xiehui [Hang County Medical Practitioners and Workers Association], "Hangxian wunian lai jiuyi gongzuo zongjie" [Work Summary of Old-Style Doctor Work in Hang County over the Past Five Years], 1954, YHA, vol. 13-5-201.

22. Ibid.

23. Karen Marcia Goodkin, "In Mao's Shadow: Local Health System Praxis, Process, and Politics in Deng Xiaoping's China" (PhD Diss., University of Connecticut, 1998), 141.

24. Xu Yuangen, ed., *Fuyangxian weishengzhi* [Fuyang County Health Gazetteer] (Beijing: Zhongguo yiyao keji chubanshe, 1991), 330; Shao Jungen, interview, March 24, 2004.

25. Chen Hongting, interview, April 16–20, 2004.

26. Shao Jungen, interview, November 20, 2009.

27. Chen Zhicheng, interview, January 6, 2005.

28. Hangxian weisheng gongzuozhe xiehui, "Hangxian wunian lai jiuyi gongzuo zongjie."

29. Union clinics located in district seats were assigned to district health clinics or hospitals, which were responsible for managing and guiding all commune clinics. In some areas, county health bureaus also assigned a few medical staff to work at union clinics. Nonetheless, both township union clinics and district health clinics belonged to township-level units in the three-tier medical system of rural China.

30. Yu Guangyan, ed., *Chun'anxian weishengzhi* [Chun'an County Health Gazetteer] (Chun'an: Chun'anxian renmin zhengfu jiguang yinshuachang, 1998), 449–54.

31. David Lampton, "Health Policy during the Great Leap Forward," *China Quarterly* 60 (December 1974), 668–98.

32. Chen Hongting, interview, April 16–20, 2004.

33. Chen Hongting, interview, March 25, 2006. See also Xu, *Fuyangxian weishengzhi*, 51.

34. Zhu Shouhua, interview, December 26, 2004.

35. Sheilam M. Hillier and J. A. Jewell, "Chinese Traditional Medicine and Modern Western Medicine: Integration and Separation in China," in *Health Care and Traditional Medicine in China, 1800–1982*, ed. Sheilam M. Hillier and J. A. Jewell (London; Boston: Routledge & Kegan Paul, 1983), 313.

36. "Jiaqiang lingdao, zuohao lianhe zhensuo zhengdun gongzuo" [Strengthening leadership and adjusting the work of union clinics], *Zhejiang weisheng tongxun* [Zhejiang Health Correspondence], May 5, 1957.

37. Hangxian weisheng gongzuozhe xiehui, "Hangxian wunian lai jiuyi gongzuo zongjie."

38. Weishengbu [Ministry of Health], "Guanyu jiaqiang jiceng weisheng zuzhi lingdao de zhishi" [Instructions on enhancing the leadership of bottom-level health organizations], August 7, 1957, *Guowuyuan gongbao* [State Council Bulletin] (1957): 743–47.

39. Zhonghua renmin gongheguo weishengbu [Ministry of Health of the People's Republic of China], "Guanyu tiaozheng nongcun jiceng weisheng zuzhi wenti de yijian" [Instructions on readjusting bottom-level rural health organizations], July 13, 1962, JSA, vol. 3119-725-830; Lin'anxian weishengzhi bianzhuan weiyuanhui [Editorial board of Lin'an County Health Gazetteer], ed., *Lin'anxian weishengzhi* [Lin'an County Health Gazetteer] (Lin'an: Lin'anxian weishengju, 1992), 107–11; and Yu, *Chun'anxian weishengzhi*, 158.

40. Chen Hongting, interview, April 20, 2004.

41. Chen Zhicheng, interview, January 6, 2005.

42. For details of the changing process of the rural medical system in 1958–64, see Xiaoping Fang, "The Global Cholera Pandemic Reaches Chinese Villages: Population Mobility, Political Control, and Economic Incentives in Epidemic Prevention, 1962–1964" (Modern Asian Studies, forthcoming).

43. Zhonghua renmin gongheguo weishengbu, "Guanyu tiaozheng nongcun jiceng weisheng zuzhi wenti de yijian."

44. Chen Hongting, interview, April 20, 2004; Zhu Shouhua, interview, December 26, 2004.

45. "Fahui geti kaiyeyi de liliang" [Fulfill private medical practitioners' role], *Xinzhongyiyao* [New Chinese Medicine] 8, 5 (1960): 243–44.

46. Yu, *Chun'anxian weishengzhi*, 46–47.

47. Ibid., 227.

48. Ibid.

49. Jiang Zilin, interview, January 19, 2005.

50. Chen Zhicheng, interview, January 6, 2005.

51. Zhejiangsheng renmin zhengfu weishengting [Health Bureau of the Zhejiang Province People's Government], "Guanyu yi huzhu hezuo wei zhongxin kaizhan nongcun weisheng gongzuo de zhishi" [Instructions on conducting rural health work through focusing on mutual aid and cooperation], September 1954, ZJA, vol. J165-4-21.

52. Zhejiangsheng renmin zhengfu weishengting [Health Bureau of the Zhejiang Province People's Government], "Guanyu xunlian guoying nongchang nongyeshengchan hezuoshe baojianyuan gongzuo de zhishi" [Instructions on training healthcare workers for the state-owned agricultural cooperatives], December 1954, ZJA, vol. J165-4-100.

53. Jiang Jingting [Mr. Cat-Dog], interview, April 20, 2004.

54. Sun Kuijin, interview, May 12, 2004.

55. Yuhangxian weishengju weishengzhi bianzhuanzu, *Yuhangxian weishengzhi*, 247.

56. Yuhangxian weishengju [Yuhang County Health Bureau], "Yuhangxian 1961 nian sibing fangzhi ji shidian diaocha xiaojie" [Investigative summary of the prevention of four diseases and experimental work in Yuhang County in 1961], January 7, 1962, YHA, vol. 42-1-16.

57. Chen Hongting, interview, April 20, 2004. Regarding resistance to submitting stool samples, see Li Yushang, "The Elimination of Schistosomiasis in Jiaxing and Haining Counties, 1948–1958," in Leung and Furth, *Health and Hygiene in Chinese East Asia*, 218.

58. Chen Hongting, interview, June 9, 2004.

59. Hangzhoushi weishengju [Hangzhou Prefectural Health Bureau], "Hangzhou diqu chuhai miebing gongzuo qingkuang he jinhou yijian" [Current situations and further instructions on exterminating pests and eliminating diseases in Hangzhou Prefecture], October 1965, HZA, vol. 87-3-101.

60. Dai Jiahe, "Zai shiwei weisheng gongzuo huiyi shang de fayan" [Speech at the Health Work Meeting of the Prefectural Party Committee], October 1965, HZA, vol. 87-3-101.

61. Peter Wilenski, *The Delivery of Health Services in the People's Republic of China* (Ottawa: International Development Research Centre, 1976), 7.

62. Zhonggong zhongyang wenxian yanjiushi [Literature Research Office of the Central Committee of the Chinese Communist Party], ed., *Jianguo yilai zhongyao wenxian xuanbian* [Collected important documents since the founding of the People's Republic of China], vol. 3 (Beijing: Zhongyang wenxian chubanshe, 1992), 241–43.

63. Laodong renshibu laodong kexue yanjiusuo [Labor Research Institute of the Ministry of Labor and Personnel], ed., *Zhonghua renmin gongheguo laodong fagui xuanbian* [Collected labor laws and regulations of the People's Republic of China] (Beijing: Laodong renshi chubanshe, 1988), 393.

64. Nathan Sivin, "Editor's Introduction," in *Science and Civilisation in China*, vol. 6, *Biology and Biological Technology, Part VI: Medicine* (Cambridge: Cambridge University Press, 2000), 29.

65. In China, according to the household registration system established in 1958, the whole population was divided into two groups: those with an agricultural (rural) household identity and those with a nonagricultural (urban) household identity. The former encompassed commune members living in the villages, who were denied a whole range of welfare benefits granted by the state. The latter referred to cadres, factory workers, and employees in state-owned enterprises and agencies. See Fei-ling Wang, *Organizing through Division and Exclusion: China's Hukou System* (Stanford, CA: Stanford University Press, 2005).

66. Xu, *Fuyangxian weishengzhi*, 76, 89.

67. Weishengbu [Ministry of Health], "1961 nian weisheng jiben jianshe jihua anpai" [Investment arrangement for health infrastructure construction], December 1962, JSA, vol. 3119-783-901.

68. Mao Zedong, *Jianguo yilai Mao Zedong wengao* [Mao Zedong manuscript since the founding of the People's Republic of China] (Beijing: Zhongyang wenxian chubanshe, 1992), vol. 11, 318–19.

69. Zhejiangsheng weishengting [Zhejiang Province Health Department], "Guanyu ba weisheng gongzuo de zhongdian fangdao nongcun qu de huibao" [Report on the implementation of "stress rural areas in medical and health work"], 1965, ZJA, vol. J165-15-19.

70. Weishengbu [Ministry of Health], "Quanguo bannong banyi peiyang gongzuo zuotanhui jiyao" [Minutes of national meeting of "half-peasant, half-doctor" training work], March 1966, JSA, vol. 3119-1124-1297.

71. Hong Jinglin, interview, January 9, 2005; and Niu Shuiying, interview, January 11, 2005.

72. Mao's criticism was not fully published and disseminated in 1965. Indeed, not until the outbreak of the Cultural Revolution did the Red Guards fully disclose it as the "June 26 directive." See Zhu Chao, *Xin zhongguo yixue jiaoyushi* [The history of

medical education in new China] (Beijing: Beijing yike daxue, Zhongguo xiehe yike daxue lianhe chubanshe, 1990), 112–20.

73. Qin Xiangguan, interview, March 26–April 2, 2004.

74. Suzanne Pepper, *Radicalism and Education Reform in 20th Century China: The Search for an Ideal Development Model* (New York: Cambridge University Press, 1996), 157–352.

75. "Cong Shanghai jichuangchang kan peiyang gongcheng jishu renyuan de daolu" [The path toward training technicians from the Shanghai tool plant], *RMRB*, July 22, 1968.

76. He Gongxin, "Pinxiazhongnong shengzan zhege chijiao yisheng: Ji jinshanxian youxiu weishengyuan Hu Lianhua" [Poor and lower-middle peasants applaud this barefoot doctor: The story of excellent health care worker Hu Lianhua], *Xinmin wanbao* [Xinmin Evening News], September 5, 1965.

77. Fang Shunxi, interview, May 9, 2004.

78. "Cong chijiao yisheng de chengzhang kan yixue jiaoyu geming de fangxiang: Shanghaishi de diaocha baogao" [Fostering a revolution in medical education through the growth of the barefoot doctors: An investigative report from Shanghai municipality], *RMRB*, September, 14, 1968.

79. During the Cultural Revolution, according to the official description and definition, "large numbers of socialist new things have emerged on the various fronts following fierce struggles between the two classes, the two roads, and the two lines. These socialist new things are conducive to reducing the three major differences between mental and manual labor, and to restricting and reducing bourgeois rights. They represent the direction of historical development." Other "newly emerged things" included model revolutionary theatrical works, revolutionary committees, May 7 cadre schools, and educated youth, etc. See David Bonavia, "The Fate of the 'New Born Things' of China's Cultural Revolution," *Pacific Affairs* 51, no. 2 (Summer 1978): 177–94.

80. Present scholarship argues that the cooperative medical service had first been implemented during the Agricultural Collectivization campaign and promoted nationwide during the Great Leap Forward campaign. According to Zhou Shouqi, the percentage of villages implementing cooperative medical services reached 10 percent in 1958, 32 percent in 1960, and 46 percent in 1962. Later discussions on the cooperative medical service mainly cite Zhou's statistic data. See Zhou Shouqi, Gu Xingyuan, and Zhu Aorong, "Zhongguo nongcun jiankang baozhang zhidu de yanjiu jinzhan" [The progress of research on China rural health-care institutions], *Zhongguo nongcun weisheng shiye guanli* [China Rural Health Management] 14, no. 9 (1994): 8; and Wang, "Xuexi jizhi yu shiying nengli," 111–33. However, the available statistical data in the health gazetteers of Hangzhou Prefecture and nine other provinces (Heilongjiang, Qinghai, Fujian, Gansu, Hubei, Jiangsu, Anhui, Sichuan, and Yunnan) indicate that the cooperative medical service was implemented sporadically in very limited areas before the mid-1960s. Within Hangzhou Prefecture, there was no cooperative medical service during the Great Leap Forward campaign. Of these nine provinces, only the health gazetteers of Hubei, Jiangsu, Sichuan, and Yunnan indicated that the cooperative medical service had been implemented during this period. More importantly, the cooperative medical service had ceased to function nationwide by 1962 because of economic retrenchment, so Zhou Shouqi's

claim that coverage had reached 46 percent of China's villages by that year is questionable. See Hangzhoushi weishengju Hangzhoushi weishengzhi bianji weiyuanhui [Editorial board of Hangzhou Prefecture Health Gazetteer of Hangzhou Prefecture Health Bureau], ed., *Hangzhoushi weishengzhi* [Hangzhou Prefecture Health Gazetteer] (Hangzhou: Hangzhoushi weishengju, 2000), 84–85; Hubeisheng difangzhi bianzhuan weiyuanhui [Editorial board of Hubei Province Local Gazetteer], ed., *Hubei shengzhi: Weisheng* [Hubei Province Gazetteer: Health] (Wuhan: Hubei renmin chubanshe, 2000), vol. 2, 1123; Jiangsusheng difangzhi bianzhuan weiyuanhui [Editorial board of the Jiangsu Province Local Gazetteer], ed., *Jiangsu shengzhi: Weishengzhi* [Jiangsu Province Gazetteer: Health] (Nanjing: Jiangsu guji chubanshe, 1999), 115–18; Sichuansheng yiyao weishengzhi bianzhuan weiyuanhui [Editorial board of the Sichuan Province Pharmaceutical and Health Gazetteer], ed., *Sichuansheng yiyao weishengzhi* [Sichuan Province Pharmaceutical and Health Gazetteer] (Chengdu: Sichuan kexue jishu chubanshe, 1991), 296; and Yunnansheng difangzhi bianzhuan weiyuanhui [Editorial board of Yunnan Province Local Gazetteer], ed., *Yunnan shengzhi: Weishengzhi* [Yunnan Province Gazetteer: Health Gazetteer] (Kunming: Yunnan renmin chubanshe, 2002), 123–24.

81. Regarding rural education in the Cultural Revolution, see Dongping Han, *The Unknown Cultural Revolution: Education Reforms and Their Impact on China's Rural Development* (New York: Garland, 2000).

82. "Guanyu jiang gongban xiaoxue fangdao dadui lai ban de jianyi" [Suggestions that state-run primary schools should be run by production brigades], *RMRB*, November 14, 1968.

83. Jean C. Robinson, "Decentralization, Money, and Power: The Case of People-Run Schools in China," *Comparative Education Review* 30, no. 1 (February 1986): 82.

84. "Shenshou pinxiazhongnong huanying de hezuo yiliao" [Cooperative medical service warmly welcomed by poor and lower-middle peasants], *RMRB*, December 5, 1968.

85. Zheng Zhihua, *Leyuan xiongfeng* [Glorious wind of Leyuan] (Hong Kong: Tianma tushu youxian gongsi, 2003), 9–26.

86. Ibid., 29–30.

87. "Shenshou pinxiazhongnong huanying de hezuo yiliao," *RMRB*, December 5, 1968.

88. For example, the *People's Daily* published a total of thirty-nine reports with "cooperative medical service" in their titles from December 5, 1968, to December 21, 1969, and thirty reports with "barefoot doctors" in their titles from September 14, 1968, to December 27, 1969. For more details, see "Renmin ribao quanwen shujuku guangpan, 1946–2008" [CD-ROM of Full Text Database of the *People's Daily*, 1946–2008].

89. Shaoxingshi weishengju geweihui [Revolutionary Committee of the Shaoxing Prefecture Health Bureau], "Gonggu he fazhan hezuo yiliao, jixu gaohao nongcun weisheng geming" [Consolidating and developing the cooperative medical service, furthering the rural health revolution], 1973, SXA, vol. GC13-61-36-3-5-11.

90. Qin Xiangguan, interview, March 26–April 2, 2004.

91. "Chuanshaxian Jiangzhen gongshe chijiao yisheng Wang Guizhen zai longzhong jinian Maozhuxi pishi chijiao yisheng diaocha baogao yizhounian dahui shang de fayan" [Jiangzhen commune barefoot doctor Wang Guizhen's Speech at the meeting for the first anniversary of Chairman Mao's written instructions on the barefoot doctor investigative report], September 4, 1969, SHA, vol. 13242-2-77.

92. Hangzhoushi weishengju [Hangzhou Prefecture Health Bureau], ed., *Hangzhoushi weisheng gongzuo dashiji, 1949–2000* [Chronicle of Health Work in Hangzhou, 1949–2000] (Hangzhou: Hangzhoushi weishengju, 2002), 57.

93. "Jiangcun gongshe dangwei jieji douzheng he liangtiao daolu douzheng de wenti" [The issues of class struggle and the struggle between the two lines in the Jiang Village Commune Chinese Communist Party Committee], July 17, 1969, YHA, vol. 148-1-132.

94. Weng Guofa, "Jiangcun gongshe dangwei dierci buchong jiancha baogao" [The second complementary self-criticism by the Jiang Village Commune Party Committee], October 7, 1966, YHA, vol. 148-1-133.

95. Red Storm (*hongbao*) and United Headquarters (*lianzong*) were two opposing rebel factions in Zhejiang Province in the early days of the Cultural Revolution. They mainly disagreed over which provincial leaders merited support and which deserved repudiation. For example, Red Storm supported the provincial party secretary at the time, Jiang Hua, while United Headquarters wanted to seize power and overthrow Jiang. The two factions sent members all over Zhejiang to disseminate their viewpoints and seek support, while establishing organizations and undertaking physical struggles. For details, see Keith Forster, *Rebellions and Factionalism in a Chinese Province, Zhejiang, 1966–1976* (Armonk, NY: M. E. Sharpe, 1990); and Zhejiang fangzhi bianjibu [Editorial board of Zhejiang Province Gazetteer], ed., *Zhejiang wenge jishi* [Chronicle of the Cultural Revolution in Zhejiang] (Hangzhou: Zhejiang fangzhi bianjibu, 1989).

96. Shen Xianbing, interview, January 10, 2005.

97. Xu Aher, interview, January 10, 2005; and Zhou Yonggan, interview, January 7, 2005.

98. Zhu Shouhua, interview, January 5, 2005; and Chen Hongting, interview, January 7, 2005; Zhou Yonggan, interview, January 7, 2005.

99. Xu Aher, interview, January 10, 2005.

100. Chen Zhicheng, interview, January 6, 2005.

101. Shen Qingyang, interview, January 19, 2005; Shen Xianbing, interview, January 10, 2005; and Xu Aher, interview, January 13, 2005.

102. "Gedadui guanyu shouchahu dengji he pidou daigaomao dengji" [Registration of households searched and commune members criticized and put on dunce caps in each brigade], September 26, 1966, YHA, vol. 148-1-138.

103. Shen Xianbing, interview, January 10, 2005.

104. Xu Zhiming, interview, January 13, 2005.

105. Zhou Yonggan, interview, November 6, 2009.

106. Chen Hongting, interview, January 7, 2005; Chen Hongting's adopted daughter, interview, January 7, 2005; and Xu Aher, interview, January 7, 2005.

107. Chen Zhicheng, interview, January 6, 2005.

108. Luo Linyuan, interview, January 5, 2005.

109. Shen Xianbing, interview, January 10, 2005.

110. Xiaoshan weishengju [Xiaoshan County Health Bureau], ed., *Xiaoshan weishengzhi* [Xiaoshan County Health Gazetteer] (Hangzhou: Zhejiang daxue chubanshe, 1989), 55.

111. Chun'anxian weishengju geweihui [Revolutionary committee of the Chun'an County Health Bureau], "Chun'anxian gongshe (zhen) weishengsuo caiwu guanli

banfa" [Financial regulations for commune (township) clinics in Chun'an County], December 29, 1973, CAA, vol. 36-1-49.

112. Shaoxingshi weishengju geweihui, "Gonggu he fazhan hezuo yiliao, jixu gaohao nongcun weisheng geming."

113. Chun'anxian weishengju geweihui [Revolutionary Committee of the Chun'an County Health Bureau], "Guanyu youguan gongshe weishengsuo bufen yiwu renyuan you nongyehu zhuanwei guojia gongying liangshi de pifu" [Approval for allowing some commune health clinic doctors to enjoy state foodstuff supplies], April 11, 1971, CAA, vol. 36-1-46.

114. Yu, *Chun'anxian weishengzhi*, 227; Yuhangxian weishengju weishengzhi bianzhuanzu, *Yuhangxian weishengzhi*, 80; Xu, *Fuyangxian weishengzhi*, 68–69; Lin'anxian weishengzhi bianzhuan weiyuanhui, *Lin'anxian weishengzhi*, 132; Fan Zhangyou, ed., *Tonglu xianzhi* [Tonglu County Gazetteer] (Hangzhou: Zhejiang renmin chubanshe, 1991), 694; and Yan, *Jiandexian yiyao weishengzhi*, 70.

115. "Guangdongsheng qujiangxian qunxindadui jianchi hezuo yiliao zhidu shiyinian de qingkuang diaocha" [Investigative report of Qunxing production brigade, Qujiang County, Guangdong Province, persisting in implementing cooperative medical services for 11 years], *RMRB*, January 11, 1969.

116. Shen Qingyang, ed., *Yuhangxian jiangcunxiang xueyi de tulangzhong* [Folk healers in Jiang Village Township, Yuhang County] (Jiang Village, 2009), 93.

117. Hong Jinglin, interview, January 11, 2005.

118. Jiang Zilin, interview, January 24, 2005; and Yuhangxian jiangcun renmin gongshe geming weiyuanhui [Revolutionary committee of Jiang Village People's Commune, Yuhang County], "Guanyu chaichu jianggongmiao jianzao gongshe jixiehua xiupeichang de qingqiu baogao" [Request for approval to dismantle Lord Jiang Temple to build machinery repair factory], April 14, 1968, YHA, vol. 148-1-162.

119. Lucas, *Chinese Medical Modernization*, 131–32.

120. Zhejiangsheng Hangzhoushi geming weiyuanhui [Revolutionary committee of Hangzhou Prefecture, Zhejiang Province], "Guanyu benshi manshi zhongyi xuetuo fenpei wenti de tongzhi" [Notice on assigning apprentices who have finished the course of study within the prefecture], July 30, 1969, HZA, vol. 132-3-144.

121. Wu Jungen, interview, April 6, 2004.

122. Zhejiangsheng Hangzhoushi geming weiyuanhui [Revolutionary Committee of Hangzhou Prefecture, Zhejiang Province], "Guanyu shishu yiliao weisheng danwei yiwu renyuan xiafang nongcun de yijian baogao" [Report on sending down the medical staff of prefecture-affiliated hospitals to the countryside], December 23, 1971, CAA, vol. 87-3-142.

123. Sulamith Heins Potter and Jack M. Potter, *China's Peasants: The Anthropology of a Revolution* (Cambridge: Cambridge University Press, 1990), 303.

124. Hangzhoushi weishengju geweihui zhenggongzu [Political Work Team of the Revolutionary Committee of the Hangzhou Prefecture Health Bureau], "Tuchu zhengzhi, jiejue sige zenmeban" [Highlighting Politics and Solving Four "How-to-Dos"], *Zhenggong jianbao* [Political Work Bulletin], December 27, 1971, HZA, vol. 87-1-146.

125. Wu Jungen, interview, April 6, 2004.

126. Hangzhoushi weishengju geweihui zhenggongzu [Political work team of the revolutionary committee of the Hangzhou Prefecture Health Bureau], "Guzhu ganjin, lizheng shangyou, duokuaihaosheng di jianshe shehuizhuyi" [Gather all forces,

strive to build socialism richly, rapidly, and critically], *Zhenggong jianbao* [Political Work Bulletin], July 18, 1970, HZA, vol. 87-3-130.

127. For brief descriptions of the sending of urban doctors to the countryside, see Gail Henderson and Myron Cohen, *The Chinese Hospital: A Socialist Work Unit* (New Haven, CT: Yale University Press, 1984), 37–38.

128. Zhejiangsheng Hangzhoushi geming weiyuanhui [Revolutionary committee of Hangzhou Prefecture, Zhejiang Province],"Guanyu yiwu renyuan xiafang gongzuo yijian baogao" [Report concerning the sending down of medical personnel to rural areas], July 7, 1971, HZA, vol. 87-3-142; "Hangzhoushi geweihui guanyu shishu yiliao weisheng danwei yiwu renyuan xiafang nongcun de yijian de baogao" [Report of the revolutionary committee of Hangzhou Prefecture on sending medical personnel from prefecture-affiliated medical and health units to rural areas], December 23, 1971, HZA, vol. 87-3-142; "Guanyu Hangzhoushi weisheng xitong guanche liuerliu zhishi xiafang yiwu renyuan de qingkuang he jige wenti de qingshi baogao" [Request for instructions on implementing the June 26 directive to send down medical personnel and a few problems in Hangzhou Prefecture], September 18, 1972, HZA, vol. 87-3-142; and "Shengwei bangongshi zhangtongzhi laidian" [Call coming from Comrade Zhang of the Provincial Party Committee Office], September 16, 1972, HZA, vol. 87-3-142.

129. Yu, *Chun'anxian weishengzhi*, 20; and Xu, *Fuyangxian weishengzhi*, 17.

130. Yu, *Chun'anxian weishengzhi*, 68; and Xu, *Fuyangxian weishengzhi*, 18.

131. Zhou Yonggan, interview, January 7, 2005.

Chapter Two

1. Leung, "Medical Instruction and Popularization in Ming-Qing China," 130–52. For the latest discussion on medical knowledge transmission, see Hinrichs, "New Geographies of Chinese Medicine," 303–8.

2. Wu Yiyi, "A Medical Line of Many Masters: A Prosopographical Study of Liu Wansu and His Disciples from the Jin to the Early Ming," *Chinese Science* 11 (1993–94): 36–65; Nathan Sivin, "Text and Experience in Classical Chinese Medicine," in *Knowledge and the Scholarly Medical Traditions*, ed. Don Bates (Cambridge: Cambridge University Press, 1995), 194; Angela Ki Che Leung, "Mingdai shehui zhong de yiyao" [Medicines and pharmaceuticals in Ming society], *Faguo hanxue* [French Sinology] 6 (2002): 349–52; and "Medical Learning from the Song to the Ming," in *The Song-Yuan-Ming Transition in Chinese History*, ed. Paul Jakov Smith and Richard Von Glahn (Cambridge, MA: Harvard University Asia Center, 2003), 386.

3. Jiang Zhushan, "Wanming Jiangnan Qi Biaojia jiazu de richang shenghuoshi: Yi yibing guanxi weili de tantao" [The daily life of the Qi Biaojia family in late Ming Jiangnan: A focus on doctor-patient relations], *Dushi wenhua yanjiu* [Urban Culture Studies] 1 (Shanghai: Sanlian shudian, 2006), 181–212.

4. Scheid, *Chinese Medicine in Contemporary China*, 119; and Liu Jingzhen and Li Bozhong, "Duotai, biyun, yu jueyu—Song, Yuan, Ming, Qing shiqi jiangzhe diqu de jueyu fangfa jiqi yunyong yu chuanbo" [Abortion, contraception and sterilization: Sterilization methods and application in Jiangsu and Zhejiang areas in the Song-Yuan-Ming-Qing periods], *Zhongguo xueshu* [China Scholarship] 1 (2000): 71–99.

5. Yi-Li Wu, "Transmitted Secrets: The Doctors of Low Yangzi Region in Popular Gynecology in Late Imperial China" (PhD diss., Yale University, 1998), 78.

6. For ways of becoming folk healers, see David Landy, *Culture, Disease, and Healing: Studies in Medical Anthropology* (New York: Macmillan, 1977), 416–17.

7. Yang and Shi, *Xinchangxian weishengzhi*, 161.

8. Croizier, *Traditional Medicine in Modern China*, 87; and Wu, *Plague Fighter*, 571.

9. Wu, *Plague Fighter*, 567.

10. Scheid, *Currents of Tradition in Chinese Medicine*, 125–26.

11. Chen Hongting, interview, January 7, 2005.

12. Shen, *Yuhangxian jiangcunxiang xueyi de tulangzhong*, 93.

13. Scheid, *Chinese Medicine in Contemporary China*, 169; and Croizier, *Traditional Medicine in Modern China*, 181.

14. Scheid, *Chinese Medicine in Contemporary China*, 169; and Shao Jing, "Hospitalizing Traditional Chinese Medicine: Identity, Knowledge and Reification" (PhD diss., University of Chicago, 1999), 109.

15. Chen Zhicheng, interview, November 6, 2009.

16. Niu Shuiying, interview, June, 2004; and Luo Zhengfu, interview, November 23, 2009.

17. Zhang Zaitong and Xian Rijin, eds., *Minguo yiyao weisheng fagui xuanbian, 1912–1948* [Collection of medical and health regulations of the Republic of China, 1912–1948] (Jinan: Shangdong daxue chubanshe, 1990), 259.

18. Qiu Shiting, ed., "1929 nian fandui feizhi zhongyi zhongyao de douzheng" [The struggle against the abolishment of Chinese medicine and Chinese pharmaceuticals in 1929], in *Hangzhou wenshi ziliao* [Hangzhou Cultural and Historical Data], vol.7, ed. Zhengxie Hangzhoushi weiyuanhui wenshi ziliao gongzuo weiyuanhui [The cultural and historical data committee of Hangzhou Prefecture political consultative committee](Hangzhou: Zhengxie Hangzhoushi weiyuanhui wenshi ziliao gongzuo weiyuanhui, 1986), 84–85.

19. "Hangshifu zhongshi renming yanjin zhongyi yong xiyao" [Hangzhou City Government cherishes human life and strictly bans the use of western medicine by Chinese medicine doctors], *Guangji yikan* [Guangji Hospital Medical Journal] 11, no. 3 (1934): 5.

20. Provisional Regulations Governing Physicians, approved on April 18, 1951, and promulgated on May 1, 1951, cited in Tao-tai Hsia, "Law on Public Health," in *Medicine and Public Heath in the People's Republic of China*, ed. Joseph R. Quinn (Bethesda, MD: National Institutes of Health, 1972), 124–25.

21. Scheid, *Chinese Medicine in Contemporary China*, 69.

22. Weishengbu renmin geming junshi weiyuanhui weishengbu [Ministry of Health and Health Department of People's Revolutionary Military Committee], "Chunji fangyi gongzuo de zhishi" [Instructions on epidemic prevention work in spring], in *Zhongyang renmin zhengfu faling huibian (1949–1950)* [Collection of law documents of the central government, 1949–1950], ed. Zhongyang renmin zhengfu fazhi weiyuanhui [The Legal Affairs Committee of the Central Government] (Beijing: Falü chubanshe, 1982), 636; Scheid, *Chinese Medicine in Contemporary China*, 69.

23. Taylor, *Chinese Medicine in Early Communist China*, 47; and Shao, "Hospitalizing Traditional Chinese Medicine," 84.

24. Weishengbu renmin geming junshi weiyuanhui weishengbu, "Chunji fangyi gongzuo de zhishi," 636; Scheid, *Chinese Medicine in Contemporary China*, 69–70.

25. In late 1953, the Ministry of Health was criticized for its policies on Chinese medicine because the licensing and recruitment regulations for Chinese medicine doctors seriously restricted their medical practice. In July 1954, Mao put forward the idea of "Western medicine studying Chinese medicine" to eradicate the boundaries between Chinese and Western medicine and form a unified Chinese medicine. Soon various training classes of "Western medicine studying Chinese medicine" were established throughout China. Meanwhile, the previous regulations on Chinese medicine doctors were abolished, China Academy of Traditional Chinese Medicine and Chinese medicine hospitals were founded, and Chinese medicine was integrated into Western medical universities, colleges, schools, hospitals, etc. Mao first proposed the "integration of Chinese and Western medicine" (*zhongxiyi jiehe*) in 1956, and it became the guiding principle from then onward. During the Cultural Revolution, the integration of Chinese pharmaceuticals and treatment methods with Western diagnostic techniques, treatment, and pharmaceuticals was further promoted and advocated. After 1980, the Ministry of Health listed Chinese medicine, Western medicine, and the integration of the two as the three great powers of Chinese medical system. However, the integration of Chinese and Western medicine is usually regarded as a branch of Chinese medicine. See Taylor, *Chinese Medicine in Early Communist China*, 30–150; Scheid, *Chinese Medicine in Contemporary China*, 65–88; and Lampton, *Politics of Medicine*, 112.

26. Miriam Gross, "Chasing Snails: Anti-Schistosomiasis Campaigns in the People's Republic of China" (PhD diss., University of California, San Diego, 2010), 364.

27. Zhejiangsheng weishengting [Zhejiang Provincial Health Bureau], "Guanyu dierpi xunhui yiliaodui gongzuo qingkuang" [Report on the work of the second batch of sent-down doctors from urban areas], 1965, ZJA, vol. J165-15-59.

28. According to Hsu, biomedicine subjects accounted for 23 percent of total lectures in the five-year training of students of traditional medicine students. See Elizabeth Hsu, "The Medicine from China Has Rapid Effects: Chinese Medicine Patients in Tanzania," *Anthropology & Medicine* 9, no. 3 (2002): 292–93.

29. Weishengbu dangzu [Ministry of Health party leadership group], "Guanyu xiyi xue zhongyi lizhiban qingkuang chengji he jingyan gei zhongyang de baogao" [Report submitted to the central committee of the Chinese Communist Party on situations, achievements, and lessons of the class of "western medicine doctors leave their profession to study Chinese medicine"], *Renmin baojian* [People's Health Care] 1 (1959): 1.

30. Lampton, *Politics of Medicine*, 114, 171.

31. Hong Jinglin, interview, January 11, 2005; Niu Shuiying, interview, January 11, 2005; and Chen Zhicheng, interview, January 6, 2005.

32. Fuyangxian weishengju [Fuyang County Health Bureau], "Guanyu peixun chijiao yisheng, shixing hezuo yiliao de gongzuo baogao" [Report on training barefoot doctors and implementing cooperative medical services], May 22, 1969, FYA, vol. 74-1-25.

33. Yuhangxian weishengju [Yuhang County Health Bureau], "Yuhangxian lingdao zai quanxian hezuo yiliao chijiao yisheng daibiao dahui shang de zongjie jianghua" [The summary speech by Yuhang County leaders at the county cooperative medical services and barefoot doctor representative meeting], November 17, 1974, YHA, vol. 42-1-88.

34. Zhang Ahhua, interview, April 20, 2004.

35. Zheng Xuedong, interview, March 25, 2007.

36. Shen Guanrong, interview, May 27, 2004.

37. Yuhangxian weishengju [Yuhang County Health Bureau], "Xuexi maozhuxi guanyu lilun wenti de zhishi, jinyibu banhao hezuo yiliao: Yuhangxian hezuo yiliao qingkuang huibao" [Study Chairman Mao's theoretic instructions and further implement cooperative medical service: Report of cooperative medical service in Yuhang County], 1973–74, YHA, vol. 150-1-52.

38. Hunansheng Anxiangxian weishengju [Anxiang County Health Bureau, Hunan Province], "Shixing kaohe fazheng, wending tigao chijiao yisheng" [Holding examination and issuing certificates, maintaining and improving barefoot doctors], *Chijiao yisheng zazhi* [Journal of Barefoot Doctors] 12 (1978): 1.

39. Chen Zhicheng, interview, November 6, 2009; and Chen Hongting, interview, March 2004.

40. Zheng Xuedong, interview, March 26, 2004.

41. Nathan Sivin, "Editor's Introduction," 29; and Furth, *Flourishing Yin*, 266–300.

42. Victoria B. Cass, "Female Healers in the Ming and the Lodge of Ritual and Ceremony," *Journal of the American Oriental Society* 106, no. 1 (January–March 1986): 233–40; Leung, "Women Practicing Medicine in Pre-Modern China," in *Chinese Women in the Imperial Past: New Perspectives*, ed. H. Zurndorfer (Leiden: Brill Academic, 1999), 101–34; and "Medical Learning from the Song to the Ming," 390–91.

43. Furth, *Flourishing Yin*, 295–96; and Bray, "Chinese Medicine," 744.

44. Unschuld, *Medical Ethics in Imperial China*, 77, 80.

45. Furth, *Flourishing Yin*, 245; Chao, "Medicine and Society in Late Imperial China," 293; and Bray, *Technology and Gender*, 321.

46. Jin Wenguan, "Tantan xiangcun funü de weisheng wenti" [On the issue of rural women's health], *Chusheng yuekan* [The sound of the hoe monthly] 1, no. 7 (1935): 11.

47. C. C. Chen, "Ting Hsien and the Public Health Movement in China," *The Milbank Memorial Fund Quarterly* 15, no. 4 (October 1937): 386. See also the Chinese clinical examination described by a Western physician, Florence Bretelle Establet, "Resistance and Receptivity: French Colonial Medicine in Southwest China, 1893–1930," *Modern China* 25, no. 2 (April 1999): 196.

48. Granny He, interview, May 2004.

49. Gail Hershatter, "Birthing Stories: Rural Midwives in 1950s China," in *Dilemmas of Victory: The Early Years of the People's Republic of China*, ed. Jeremy Brown and Paul G. Pickowicz (Cambridge, MA: Harvard University Press, 2007), 337–58; and Joshua Goldstein, "Scissors, Surveys, and Psycho-Prophylactics: Prenatal Health Care Campaigns and State Building in China, 1949–1954," *Journal of Historical Sociology* 11, no. 2 (June 1998): 153–84.

50. Angela Ki Che Leung, "Dignity of the Nation, Gender Equality, or Charity for All? Options for the First Modern Chinese Women Doctors," in *the Dignity of Nations: Equality, Competition, and Honor in East Asian Nationalism*, ed. Sechin Y. S. Chien and John Fitzgerald (Hong Kong: Hong Kong University Press, 2006), 73.

51. Yuhangxian weishengju [Yuhang County Health Bureau], "Yuhangxian hezuo yiliao zanxing guanli banfa" [Temporary regulations on Yuhang County cooperative medical service], October 23, 1978, SDA.

52. Chen Zhikun, interview, May 14, 2004.

53. Luo Zhengfu, interview, November 23, 2009.

54. Hangzhoushi weishengju Hangzhoushi weishengzhi bianji weiyuanhui, *Hangzhoushi weishengzhi*, 84–87.

55. Judith Banister, *China's Changing Population* (Stanford, CA: Stanford University Press, 1987), 67.

56. Between 1949 and 1976, often called the Maoist period, sex was a taboo topic. People's personal lives were subject to state and work unit scrutiny, and puritanical interventions were common. Records from the medical sector provide us with remarkable evidence of the mechanisms for disciplining individuals engaged in adultery, premarital sex, premarital cohabitation, and sexual harassment. In the event of sexual indiscretions between male physicians and their female colleagues (doctors, nurses, pharmacists, etc.) or patients, male physicians were severely punished through public criticism, dismissal from their posts, and criminal prosecution. See Xiaoping Fang, "Sexual Misconduct and Punishment in Chinese Hospital in the 1960s and 1970s," *Nan nü: Men, Women, and Gender in China* 14, no. 2 (2012): 1–35.

57. Chen Zhicheng, interview, October 9, 2010. See also Ren Yingqiu, "Wo dui zhongyi jinxiu jiaoyu jidian bu chengshu de yijian" [My preliminary views on further training for practitioners of Chinese medicine], *Beijing Zhongyi* [Beijing Journal of Chinese Medicine] 3, no. 3 (1954): 10–14.

58. Yan Yunxiang, "Rural Youth and Youth Culture in North China," *Culture, Medicine, and Psychiatry* 23, no. 1 (March 1999): 86.

59. Zheng Xuedong, interview, March 17, 2004.

60. Zhu Shouhua, interview, January 5, 2005.

61. Huanshan renmin yiyuan [Huanshan People's Hospital], "Fuyangxian chijiao yisheng fuxun dengjibiao" [Registration forms for Fuyang County barefoot doctor retraining class], October 1978, FYA, vol. 74-3-29; Gaoqiao renmin yiyuan [Gaoqiao People's Hospital], "Qingyunqu 1981 nian diyiqi chijiao yisheng peixunban huamingce" [Roster of the first barefoot doctor training class in Qingyun District in 1981], April 9, 1981, FYA, vol. 74-3-29.

62. Wang Sijun and Wang Ruizi, eds., *Zhongguo renkou: Zhejiang fence* [China population: Zhejiang] (Beijing: Zhongguo caizheng jingji chubanshe, 1988), 348.

63. Luo Zhengfu, interview, November 23, 2009.

64. Zhou Yonggan, interview, May 21, 2004.

65. Xu Shuilin, interview, November 5, 2009.

66. Shen Guanrong, interview, May 25, 2004.

67. Chen Zhicheng, interview, January 6, 2005.

68. Luo Zhengfu, interview, November 23, 2009.

69. Shen, *Yuhangxian jiangcunxiang xueyi de tulangzhong*, 93; and Jiang Sheng'e, interview, November 11, 2009.

70. Wu, "Medical Line of Many Masters," 36–65.

71. Marta Hanson, "Merchants of Medicine: Huizhou Mercantile Consciousness, Morality, and Medical Patronage in Seventeenth-Century China," in *East Asian Science: Tradition and Beyond*, ed. Keizô Hashimoto, Catherine Jami, and Lowell Skar (Osaka: Kansai University Press, 1995), 208.

72. Leung, "Medical Learning from the Song to the Ming," 396.

73. The National Library of China, accessed June 1, 2012, http://opac.nlc.gov. cn/F.

74. There were twenty kinds of books for rural health workers published from 1949 to 1969, before the advent of the barefoot doctors. For the titles with the key words "barefoot doctors" in the section for books and journals, see http://opac.nlc. gov.cn/F (accessed June 1, 2012).

75. There were two series of barefoot doctor textbooks during the 1970s: one for southern China and another for northern China because of the variations in climatic and geographic conditions, which had a bearing on disease.

76. *Gongnong yiliao weisheng shouce* [Worker and peasant health manual] (Hangzhou: Hangzhoushi weisheng geming weiyuanhui, 1969), ed. Hangzhoushi disan renmin yiyuan ji hongyi peixunban jiaocai bianweihui [Hangzhou City No. 3 People's Hospital and editorial board of red doctor training class textbooks]; and *Chijiao yisheng shouce* [Barefoot doctor's manual] (Shanghai: Shanghai kexue jishu chubanshe, 1969), ed. Shanghaishi zhongyi xueyuan, Zhejiangsheng zhongyi xueyuan, Zhejiangsheng zhongyi yanjiuyuan [Shanghai Chinese Medicine College, Zhejiang Chinese Medicine College, and Zhejiang Chinese Medicine Research Institute].

77. Chun'anxian weishengju [Chun'an County Health Bureau], "Guanyu fagei chijiao yisheng peixun jiaocai de tongzhi" [Notice on issuing barefoot doctor training textbooks], November 27, 1974, CAA, vol. 36-1-51.

78. Chen Yongyuan, "Nuli zuohao faxing gongzuo, ba chijiao yisheng zazhi songdao chijiao yisheng shouli" [Try to do circulation work well, send the *Journal of Barefoot Doctors* to the hands of barefoot doctors], *Chijiao yisheng zazhi* [Journal of Barefoot Doctors] 34, no. 10 (1976): 14.

79. Farquhar, "Market Magic," 239.

80. White, "Deciphering 'Integrated Chinese and Western Medicine,'" 1333–47.

81. Shanghaishi zhongyi xueyuan, *Chijiao yisheng shouce*, 75–131, 562–81.

82. Ibid., 582–648.

83. Wang Guizhen, "Tiancailun jiu shi fupilun" [Genius theory is restoration theory], *Chijiao yisheng zazhi* [Journal of Barefoot Doctors] 4 (1974): 7.

84. Shao Jungen, interview, November 20, 2009.

85. Scheid, *Chinese Medicine in Contemporary China*, 73.

86. Shen Guanrong, interview, May 27, 2004.

87. Chuanshaxian weishengju [Chuansha County Health Bureau], "Guanyu chijiao yisheng dangqian xianzhuang he gaijin yijian de qingshi baogao" [Report on the current situations of barefoot doctors and suggested improvements], August 1979, PDA, vol. 84-3-29.

88. Gong Youlong and Chao Limin, "Shanghaixian de chijiao yisheng" [Barefoot doctors in Shanghai County], *Shanghai diyi yixueyuan xuebao* [No.1 Shanghai Medical College Journal] 1 (1982): 76.

89. Zhejiangsheng weishengting [Zhejiang Province Health Department], ed., *Nongcun weishengyuan keben* [Rural health worker's textbook] (Hangzhou: Zhejiang renmin chubanshe, 1966); Shanghaishi diyi remin yiyuan erke [Pediatrics Department of Shanghai Municipal No. 1 People's Hospital], ed., *Ertong changyong yaowu* [Common medicines for children] (Shanghai: Shanghai kexue jishu chubanshe, 1966); Hangzhoushi weisheng fangyizhan [Hangzhou Prefecture Sanitation and Epidemic-Prevention Station], ed., *Jiji yufang huxidao chuanranbing* [Actively

preventing infectious respiratory diseases] (Hangzhou: Hangzhoushi weisheng fangyizhan geweihui, 1970); Zhejiangsheng geweihui shengchan zhihuizu weishengju [Health Bureau of the Production Directing Team of Zhejiang Province Revolutionary Committee], ed., *Zhejiang minjian changyong caoyao* [Common folk herbal medicines in Zhejiang Province], vol. 3 (Hangzhou: Zhejiang renmin chubanshe, 1970–72); Hangzhoushi weisheng fangyizhan geming weiyuanhui [Revolutionary Committee of Hangzhou Prefecture Sanitation and Epidemic-Prevention Station], ed., *Nongyao shiyong yu zhongdu fangzhi* [Pesticide use and poisoning prevention] (Hangzhou: Hangzhoushi weisheng fangyizhan geweihui, 1971); Zhejiangsheng weisheng xuanchuan xiezuozu [Zhejiang Province Health Propaganda Coordinating Team], ed., *Weisheng fangyi shouce* [Sanitation and epidemic-prevention manual] (Hangzhou: Zhejiangsheng weisheng xuanchuan xiezuozu, 1974); Chuanshaxian jiangzhen gongshe chijiao yisheng [Barefoot doctors of Jiangzhen Commune, Chuansha County], ed., *Chijiao yisheng changyong yaowu* [Common medicines prescribed by barefoot doctors](Shanghai: Shanghai renmin chubanshe, 1975); and Hangzhoushi jihua shengyu bangongshi [Hangzhou Prefecture Family Planning Office], ed., *Renkou fei kongzhibuxing* [The population must be controlled] (Hangzhou: Hangzhoushi jihua shengyu bangongshi, 1978).

90. Christopher Houng Chin Khng, "Trends in the Utilization of Traditional Chinese Medicines in Rural China: A Case Study of Yuhang County, Zhejiang Province" (master's thesis, Faculty of Graduate Studies, University of Guelph, 2001), 75.

91. Barefoot doctors were renamed "village doctors" in 1985.

92. Chun'anxian weishengju [Chun'an County Health Bureau], "Guanyu xuetugong peixun qijian buzhufei de tongzhi" [Notice on subsidies paid to apprentices during the training period], September 9, 1976, CAA, vol. 36-1-53.

93. Xu Xiaoqun, "National Essence vs. Science: Chinese Native Physicians' Fight for Legitimacy, 1912–1937," *Modern Asian Studies* 31, no. 4 (October 1997): 847–78.

94. Ren Zhentai, ed., *Hangzhou shizhi* [Hangzhou Prefectural Gazetteer], vol. 1 (Beijing: Zhonghua shuju, 1995), 300; and Miao Yubing, "Jiefangqian Hangzhoushi de difang weisheng yiliao" [Local health and medicine in Hangzhou before liberation], in *Hangzhou wenshi zilliao* [Hangzhou Cultural and Historical Data], vol. 6, ed. Zhengxie Hangzhoushi weiyuanhui wenshi ziliao gongzuo weiyuanhui [The Cultural and Historical Data Committee of Hangzhou Prefecture Political Consultative Committee] (Hangzhou: Zhengxie Hangzhoushi weiyuanhui wenshi ziliao gongzuo weiyuanhui, 1988): 77.

95. Hangzhoushi weishengju [Hangzhou Prefecture Health Bureau], "Zhonggong Hangzhoushi weishengju dangzu guanyu guance zhonggong zhongyang (1978) 56 hao wenjian de yijian" [Party Leadership Group of Hangzhou Prefecture Health Bureau's instructions on implementing no. 56 file of the Central Committee of Chinese Communist Party (1978)], February 28, 1979, CAA, vol. 1-2-299. For the research on prestigious old Chinese medicine doctors, see Jun Wang, "A Life History of Ren Yingqiu: Historical Problems, Mythology, Continuity and Difference in Chinese Medical Modernity" (PhD diss., University of North Carolina at Chapel Hill, 2003).

96. Zhonggong weishengbu dangzu [Party Leadership Group of the Ministry of Health], "Guanyu renzhen guance dang de zhongyi zhengce, jiejue zhongyi duiwu houji faren wenti de baogao" [Report on seriously implementing the party's Chinese medicine policies and solving the issue of no qualified successors], August 25, 1978, CAA, vol. 1-2-224.

97. Hangzhoushi weishengju, "Zhonggong Hangzhoushi weishengju dangzu guanyu guance zhonggong zhongyang (1978) 56 hao wenjian de yijian."

Chapter Three

1. Yuhangxian diming weiyuanhui, *Yuhangxian dimingzhi*, 256.

2. Zheng Simin, *Jishengchongbing zhishi* [Knowledge of parasitic diseases] (Shanghai: Shanghai renmin chubanshe, 1973), 10.

3. Jianshe weiyuanhui diaocha Zhejiang jingjisuo [Zhejiang Institute of Economics Survey of Construction Commission], *Zhejiang Lin'an nongcun diaocha* [Rural survey of Lin'an County, Zhejiang Province] (Hangzhou: Jianshe weiyuanhui diaocha Zhejiang jingjisuo, 1931), 59–61.

4. Zhejiang xuexichongbing fangzhishi bianweihui [Editorial board of the history of schistosomiasis prevention and treatment in Zhejiang Province], ed., *Zhejiang xuexichongbing fangzhishi* [The history of schistosomiasis prevention and treatment in Zhejiang Province] (Shanghai: Shanghai kexue jishu chubanshe, 1992), 22; and Zheng, *Jishengchongbing zhishi*, 10.

5. Zhang Binhua, ed., *Chongfu Zhenzhi* [Chongfu Township Gazetteer] (Shanghai: Shanghai shudian chubanshe, 1994), 244.

6. Hubeisheng Changyangxian hejiaping gongshe [Hejiaping Commune, Changyang County, Hubei Province], "Fangshou fadong qunzhong, renzhen gaohao nongcun de liangguan wugai" [Fully Mobilize the Masses and Seriously Undertake "Two Controls and Five Reforms"], *Zhongguo linchuang yisheng* [Journal of Chinese Physicians] 12 (1976): 5.

7. Wang Xiaolan, "Gouchongbing gaishu" [General survey of hookworm knowledge], *Yiyao shijie* [Medicine and the Pharmaceutical World] 6, no. 2 (1951): 32–34.

8. Zheng, *Jishengchongbing zhishi*, 57.

9. Nanfang shisan shengshi "liangguang" "wugai" xuexiban [Training class on "Two Controls" and "Five Reforms" class for thirteen provinces and municipalities in Southern China], ed., *Nanfang nongcun weisheng "liangguan""wugai" ziliao huibian* [Compiled documents of "Two Controls" and "Five Reforms" in rural Southern China] (Beijing: Renmin weisheng chubanshe, 1975).

10. Wang Kewu, Wang Lieting, and He Songtang, eds., *Zhejiang nüeji kongzhi* [Malaria control in Zhejiang] (Hangzhou: Zhejiangsheng weisheng fangyizhan, 1993), 6.

11. Huang Yuguang, "Xiaxiang qiyue jiaoyu shen" [The profound education I received in the countryside over the past seven months], *HZRB*, November 2, 1965.

12. Lin'anxian weishengzhi bianzhuan weiyuanhui, *Lin'anxian weishengzhi*, 271.

13. Wang Kewu, Wang Lieting, and He Songtang, *Zhejiang nüeji kongzhi*, 46.

14. Li Jinghan, *Zhongguo nongcun wenti* [China's rural issues] (Changsha: Shangwu yishuguan, 1939), 103.

15. Hangzhoushi Tingzhi renmin gongshe baojianyuan [Health clinic of Tingzhi People's Commune, Hangzhou City], "Tingzhi renmin gongshe dang'an lishi ziliao huibian, 1949–1958" [Compiled historical data of Tingzhi People's Commune, 1949–1958], April 24, 1959, YHA, vol. 42-1-3.

16. "Yiliaodui xiaxiang zuodao changliushui bu duanxian" [Medical teams should be sent to the countryside continuously], *HZRB*, June 27, 1974.

17. Zhang Weizhong, interview, May 7, 2004.

18. Zheng, *Jishengchongbing zhishi*, 76.

19. Wei Dongpeng, "Transmission and Natural Regulations of Infection with Ascaris Lumbricoides in Rural Community in China," *Journal of Parasitology* 84, no. 2 (April 1998): 252–58.

20. Hangzhoushi Tingzhi renmin gongshe baojianyuan, "Tingzhi renmin gongshe dang'an lishi ziliao huibian."

21. Hangzhoushi weisheng fangyizhan [Hangzhou Prefecture Sanitation and Epidemic Prevention Station], *Yiqing ziliao huibian, 1950–1979* [Compiled data on epidemic diseases, 1950–1979] (Hangzhou: Hangzhoushi fangyizhan, 1982), preface.

22. Hangzhoushi weisheng fangyizhan, *Yiqing ziliao huibian, 1950–1979*, 2.

23. Ren, *Hangzhou shizhi*, 1:462.

24. In 1950, the People's Liberation Army stationed in Fujian and Zhejiang undertook a course in amphibious training to prepare for the military unification of Taiwan. However, large numbers were infected by schistosomiasis and became incapacitated by the liver disease it causes. The plan was finally aborted. See Edward Earl Rice, *Mao's Way* (Berkeley: University of California Press, 1972), 149–50; and Gross, "Chasing Snails," 64–65.

25. By 1983, death caused by acute infectious diseases was no longer one of the top ten factors. See Yuhangxian weishengju weishengzhi bianzhuanzu, *Yuhangxian weishengzhi*, 234–35.

26. The available statistic data indicate that acute infectious diseases ranked ninth among causes of death in both Fuyang and Jiande Counties, and seventh in Xiaoshan and Lin'an Counties in 1974–76. See Xu, *Fuyangxian weishengzhi*, 323; Xiaoshanshi weisheng fangyizhan [Xiaoshan City Sanitation and Epidemic-Prevention Station], ed., *Xiaoshan weisheng fangyizhi* [Xiaoshan City Sanitation and Epidemic-Prevention Gazetteer] (Xiaoshan: Xiaoshanshi weisheng fangyizhan, 1996), 224; Yan, *Jiandexian yiyao weishengzhi*, 155; and Lin'anxian weishengzhi bianzhuan weiyuanhui, *Lin'anxian weishengzhi*, 315.

27. Zhang Ahniu, interview, January 23, 2005.

28. Zheng Jinzhu, interview, November 19, 2009.

29. Yuhangxian weishengju weishengzhi bianzhuanzu, *Yuhangxian weishengzhi*, 249.

30. Ibid., 254.

31. See Blumenthal and Hsiao, "Privatization and Its Contents," 1165–69; and Gail Henderson, "Issues in the Modernization of Medicine in China," in *Science and Technology in Post-Mao China*, ed. Denis Fred Simon and Merle Goldman (Cambridge, MA: Harvard University Press, 1989), 200–201.

32. Li Yushang, "The Elimination of Schistosomiasis in Jiaxing and Haining Counties, 1948–1958," 205–6.

33. Xu Xifan, "Fangzhizhu xuexichongbing" [Preventing schistosomiasis], *Dongnan ribao* [Southeastern Daily]. December 12, 1948.

34. Mobo C. F. Gao, *Gao Village: A Portrait of Rural Life in Modern China* (Honolulu: University of Hawai'i Press, 1999), 133.

35. Maurice Meisner, *Mao's China: A History of the People's Republic* (New York: Free Press, 1977), 235.

36. Village women who participated in agricultural production in the people's commune era still admire the "happiness" of their mothers and grandmothers before "liberation," and deplored the hardship of manual labor during the collective era.

37. Chen Zhicheng, interview, November 6, 2009; Yan, *Jiandexian yiyao weishengzhi,* 107–8.

38. Zhu Deming, "Jindai Hangzhou zhongyaodian gouchen" [The history of Chinese medicine shops in modern Hangzhou], *Zhonghua yishi zazhi* [Chinese Journal of Medical History] 36, no. 4 (October 2006): 243.

39. Wu Shichun, ed., *Qianhong cunzhi* [Qianhong Village Gazetteer] (Yiwu: Qianhong cunzhi bianzhuan weiyuanhui, 1996), 150.

40. Angela Ki Che Leung argues that the wide distribution of private medicine shops indicates that a nationwide commercialization of medicine was steadily prevalent from the fifteenth century onward, in addition to medicine peddlers. See Leung, "Mingdai shehui zhong de yiyao," 354. See also Fan Rusen and Ji Tianshu, "Jindai beifang yaoping gongying tixi de jiangou" [The development of pharmaceutical supply and marketing systems in modern north China], *Zhongguo lishi dili lunchong* [Collections of Essays on Chinese Historical Geography] 18, no. 2 (June 2003): 104–13; and Liu Luya, "Jiuzhongguo de zhiyaoye" [The pharmaceutical industry in the old China], *Lishi dang'an* [Historical Archives] 2 (1995): 105–12.

41. For sales strategies and pharmaceutical consumption in urban areas in modern China, see Sherman Cochran, *Chinese Medicine Men: Consumer Culture in China and Southeast Asia* (Cambridge, MA: Harvard University Press, 2006).

42. Qiao Qiming, *Zhongguo nongcun shehui jingjixue* [Social economics of rural China] (Shanghai: Shanghai shudian, 1992), 308–9.

43. From 1881 to 1926, Duncan David Main, another British missionary doctor, was in charge of this hospital. See Xiaoping Fang, "Dedicated to a Medical Career in the 'Heaven Below': Duncan David Main's Correspondence, 1914–1926," Research Report, Rockefeller Archive Center (RAC), 2008.

44. Hangzhou yiyao shangyezhi bianzhuan weiyuanhui [Editorial board of Hangzhou Pharmaceutical Commerce Gazetteer], ed., *Hangzhou yiyao shangyezhi* [Hangzhou Pharmaceutical Commerce Gazetteer] (Beijing: Zhongguo qingnian chubanshe, 1990), 9.

45. Xu, *Fuyangxian weishengzhi,* 329–30; Wang Qing, ed., *Yuhang shizhi* [Yuhang City Gazetteer] (Beijing: Zhonghuashuju, 2000), 173; Zhou Jinkui, ed., *Jiande xianzhi* [Jiande County Gazetteer] (Hangzhou: Zhejiang renmin chubanshe, 1986), 710–11; and Chun'an xianzhi bianzhuan weiyuanhui [Editorial board of Chun'an County Gazetteer], ed., *Chun'an xianzhi* [Chun'an County Gazetteer] (Shanghai: Hanyu dacidian chubanshe, 1990), 608.

46. Zhejiangsheng yiyaozhi bianzhuan weiyuanhui [Editorial board of Zhejiang Province Pharmaceutical Gazetteer], ed., *Zhejiangsheng yiyaozhi* [Zhejiang Province Pharmaceutical Gazetteer] (Beijing: Fangzhi chubanshe, 2003), 346.

47. Shi Fu, ed., *Jinhua xianzhi* [Jinhua County Gazetteer] (Hangzhou: Zhejiang renmin chubanshe, 1992), 648.

48. Shao Jungen, interview, November 20, 2009.

49. For more on pharmaceuticals in modern Zhejiang, see Zhu Deming, *Zhejiang yiyaoshi* [The history of medicine and pharmaceuticals in Zhejiang] (Beijing: Renmin junyi chubanshe, 1999), 80–115.

50. *Gongsi heying* (state-private joint ownership) was the principal form adopted during the socialist transformation of capitalist enterprises in China in the mid-1950s. See Qi Moujia, ed., *Dangdai zhongguo de yiyao shiye* [Pharmaceuticals in contemporary China] (Beijing: Zhongguo shehui kexue chubanshe, 1988), 284–88.

51. Chen Zhicheng, interview, November 6, 2009.

52. Yu Hui, "Zhongguo zhengfu yaoye guanzhi zhidu xingcheng zhangai de fenxi" [The analysis of obstacles formed by Chinese government pharmaceutical management institutions], *Guanli shijie* [Management World], Part I, 5 (1997): 126–35; Part II, 6 (1997): 87–95.

53. Hangzhou yiyao shangyezhi bianzhuan weiyuanhui, *Hangzhou yiyao shangyezhi*, 127.

54. Shao Jungen, interview, November 20, 2009.

55. Hangzhou yiyao shangyezhi bianzhuan weiyuanhui, *Hangzhou yiyao shangyezhi*, 124.

56. Yuhangxian weishengju [Yuhang County Health Bureau], "Sheng guiding diyipi zhongxi chengyao xiaxiang pinzhongbiao" [Inventory of the first batch of Chinese and Western patent medicines sent to the countryside on the orders of the provincial government], October 21, 1965, YHA, vol. 42-1-29.

57. "Guanyu kaizhan zhongxi chengyao xiaxiang shidian qingkuang de baogao" [Report on pilot work of Chinese and Western medicines sent to the countryside], October 21, 1965, YHA, vol. 42-1-29.

58. Hangzhou yiyao shangyezhi bianzhuan weiyuanhui, *Hangzhou yiyao shangyezhi*, 125.

59. Shen Xianbing, interview, January 10, 2005.

60. Luo Zhengfu, interview, November 23, 2009.

61. Zhongguo yaocai gongsi, Zhongguo yiyao gongsi, Zhejiang Jiande gongsi [Pharmaceutical company of Jiande County Zhejiang Province of China *materia medica* company and China pharmaceutical company], "1965 nian gongzuo zongjie" [Work summary of 1965], January 30, 1966, JDA, vol. 31-3-12.

62. Chun'anxian weishengju geweihui, Chun'anxian shangyeju geweihui [Revolutionary Committee of Chun'an County Health Bureau, Revolutionary Committee of Chun'an County Commerce Bureau], "Guanyu tiaozheng yiyao shangpin pizhuan shouxufei de tongzhi" [Instruction on adjusting commission charges on wholesale pharmaceuticals], December 24, 1971, CAA, vol. 36-1-46.

63. Shen Xianbing, interview, January 9, 2005; Chen Zhicheng, interview, January 10, 2005; and Luo Aijuan, interview, March 26, 2007.

64. Zhongguo yiyao gongsi [China Pharmaceutical Company], ed., *Zhongguo yiyao shangye shigao* [The history of pharmaceutical commerce in China] (Shanghai: Shanghai shehui kexueyuan chubanshe, 1990), 367.

65. Chun'anxian weishengju, Chun'anxian shangyeju [Chun'an County Health Bureau, Chun'an County Commerce Bureau], "Guanyu paiyuan canjia zhongxi yaopin qixie zhanxiao de tongzhi" [Instruction on assigning staff to attend Chinese and Western medicine and medical machinery exhibition], April 1, 1979, CAA, vol. 36-1-57.

66. Wang Wenzhi, ed., *Fuyang xianzhi* [Fuyang County Gazetteer] (Hangzhou: Zhejiang renmin chubanshe, 1993), 218.

67. Though still very expensive by late 1950s, the use of antibiotics had been increasing steadily. Compared with 1952, the use of antibiotics in the whole China increased by 580 percent. These antibiotics were very effective in clinical treatment. For example, before the application of antibiotics in China, the mortality rate of acute appendicitis complicated by peritonitis reached 5–10 percent. After antibiotics were applied, the rate dropped to only 0.5 percent. See Meng Qian, "Heli shiyong kangshengshu" [Use antibiotics properly], *RMRB*, February 24, 1957.

68. "Zhongxi jiehe, tuyang jiehe, renzhen banhao hezuo yiliao" [To combine Chinese and Western, combine folk and foreign, and implement cooperative medical services seriously], *RMRB*, January 31, 1969.

69. "Weida lingxiu maozhuxi shenqie guanhuai guangda geming renmin zai quanguo fanwei nei shixian yaopin quanmian dafudu jiangjia" [Great Leader Chairman Mao takes care of the vast masses of revolutionary people and implements complete and large-scale price reduction], *RMRB*, September 25, 1969.

70. Zhongguo yiyao gongsi, *Zhongguo yiyao shangye shigao*, 273.

71. "Woguo yiyao gongye you henda de fazhan" [Our nation's pharmaceutical industry has advanced by great strides], *HZRB*, February 28, 1972.

72. "Weida lingxiu maozhuxi shenqie guanhuai guangda geming renmin zai quanguo fanwei nei shixian yaopin quanmian dafudu jiangjia," *RMRB*, September 25, 1969; Zhongguo yiyao gongsi, *Zhongguo yiyao shangye shigao*, 362.

73. Shen Xianbing, interview, January 10, 2005.

74. Ibid.

75. Luo Zhengfu, interview, November 23, 2009.

76. Hong Jinglin, interview, November 10, 2009.

77. Xiaoshanshi weisheng fangyizhan, *Xiaoshan weisheng fangyizhi*, 52.

78. Carol Benedict, "Bubonic Plague in Nineteenth-Century China," *Modern China* 14, no. 2 (April 1988): 138.

79. Yan, *Jiandexian yiyao weishengzhi*, 144.

80. For more information on the research into and invention of the measles vaccine, see Scott B. Halstead and Yu Yong-xin, "Human Viral Vaccines in China," in *Science and Medicine in Twentieth-Century China: Research and Education*, ed. John Z. Bowers, J. William Hess, and Nathan Sivin (Ann Arbor, MI: Center for Chinese Studies, University of Michigan, 1988), 144–46.

81. Lin'anxian weishengzhi bianzhuan weiyuanhui, *Lin'anxian weishengzhi*, 257–58.

82. Xiaoshan weishengju, *Xiaoshan weishengzhi*, 163; and Yuhangxian weisheng fangyizhan [Yuhang County Sanitation and Epidemic-Prevention Station], ed., *Yuhangxian weisheng fangyizhi* [Yuhang County Sanitation and Epidemic Prevention Gazetteer] (Hangzhou: Zhejiangsheng Yuhangxian weisheng fangyizhan, 1990), 58.

83. Lin'anxian weishengzhi bianzhuan weiyuanhui, *Lin'anxian weishengzhi*, 26.

84. Hangzhoushi weisheng fangyizhan, *Yiqing ziliao huibian, 1950–1979*, 12.

85. Shen Xianbing, interview, January 10, 2005.

86. Fuyang jihua shengyu weiyuanhui [Fuyang County Family Planning Committee], "Guanyu quanguo shixing mianfei gongying biyunyao he biyun gongju de jinji lianhe tongzhi" [Emergent joint notice on supplying free prophylactics and

contraceptives nationwide], January 1974, FYA, vol. 74-3-13; Yu Fuquan, interview, May 12, 2004.

87. Fuyangxian weishengju geming weiyuanhui [Revolutionary committee of the Fuyang County Health Bureau], "Guanyu diaobo gei bufen gongshe fanghuan quhuan shoushu qixie de tongzhi" [Notice on supplying IUD instruments to some commune clinics], December 27, 1973, FYA, vol. 74-3-10.

88. Sidel and Sidel, *Serve the People*.

89. "1972 nian weisheng gongzuo yijian" [Instructions on Health Work in 1972], April 1, 1972, CAA, vol. 36-1-48.

90. "Shenshou pinxia zhongnong huanying de hezuo yiliao," *RMRB*, December 5, 1968.

91. "Weida lingxiu maozhuxi shenqie guanhuai geming renmin, quanguo fanwei nei shixian yaopin quanmian dafudu jiangjia" [Great Leader Chairman Mao takes care of the vast masses of revolutionary people and implements complete and large-scale price reduction], *RMRB*, September 25, 1969.

92. Hangzhou yiyao shangyezhi bianzhuan weiyuanhui, *Hangzhou yiyao shangyezhi*, 11.

93. Zhongguo yiyao gongsi, *Zhongguo yiyao shangye shigao*, 32.

94. Zheng Chunyan, interview, March 23, 2004.

95. Zhonggong Anxi gongshe dangwei [The Anxi Commune Committee of the Communist Party of China], "Zai douzhengzhong jianchi tuiguang zhongcaoyao" [Promoting Chinese herbal medicine in the struggles], April 11, 1975, YHA, vol. 42-1-51.

96. Zhejiangsheng geweihui shengchan zhihuizu weishengju, *Zhejiang minjian changyong caoyao*.

97. Yan, *Jiandexian yiyao weishengzhi*, 125–33; Yu, *Chun'anxian weishengzhi*, 347–54; Xu, *Fuyangxian weishengzhi*, 255–60; Lin'anxian weishengzhi bianzhuan weiyuanhui, *Lin'anxian weishengzhi*, 344–50; and Xiaoshan weishengju, *Xiaoshan weishengzhi*, 207–9.

98. Chen Zhicheng, interview, January 6, 2005.

99. Chen Zhicheng, interview, January 5, 2005; Zhu Shouhua, interview, January 5, 2005; Xu Shuilin, interview, November 6, 2009; and Luo Zhengfu, interview, November 23, 2009.

100. "Woguo nongcun hezuo yiliao buduan gonggu fazhan" [Cooperative medical services in our country keep developing steadily], *HZRB*, September 28, 1973.

101. Chen Zhicheng, interview, January 6, 2005.

102. Ibid.

103. Shen Guanrong, interview, May 27, 2004.

104. Yu Fuquan, interview, May 12, 2005.

105. "Zhuajin jijie cai yaocai" [Lose no time in collecting herbal medicines], *Chijiao yisheng zazhi* [Journal of Barefoot Doctors] 8, no. 2 (1974): 45;

106. Shanghaishi Chuanshaxian Jiangzhen gongshe weishengyuan [Jiangzhen Commune Clinic of Chuansha County, Shanghai Municipality], ed., *Chijiao yisheng jiaocai: Gong nanfang diqu fuxun shiyong* [Barefoot doctor textbooks: For retraining in Southern China] (Beijing: Renmin weisheng chubanshe, 1974), 745–49.

107. Guangdongsheng zhiwu yanjiusuo caiyao zhishi bianxiezu [Editorial team of Knowledge of Collecting Herbal Medicine, Guangdong Province Botanical Research

Institute], ed., *Caiyao zhishi* [Knowledge of Collecting Herbal Medicine] (Guangzhou: Guangdong renmin chubanshe, 1977), 33–35.

108. Zhonggong Anxi gongshe dangwei, "Zai douzhengzhong jianchi tuiguang zhongcaoyao."

109. Mr. Cat-Dog, interview, April 20, 2004.

110. Zhonggong Anxi gongshe dangwei, "Zai douzhengzhong jianchi tuiguang zhongcaoyao."

111. Zhonggong Beijingshi Pingguxian huangsongyu gongshe huangsongyu dadui zhibu [Communist Party of China branch of the Huangsongyu Brigade, Huangsongyu Commune, Pinggu County, Beijing Municipality], "Yi dang de jiben luxian weigang, gonggu fazhan hezuo yiliao" [Take the party's basic route as guiding principle, strengthen and develop cooperative medical services], *Chijiao yisheng zazhi* [Journal of Barefoot Doctors] 2 (1974): 11.

112. Guangdong Guangzhoushi yaopin jianyansuo [The Institute for Drug Control of Guangzhou City, Guangdong Province], "Shenru nongcun, chujin zhongcaoyao zhiji zhiliang de tigao" [Going to rural areas and improving the quality of Chinese herbal medicine preparation], *Xin yixue* [New Medicine] 9, 1 (1978): 1.

113. Jiandexian weishengju [Jiande County Health Bureau], "Nongcun weisheng gongzuo jiben qingkuang" [Basic situations of rural health work], September 1974, JDA, vol. 31-4-11.

114. Luo Zhengfu, interview, November 23, 2009.

115. Yan Shengyu, interview, May 27, 2007.

116. Yan, *Jiandexian yiyao weishengzhi*, 125.

117. Zhu Shouhua, interview, January 5, 2005.

118. Hengjin Dong, Lennart Bogg, Clas Rehnberg, and Vinod Diwan, "Drug Policy in China: Pharmaceuticals Distribution in Rural Areas," *Social Science & Medicine* 48, no. 6 (March 1999): 777–86.

Chapter Four

1. According to Huanguang Jia's observations in Shanxi Province, the unification of the two medical systems before the Cultural Revolution was merely symbolic and superficial. Chinese medicine and Western medicine remained almost entirely separate until 1967. See Huanguang Jia, "Chinese Medicine in Post-Mao China: Standardization and the Context of Modern Science" (PhD diss., University of North Carolina, Chapel Hill, 1997), 28.

2. Chen Hongting, interview, April 2004. See also Farquhar, *Knowing Practice*, 61–146.

3. Chen Zhicheng, interview, November 6, 2009.

4. Hangzhoushi Tingzhi renmin gongshe baojianyuan, "Tingzhi renmin gongshe dang'an lishi ziliao huibian."

5. Wang, "Life History of Ren Yingqiu," 46.

6. Linqiqu weishengyuan [Linqi Districit Clinic], "Linqiqu yaozheng jiancha baogao" [Investigative report of pharmaceutical work in Linqi District], November 9, 1965, CAA, vol. 75-1-76.

7. Chun'anxian renmin weiyuanhui weishengke [Health Bureau of Chun'an County People's Committee], "Yi zhengdun gonggu tigao zhiliang, qinjian ban weisheng shiye" [Strengthening and improving medical service through adjustment, doing health work frugally], June 13, 1957, CAA, vol. 36-1-26. Pyramidon mainly treats headache, joint pain, and muscle pain, etc. For some patients, it will decrease the number of granulocytes and causeaplastic anemia. In the 1970s, it was advised that this medicine should not be prescribed as the preferred analgesic and antipyretic drug. See Chuanshaxian jiangzhen gongshe chijiao yisheng, *Chijiao yisheng changyongyaowu*, 35.

8. Lin'anxian weishengju [Lin'an County Health Bureau], "Guanyu 1966 nian weisheng gongzuo de yijian" [Instructionson health work in 1966], February 17, 1966, LAA.

9. There were a total of three films describing barefoot doctors in the 1970s: *Chunmiao*, directed by Xie Jin, Shanghai Film Factory, 1975; *Hongyu*, directed by Cui Wei, Beijing Film Factory, 1975; and *Yanmin hupan*, directed by Gao Tianhong, Changchun Film Factory, 1975. *Hongyu* was based on a novel. See Yang Xiao, *The Making of a Peasant Doctor* (Beijing: Foreign Language Press, 1976). *Yanming Hupan* tells the story of how a barefoot doctor strengthened the cooperative medical service by struggling against a bad doctor who was hiding inside the medical station in a village in northeastern China.

10. Ge Zichang, "Zhongguo diyige nü chijiao yisheng de quzhe rensheng" [The intricate life of the first Chinese female barefoot doctor], *Guizhou wenshi tiandi* [Guizhou Literature and History World] 2 (2001): 33.

11. Zhang Xun, "Wuchan jieji wenhua dageming de zange: Ping caise gushipian Chunmiao" [The paean of the great proletariat cultural revolution: Comments on color movie *Chunmiao*], *ZJRB*, December 2, 1975.

12. Stanley Joel Reiser, *Medicine and the Reign of Technology* (Cambridge: Cambridge University Press, 1978), 1.

13. Bray, *Technology and Gender*, 313.

14. Kleinman, *Patients and Healers in the Context of Culture*, 262.

15. Xu Peichun, interview, May 14, 2004.

16. Yan Shengyu, interview, May 26, 2004.

17. Xu Peichun, interview, May 13, 2004.

18. Yan Shengyu, interview, May 26, 2004.

19. Chao, *Medicine and Society in Late Imperial China*, 158.

20. See Cullen, "Patients and Healers in Late Imperial China," 120; Lu Gwei-djen and Joseph Needham, *Celestial Lancets: A History and Rationale of Acupuncture and Moxa* (New York: Cambridge University Press, 1980), 160; Furth, *Flourishing Yin*, 277; and Chao, *Medicine and Society in Late Imperial China*, 159–60.

21. Hangxian weisheng gongzuozhe xiehui [Hang County Medical Practitioners and Workers Association], "Zhongyi daibiao dahui zongjie" [Summary of the Chinese medicine doctors' meeting], May 1955, YHA, vol. 13-5-106.

22. Zhou Ruhan, ed., *Yuhang xianzhi* [Yuhang County Gazetteer] (Hangzhou: Zhejiang renmin chubanshe, 1990), 768.

23. Xu Peichun, interview, May 13, 2004.

24. Shao Jungen, interview, November 20, 2009.

25. Xu Peichun, interview, May 14, 2004.

26. Ibid.

27. Zhou Yonggan, interview, November 6, 2009.

28. Xu Peichun, interview, May 15, 2004.

29. Xu Peichun, interview, May 14, 2004.

30. Yan Shengyu, interview, May 26, 2004.

31. Zhonggong Yuhangxian weishengju zongzhi [Yuhang County Committee Branch of the Communist Party of China], "Dali tuiguang shiyong zhongcaoyao, gonggu he fazhan hezuo yiliao" [Promoting Chinese herbal medicines vigorously, strengthening and developingthe cooperative medical services], April 15, 1975, YHA, vol. 150-1-52.

32. Zhonggong fuyang xianwei [Fuyang County Committee of the Communist Party of China], "Guanyu yushan gongshe gonggu he fazhan hezuo yiliao de diaocha baogao" [Investigative report on how Yushan Commune strengthens and develops its cooperative medical service], May 1972, FYA, vol. 74-3-11.

33. Xu Peichun, interview, May 14, 2004; and Yan Shengyu, interview, May 26, 2004.

34. Fang Jianxin, interview, December 23, 2005.

35. Yan Shengyu, interview, May 26, 2004.

36. Zheng Xuedong, interview, December 3, 2005.

37. "Jianchi luxian douzheng, gonggu hezuo yiliao" [Stay on the path of struggle and strengthen the cooperative medical service], *HZRB*, July 5, 1972.

38. Yan Shengyu, interview, May 26, 2004.

39. Fang Shunxi, interview, May 9, 2004.

40. Xu Peichun, interview, May 13, 2004.

41. Yuhangxian weishengju, "Xuexi maozhuxi guanyu lilun wenti de zhishi, jinyibu banhao hezuo yiliao."

42. Fuyangxian weishengju [Health Bureau of Fuyang County], "Quansheng weisheng gongzuo huiyi wenjian: Jixu gonggu he fazhan hezuo yiliao" [Files of the provincial health work meeting: To further strengthen and develop cooperative medical services], May 1980, FYA, vol. 74-3-26.

43. Fang Benpei, interview, December 4, 2005.

44. Li and Xu, "Yiliao weishengwang," 94.

45. Yuhangxian weishengju [Yuhang County Health Bureau], "Guanyu juban nongcun yishiban de jidian yijian" [A few instructions on convening training courses for rural doctors], October 27, 1986, SDA.

46. For more on diagnosis and healing through the integration of Chinese and Western medicine, see Volker Scheid, "Shaping Chinese Medicine: Two Cases from Contemporary China," in *Innovation in Chinese Medicine*, ed. Elisabeth Hsu (Cambridge: Cambridge University Press, 2001), 370–404; and*Chinese Medicine in Contemporary China*, 150–51, 227, 254.

47. Luo Aijuan, interview, April 15, 2007.

48. Bradley P. Stoner, "Understanding Medical Systems: Traditional, Modern, and Syncretic Health Care Alternatives in Medically Pluralistic Societies," *Medial Anthropology Quarterly* 17, no. 2 (February 1986): 45; and Charles Leslie, *Asian Medical Systems: A Comparative Study* (Berkeley: University of California Press, 1976), 6–7.

49. Shen, *Yuhangxian jiangcunxiang xueyi de tulangzhong*, 93.

50. David Landy, "Role Adaptation: Traditional Curers under the Impact of Western Medicine," *American Ethnologist* 1, no. 1 (February 1974): 103–27. The phenomenon also occurred in the remote border areas. Liu Xiaoxing found that it was common for ritual practitioners, especially the younger ones, to learn to about the use of biomedicine drugs and techniques in Chuxiong, Yunnan Province. See Liu, "Change and Continuity of Yi Medical Culture in Southwest China," 232.

51. Elisabeth Hsu, "The Reception of Western Medicine in China: Examples from Yunnan," in *Science and Empires: Historical Studies about Scientific Development and European Expansion,* vol.136, ed. Patrick Petitjean, Catherine Jami, and Anne Marie Moulin (Dordrecht, Boston: Kluwer Academic Publishers, 1992), 101; and Establet, "Resistance and Receptivity," 171–203.

52. Sean Hsiang-lin Lei also argues that "the Chinese people as a whole were too poor to act on a belief in any kind of medicine at all." See Lei, "When Chinese Medicine Encountered the State, 1928–1937," 15.

53. Shao Jungen, interview, November 20, 2009.

54. Yuhangxian weishengju, "Guanyu kaizhan zhongxi chengyao xiaxiang shidian qingkuang de baogao."

55. Roy Porter argued that social commercialization influenced the way that English villagers acquired medicines. Medicines were not solely obtained from the fields anymore, but were bought in shops instead. Roy Porter, "The Patient in England, C1660–C1800," in *Medicine in Society: Historical Essays,* ed. Andrew Wear (Cambridge: Cambridge University Press, 1992), 91–118.

56. Hangzhou yiyao shangyezhi bianzhuan weiyuanhui, *Hangzhou yiyao shangyezhi,* 182. In the villages around Hangzhou areas during the 1970s, peasants usually used a pole to carry heavy things.

57. Zhonggong Anxi gongshe dangwei, "Zai douzhengzhong jianchi tuiguang zhongcaoyao." Regarding the decoction process of *materia medica,* see Farquhar, "Eating Chinese Medicine," *Cultural Anthropology* 9, no. 4 (November 1994):476.

58. Fang Benpei, interview, April 22, 2006.

59. "Hezuo yiliao shiwunian: Lin'anxian Hengxi gongshe de diaocha" [Implementing cooperative medical service for 15 years: An investigative report into Hengxi Commune, Lin'an County], *HZRB,* June 25, 1973.

60. Zhonggong Yuhangxian weishengju zongzhi, "Dali tuiguang shiyong zhongcaoyao, gonggu he fazhan hezuo yiliao."

61. Jiang Genyu, interview, May 18, 2004.

62. In Lin Village, Fujian Province, Huang Shumin found that the villagers visited the clinic for any problem they experienced and often demanded the most expensive medicine for minor illnesses. See Huang Shumin, "Transforming China's Collective Health Care System: A Village Study," *Social Science & Medicine* 27, no. 9 (1988): 882.

63. "Lin'an Qingshan gongshe tuiguang caoyi caoyao de diaocha" [Investigative report of the promotion of herbal medicinal men and herbal medicines in Qingshan Commune, Lin'an County], *HZRB,* November 22, 1969.

64. "Xuehao wuchanjieji zhuanzheng lilun, wei hanwei maozhuxi geming weisheng luxian er fendou" [Study the proletarian dictatorship theory, strive to safeguard Chairman Mao's revolutionary health route], *Chijiao yisheng xianjin shiji huibian* [Collection of model deeds of barefoot doctors] (Beijing: Renmin weisheng chubanshe, 1974), 27.

65. Chun'an xianzhi bianzhuan weiyuanhui, *Chun'an xianzhi*, 107.

66. See also Kleinman, *Patients and Healers in the Context of Culture*, 87.

67. Ibid., 94.

68. Felix Mann, "Chinese Traditional Medicine: A Practitioner's View," *China Quarterly* 23 (July–September 1965): 31.

69. See also Mao Boying, Gao Xi, and Hong Zhongli, *Zhongguo yixue wenhuashi* [The history of Chinese medical culture] (Shanghai: Shanghai renmin chubanshe, 1994), 801; Henderson and Cohen, *Chinese Hospital*, 121; and Lei Jin, "From Mainstream to Marginal? Trends in the Use of Chinese Medicine in China from 1991 to 2004," *Social Science & Medicine* 71, no. 6 (September 2010): 1066.

70. Interestingly, in Zengbu Brigade, Guangdong Province, in southern China, where the Potters did their anthropological fieldwork, the villagers held the same comparative medical beliefs about Chinese and Western medicine. But the Potters found that "the people of Zengbu—both laymen and medical practitioners alike—believed firmly in the superiority of Chinese medicine. . . . Most of the prescriptions given by the doctor at the health clinic (and by lay practitioners in the village) were for Chinese herbs. The brigade operated a Chinese medicine herbal shop." See Potter and Potter, *China's Peasants*, 133–34.

71. Khng, "Trends in the Utilization of Traditional Chinese Medicines in Rural China," 98–102. Based on the fieldwork in Yunnan in 1989–90, Elisabeth Hsu argues that Chinese and Western medicines are both considered scientific. In contrast to traditional Chinese medicine, modern Western medicine is ascribed the characteristic of modern technology and believed to cause rapid recovery. See Hsu, "Western Medicine in Yunnan," 99. See also Kleinman, *Patients and Healers in the Context of Culture*, 194; and Farquhar, *Knowing Practice*, 20.

72. Shorter, "History of the Doctor-Patient Relationship," 789. See also George Ritzer and David Walczak, "Rationalization and the Deprofessionalization of Physicians," *Social Forces* 67, no. 1 (September 1988): 14.

73. Yan Shengyu, interview, May 26, 2004.

74. Xu Shuilin, interview, November 5, 2009.

75. World Bank, *Financing Health Care: Issues and Options for China* (Washington, DC: World Bank, 1997), 1.

76. Zhonggong Fuyang xianwei, "Guanyu yushan gongshe gonggu he fazhan hezuo yiliao de diaocha baogao."

77. "Qiongdui zenyang ban hezuo yiliao" [How a poor brigade should run the cooperative medical service], *RMRB*, May 23, 1969.

78. Fuyangxian weishengju [Fuyang County Health Bureau], "Xianwei changwei Yao Yansheng tongzhi zai xian weisheng gongzuo huiyi shang de jianghua" [The speech of the standing committee member of the County Party Committee Comrade Yao Yansheng at the county health work meeting], April 26, 1977, FYA, vol. 74-3-26.

79. Shaoxingshi weishengju geweihui, "Gonggu he fazhan hezuo yiliao, jixu gaohao nongcun weisheng geming."

80. Shanghaishi weishengju [Shanghai Municipal Health Bureau], "Shanghaishi jiaoxian hezuo yiliao shidian qingkuang baogao" [Report on experimental cooperative medical services in suburban counties of Shanghai Municipality], June 1969, SHA, vol. 13242-2-76; and Fujiansheng weishengzhi bianzhuan weiyuanhui [Editorial board of the Fujian Province Health Gazetteer], ed., *Fujiansheng weishengzhi* [Fujian

Province Health Gazetteer] (Fuzhou: Fujiansheng weishengzhi bianzhuan weiyuan-hui, 1989), 610–11.

81. Zhonggong Yuhangxian weishengju dangzongzhi [General branch of the Communist Party of China of the Yuhang County Health Bureau], "Guanyu shuangxia hou zhaokai hezuo yiliao yu chijiao yisheng daibiao dahui de qingshi baogao" [Request for convening the county cooperative medical service and bare-foot doctor representative meeting after summer harvesting and planting], July 1974, YHA, vol. 42-1-37.

82. Xiaoping Fang, "Zhongguo nongcun de chijiao yisheng yu hezuo yiliao zhidu: Zhejiangsheng fuyangxian de gean yanjiu" [Barefoot doctors and cooperative medi-cal services in rural china: A case study of Fuyang County, Zhejiang Province], *Ershiyi shiji* [Twenty-First Century] 79 (October 2003): 87–98.

83. Duckett, *The Chinese State's Retreat from Health*, 67; Zhu Ling, "Zhengfu yu non-gcun jiben yiliao baojian baozhang zhidu xuanze" [The government and options for alternative medical and health systems in rural areas], *Zhongguo shehui kexue* [Social Sciences in China], 4 (2000): 91–92; Wang, "Xuexi jizhi yu shiying nengli," 121; and Lampton, *Politics of Medicine*, 237–40.

84. Chen Zhicheng, interview, January 10, 2005.

85. Lampton argues that the number of brigades implementing cooperative med-ical services varied with the rise and fall of food grain production. See Lampton, *Politics of Medicine*, 238.

86. Fang Shunxi, interview, May 9, 2004.

87. Banister, *China's Changing Population*, 62; Hangzhoushi weishengju Hang-zhoushi weishengzhi bianji weiyuanhui, *Hangzhoushi weishengzhi*, 84–85.

88. Hangzhoushi weishengju, "Hangzhou diqu nongcun shengchan dadui shengchandui weisheng zuzhi qingkuang" [Survey of health organizations in pro-duction brigades and production teams in Hangzhou Prefecture], 1975, HZA, vol. 87-3-302; "Hangzhou diqu nongcun shengchan dadui shengchandui weisheng zuzhi qingkuang," 1976, HZA, vol. 87-3-307.

89. Shaoxingshi weishengju [Shaoxing Prefecture Health Bureau], "Guanyu sha-oxing xinchang liangxian hezuo yiliao qingkuang de diaocha baogao" [Investigative report of the cooperative medical services in Shaoxing and Xinchang Counties], June 1973, SXA, vol. GC.13-61-36-3-5-11.

90. Xu Shuilin, interview, November 5, 2009.

91. Yan, *Jiandexian yiyao weishengzhi*, 116; and Ren, *Hangzhou shizhi*, 1: 416.

92. Qi, *Dangdai zhongguo de yiyao shiye*,150–59.

93. Luo Aijuan, interview, May 24, 2011. Regarding the comparative effects of Chi-nese patent medicine and *materia medica*, see Farquhar, "Eating Chinese Medicine," 476.

94. Yan Shengyu, interview, May 22, 2011.

95. Scheid, *Chinese Medicine in Contemporary China*, 94–95.

96. Hangzhou yiyao shangyezhi bianzhuan weiyuanhui, *Hangzhou yiyao shangyezhi*, 87.

97. Shao Jungen, interview, November 20, 2009.

98. Fang Benpei, May 21, 2011.

99. Hangzhou yiyao shangyezhi bianzhuan weiyuanhui, *Hangzhou yiyao shangyezhi*, 88–89.

100. Fang Benpei, interview, May 21, 2011.

101. Zheng Jinzhu, interview, May 23, 2011.

102. Yan, *Jiandexian yiyao weishengzhi*, 112–13; and Ren, *Hangzhou shizhi*, 1: 416.

103. Huang Shuze and LinShixiao, eds., *Dangdai zhongguo de weisheng shiye* [Health development in contemporary China], vol. 2 (Beijing: Zhongguo shehui kexue chubanshe, 1986), 301–15.

104. Ibid., 301.

105. Xu Tong, "Combing Traditional Chinese Medicine and Modern Western Medicine," in *The Role of Traditional Chinese Medicine in Primary Health Care in China*, ed. O. Akerele, G. Stott, and Lu Weibo (Manila: World Health Organization, 1985), 35.

106. Yan Shengyu, interview, May 22, 2011.

107. For example, the pharmaceutical expenditure per capita in urban Hangzhou was RMB 20.68 in 1974, while the expenditure per capita in each county within the sales area of Hangzhou Chinese and Western Pharmaceutical Station was only RMB 5.43. See Hangzhou yiyao shangyezhi bianzhuan weiyuanhui, *Hangzhou yiyao shangyezhi*, 114.

108. Yan Xiaocheng, "Xuyao gaijin de jige difang" [Issues That Should Be Improved], *Chijiao yisheng zazhi* [Journal of Barefoot Doctors], 11 (1978): 46.

109. Chen, *Medicine in Rural China*, 149–50.

110. Farquhar, "Market Magic," 244.

111. Hai Wen, Wang Jian, Chen Qiulin, Zhao Zhong, and Hou Zhengang, "Nongcun weisheng fuwu tixi tantao" [Discussion on rural health service system], China Center for Economic Research and China Academy of Healty Policy, Peking University, May 12, 2003.

112. Fang Shunxi, interview, May 9, 2004.

113. Yu Fuquan, interview, May 12, 2004.

114. White, "Deciphering 'Integrated Chinese and Western Medicine,'" 1342. See also Anna Lora-Wainwright, "Using Local Resources: Barefoot Doctors and Bone Manipulation in Rural Langzhong, Sichuan Province, PRC," *Asian Medicine: Tradition and Modernity* 1, no. 2 (2005): 13.

115. Xu Shuilin, interview, November 5, 2009.

116. Yan Shengyu, interview, November 3, 2009.

117. Yan Shengyu, interview, May 22, 2011.

118. Regarding enhanced placebo effects, see Ted J. Kaptchuk, Peter Goldman, David A Stone, and William B Stason, "Do Medical Devices Have Enhanced Placebo Effects?" *Journal of Clinical Epidemiology* 53, no. 8 (2000): 786–92.

119. He Xiao, "Diaoping senlin" [Drip bottle forest], *Xinjingbao* [Beijing News], December 28, 2010.

120. Liu, "Change and Continuity of Yi Medical Culturein Southwest China," 101.

121. This mainly refers to the overuse of antibiotics and hormones. See Ding Hong, Wu Lijuan, Yuan Fang, Yang Shanfa, and Dong Wenjing, "Xiangcun yisheng kangshengsu yu jisu shiyong fenxi" [The analysis of antibiotics and hormones prescribed by village doctors], *Yixue yu zhexue* [Medicine and Philosophy] 26, no. 10 (October 2005): 33–40.

122. Dong, Bogg, Rehnberg, and Diwan, "Drug Policy in China," 784.

123. Liu Yuanli, "China's Public Health-Care System: Facing the Challenges," *Bulletin of the World Health Organization* 82, no. 7 (July 2004): 536.

124. Zhejiangsheng weishengting [Zhejiang Provincial Health Department], *Zhejiangsheng xiangcun yisheng jiben yaowu mulu* [The basic catalogue of pharmaceuticals prescribed by village doctors in Zhejiang Province], March 16, 2006.

125. Recent studies point out that the New Rural Cooperative Medical Service seemed to encourage village doctors to prescribe even more drugs and antibiotics and be even more likely to use injections. Irrational drug prescription also occurred in village health stations without the NRCMS. The incentive to sell more drugs—and more expensive drugs—existed because these village health stations are left to support themselves without government subsidies. See Xiaoyun Sun, Sukhan Jackson, Gordon A. Carmichael, and Adrian C. Sleigh, "Prescribing Behaviour of Village Doctors under China's New Cooperative Medical Scheme," *Social Science & Medicine* 68, no. 10 (May 2009): 1779.

126. Organization for Economic Cooperation and Development, *OECD Economic Survey China 2010*, vol. 2010/6 (Paris: OECD Publications, February 2010), 225.

127. Although some villagers pay for pharmaceuticals themselves, state-funded medical services cover all or part of the pharmaceuticals consumed by villagers who joined new cooperative medical service, urban residents, and other civil servants working in the government agencies, hence the high numbers involved.

128. Organization for Economic Cooperation and Development, *OECD Economic Survey China 2010*, 227.

129. White, "Deciphering 'Integrated Chinese and Western Medicine,'" 1333–47.

130. Khng, "Trends in the Utilization of Traditional Chinese Medicines in Rural China," 88.

131. Farquhar, "Eating Chinese Medicine," 476.

132. Luo Aijuan, interview, May 24, 2011.

133. Scheid, *Chinese Medicine in Contemporary China*, 108; Farquhar, "Eating Chinese Medicine," 477; *Knowing Practice*, 20; and Khng, "Trends in the Utilization of Traditional Chinese Medicines in Rural China," 135. For the application of Chinese medicine in treating SARS patients in the SARS epidemic in the spring of 2003, see Marta Hanson, "Conceptual Blind Spots, Media Blindfolds: The Case of SARS and Traditional Chinese Medicine," in Leung and Furth, *Health and Hygiene in Chinese East Asia*, 228–54.

Chapter Five

1. Sivin, *Traditional Medicine in Contemporary China*, 13.

2. Shao, "Hospitalizing Traditional Chinese Medicine," 119; and Freidson, *Profession of Medicine*, 156.

3. Dorothy Porter and Roy Porter, *Patient's Progress: Doctors and Doctoring in Eighteenth-Century England* (Oxford: Polity in Association with Basil Blackwell, 1989), 81.

4. Chen Zhicheng, interview, November 6, 2009.

5. Shao Jungen, interview, November 20, 2009.

6. Hangzhoushi Tingzhi renmin gongshe baojianyuan, "Tingzhi renmin gongshe dang'an lishi ziliao huibian."

7. Scheid, *Currents of Tradition in Chinese Medicine*, 101.

8. Yuhangxian weishengju weishengzhi bianzhuanzu, *Yuhangxian weishengzhi*, 84–85.

9. Ibid., 167.

10. Though Chinese villagers in some areas had accessed missionary hospitals or other modern-style hospitals since the late nineteenth century, they were not widely accessible for the majority of villagers. For more on Chinese patients' experience in missionary hospitals in late nineteenth- and early twentieth-century China, see Renshaw, *Accommodating the Chinese*, 139–94.

11. Lindsay Granshaw and Roy Porter, eds., *The Hospital in History* (London: Routledge, 1989), 1.

12. Chun'anxian renmin weiyuanhui weishengke [Health bureau of Chun'an County People's Committee], "Yi zhengdun gonggu tigao zhiliang, qinjian ban weisheng shiye" [Strengthening and improving medical service through adjustment, doing health work frugally].

13. Chun'anxian renmin weiyuanhui [The people's commission of Chun'an County], "Chun'anxian shehui kaiye yishi renyuan guanli zanxing tiaoli" [Temporary regulations for social medical practitioners in Chun'an County], September 28, 1963, CAA, vol. 30-1-275.

14. Fuyangxian weishengju [Fuyang County Health Bureau], "Guanyu 1962 nian weisheng gongzuo qingkuang de zongjie" [Summary of health work in 1962], January 1963, FYA, vol. 87-2-65.

15. Fuyangxian nongyang quwei [Nongyang District Committee of the Communist Party of China, Fuyang County], "Fuyangxian longyangqu 1964 nian weisheng gongzuo zongjie" [Summary of health work in Longyang District, Fuyang County in 1964], 1964, FYA, vol. 74-1-19.

16. Chun'anxian renmin weiyuanhui [People's commission of Chun'an County], "Chun'anxian liudongyi caoyaoyi guanli zanxing tiaoli" [Temporary regulations for itinerant doctors and herbal medicine peddlers in Chun'an County], April 27, 1962, CAA, vol. 30-1-275.

17. Yuhangxian weishengju weishengzhi bianzhuanzu, *Yuhangxian weishengzhi*, 153.

18. Zhejiangsheng weishengting [Zhejiang Province Health Department], "Nongcun lianhe yiliao jigou he kaiye yisheng zanxing guanli banfa" [Temporary regulations for rural union clinics and medical practitioners], 1963, ZJA, vol. J165-12-54.

19. Regarding the case records kept by Chinese medicine doctors both prior to and after 1949, see Christopher Cullen, "Yi'an (Case Statement): The Origins of a Genre of Chinese Medical Literature," in *Innovation in Chinese Medicine*, ed. Elisabeth Hsu (Cambridge: Cambridge University Press, 2001), 297–323; and Eric I. Karchmer, "Chinese Medicine in Action: On the Postcoloniality of Medical Practice in China," *Medical Anthropology* 29, no. 3 (2010): 235.

20. "Zhejiangsheng kaiye yiyaoshi renyuan guanli shixing banfa" [Temporary regulations for pharmaceutical practitioners in Zhejiang Province], January 31, 1951.

21. Shao, "Hospitalizing Traditional Chinese Medicine," 89.

22. Hangxian sandun lianhe zhensuo [Sandun Union Clinic of Hang County], "Hangxian sandun lianhe yiyuan zhangcheng, 1957" [Program of Sandun Union Clinic, Hang County], November 1957, YHA, vol. 13-5-220.

23. Hangxian Pingyao lianhe zhensuo [Pingyao Union Clinic of Hang County], "Pingyao lianhe zhensuo zhangcheng gexiang zhidu caoan" [Draft program and regulations of Pingyao Union Clinic], October 17, 1957, YHA, vol. 13-5-220.

24. Hangxian weisheng gongzuozhe xiehui, "Zhongyi daibiao dahui zongjie."

25. Chen Zhicheng, interview, November 6, 2009.

26. Yuhangxian weishengju weishengzhi bianzhuanzu, *Yuhangxian weishengzhi*, 153–54.

27. Shao, "Hospitalizing Traditional Chinese Medicine," 15.

28. Luo Zhengfu, interview, November 23, 2009. There was also some resistance to hospital treatment among schistosomiasis patients in the early stages of this process. See Gross, "Chasing Snails," 412–17.

29. "Zai gongshuqu xuexichongbing zhiliaozhan li" [At Gongshu District schistosomiasis treatment station], *HZRB,* January 8, 1956.

30. Zheng Jinzhu, interview, November 19, 2009.

31. "Ba xianyiyuan bancheng nongmin de yiyuan" [Run the county hospital asa peasants' hospital], *HZRB,* October 3, 1965.

32. Scheid, *Chinese Medicine in Contemporary China,* 120–21.

33. See also Henderson and Cohen, *Chinese Hospital,* 108.

34. Jiangcun renmin gongshe hezuo yiliao guanli weiyuanhui [The management committee of Jiang Village People's Commune cooperative medical service], "Jiangcun hezuoyiliao zhangcheng, caoan" [Jiang Village People's Commune cooperative medical service program, draft], January 1970, YHA, vol.148-1-186.

35. Weishengbu [The Ministry of Health], "Quanguo nongcun renmin gongshe weishengyuan zanxing tiaoli, caoan" [Temporary national regulations for rural people's commune clinics, draft], October 31, 1979, CAA, vol. 36-1-60.

36. Yuhangxian weishengju [Yuhang County Health Bureau], "Yuhangxian nongcun hezuo yiliao guanli banfa" [Regulations for rural cooperative medical service management], April 17, 1978, YHA, vol. 42-1-46.

37. Zhonggong Anxi gongshe weiyuanhui [Anxi commune committee of the Communist Party of China], "Huazhuxi zhiming fangxiang, hezuo yiliao buduan gonggu fazhan" [Chairman Hua pointed out the direction, cooperative medical service keeps consolidating and developing], March 1977, YHA, vol. 42-1-89.

38. Jiangcun renmin gongshe hezuo yiliao guanli weiyuanhui, "Jiangcun hezuoyiliao zhangcheng, caoan." For the patient referral systems in both rural and urban areas in 1979–80, see Henderson and Cohen, *Chinese Hospital,* 89–93.

39. The urban counterpart to this was the "sectional medical service," wherein each urban hospital was responsible for servicing all the residents in its geographic area, while each medical facility was specifically responsible for the workers in factories with which it had contracts. Workers had to obtain permission from the factory medical officer before going to the hospital. See Lampton, *Politics of Medicine,* 107; and "Health Policy during the Great Leap Forward," 675.

40. Regarding Chinese family members' role accompanying patients to the hospital, see Joseph Schneider and Wang Laihua, *Giving Care, Writing Self: A "New Ethnography"* (New York: Peter Lang, 2000), 33–59.

41. See also Renshaw, *Accommodating the Chinese,* 207. In 1979, in order to improve hospital management, the Ministry of Health asked hospitals to reduce the numbers of relatives accompanying patients, improve patients' diets, and properly organize their daily lives. See Weishengbu [The Ministry of Health], "Guanyu gaohao sanfen zhiyi zuoyou xian de weisheng shiye zhengdun jianshe de yijian" [Instructions on readjusting and developing health in one-third of counties], in *Zhonghua renmin*

gongheguo weisheng fagui xuanbian, 1978–1980 [Collected legal documents of the People's Republic of China, 1978–1980], ed. Zhonghua renmin gongheguo weishengbu bangongting [General Office of the Ministry of Health of the People's Republic of China] (Beijing: Falüchubanshe, 1982), 172.

42. Luo Aijuan, interview, March 26, 2007.

43. Zheng Chunyan, interview, May 4, 2004.

44. "Zhejiangsheng geming weiyuanhui guanyu jianshe nongcun guangbowang de jueding" [Zhejiang Province revolutionary committee's instruction concerning the establishment of the broadcast network in rural areas], *ZJRB*, May 31, 1969. See also Zhang Letian, *Gaobie lixiang: renmin gongshe zhidu yanjiu* [Farewell to ideals: A study of the people's commune system] (Shanghai: Dongfang chuban zhongxin, 1998), 439–40.

45. World Health Organization, *Primary Health Care: The Chinese Experience, the Report of an Inter-Regional Seminar* (Geneva: The World Health Organization, 1983), appendix, information sheet distributed at the seminar.

46. Yan Shengyu, interview, May 8, 2004.

47. Fang Benpei, interview, April 22, 2006.

48. Jiang Xiu, interview, April 17, 2006.

49. Yip, *Health and National Reconstruction in Nationalist China*, 190–91; Yang, *Zaizao "bingren,"* 380–94; Jing Jun, *Dingxian shiyan: Shequ yixue yu huabei nongcun* [Ding County experiment: Community medicine and rural North China] (Beijing: Department of Sociology, Tsinghua University, 2004).

50. Li Ting'an, *Zhongguo xiangcun weisheng wenti* [Chinese rural health issue] (Shanghai: Shangwu yinshuguan, 1935), 108.

51. Chen, *Medicine in Rural China*, 83.

52. Ibid.,161.

53. Ibid.

54. Yuhangxian weishengju [Yuhang County Health Bureau], "Xuexi maozhuxi guanyu lilun wenti de zhishi, jinyibu banhao hezuo yiliao" [Study Chairman Mao's directives on theoretic issues, further implement cooperative medical service], 1974, YHA, vol. 42-1-88.

55. Shao Jungen, interview, November 20, 2009.

56. Zhu Shouhua, interview, January 5, 2005.

57. Li Lanyan, "Renzhen guanche bazi fangzhen, wei jiashu fazhan weisheng shiye er fendou" [Implement the "eight-character principles" seriously and strive to develop health work quickly], July 5, 1979, FYA, vol.74-3-42.

58. Yuhangxian weishengju, "Guanyu juban nongcun yishiban de jidian yijian."

59. Fuyangxian weishengju [Fuyang County Health Bureau], "Xianwei guanyu weisheng jihua shengyu gongzuo de yijian" [The county committee of the Communist Party of China's instructions on health and family planning work], January 3, 1980, FYA, vol. 1-5-289.

60. Zhou Yonggan, interview, November 6, 2009.

61. Xu Peichun, interview, May 13, 2004.

62. Fang Benpei, interview, March 21, 2007.

63. Xiaoshanxian weishengju [Xiaoshan County Health Bureau], "Guanyu xiaoshanxian gongshe weishengyuan qingkuang de diaocha baogao" [Investigative report of Xiaoshan County commune clinics], August 12, 1972, XSA, vol. 25-1-37.

64. Xu Peichun, interview, March 24, 2004.

65. Fang Benpei, interview, March 22, 2006.

66. Xiaoshanxian weishengju, "Guanyu xiaoshanxin gongshe weishengyuan qingkuang de diaocha baogao."

67. Chen, *Medicine in Rural China*, 169.

68. Jiandexian weishengju, "Nongcun weisheng gongzuo jiben qingkuang."

69. Fuyangxian weishengju, "Xianwei changwei Yao Yansheng tongzhi zai xian weisheng gongzuo huiyi shangde jianghua."

70. Yan, *Jiandexian yiyao weishengzhi*, 84; Ren, *Hangzhou shizhi*, 1:416.

71. Weishengbu, "Quanguo nongcun renmin gongshe weishengyuan zanxing tiaoli, caoan."

72. Jia, "Chinese Medicine in Post-Mao China," 50; and Henderson and Cohen, *Chinese Hospital*, 102.

73. Zhu, "Zhengfu yu nongcun jiben yiliao baojian baozhang zhidu xuanze," 93.

74. Gao Ming and Qian Haoping, "Beida nüboshihou yao kan weishengyuan" [A woman postdoctoral fellow of Peking University would like to cancel township clinics], *Yiyao chanye zixun* [Medicine and Management Industry Information] 3, no. 7 (March 2006): 55; Wang Hongman, *Daguo weisheng zhinan: Zhongguo nongcun yiliao weisheng xianzhuang yu zhidu gaige tantao* [The dilemma of a big country: The present situation of rural health in China and discussion on system reform] (Beijing: Beijing daxue chubanshe, 2004); Joan Kaufman, "SARS and China's Health-Care Response: Better to be Both Red and Expert!" in SARS in China: Prelude to Pandemic? ed. Arthur Kleinman and James L. Watson (Stanford, CA: Stanford University Press, 2006), 58; and Organization for Economic Cooperation and Development, *OECD Economic Survey China 2010*, 222.

75. "Dangqian gedi peixun nongcun weisheng renyuan qingkuang de huibao" [Reports on current health worker training work in different locations], November 3, 1965, ZJA, vol. J165-15-126.

76. According to Henderson and Cohen's study, based on the Second Attached Hospital of Hubei Provincial Medical College in Wuhan between November 1979 and March 1980, the majority of patients (72 percent) admitted to the infectious disease ward came from urban and suburban areas of Wuhan city. Furthermore, the illnesses of urban patients were less serious than those of rural patients. See Henderson and Cohen, *Chinese Hospital*, 95, 107.

77. N. D. Jewson, "The Disappearance of the Sick-Man from Medical Cosmology," *Sociology* 10, no. 2 (1976): 225–44.

78. Leung, "Yiliaoshi yu zhongguo 'xiandaixing' wenti," 1.

Chapter Six

1. Freidson, *Profession of Medicine*, 3.

2. Li Jinghan, *Dingxian shehui gaikuang diaocha* [Social survey of Ding County] (Shanghai: Shanghai shudian, 1992), 292–95.

3. Ibid., 294.

4. Fuyangxian weishengju [Fuyang County Health Bureau], "Weisheng jianbao: Jin Guanhuan tongzhi de laixin" [Health bulletin: A letter from Comrade Jin Guanhuan], June 20, 1977, FYA, vol. 74-3-26.

5. Baise diqu weishengju dapipanzu [Baise Prefecture health bureau critique team], "Bo 'chijiao yisheng chuanxielun'" [Refute "a speech about the barefoot doctors wearing shoes"], *Guangxi weisheng* [Journal of Guangxi Health] 3 (1976): 7–8.

6. Miao Yu, "Fanji weisheng zhanxian youqin fan'anfeng" [Repulse the right-deviationist wind to reverse the verdict on health front], *ZJRB*, April 3, 1976.

7. Niu Shuiying, interview, January 8, 2005.

8. Xu Peichun, interview, May 13, 2004.

9. Fang Benpei, interview, December 3, 2005.

10. Yuhangxian weishengju, "Xuexi maozhuxi guanyu lilun wenti de zhishi, jinyibu banhao hezuo yiliao."

11. Xu Peichun, interview, May 13, 2004.

12. Unschuld, *Medical Ethics in Imperial China*, 28.

13. Chen Cunren, *Wo de yiwu shengya* [My medical career] (Guilin: Guangxi shifan daxue chubanshe, 2007), 12. Fan Shouyuan confirmed, "When they (physicians) talked with their patients, they would say such and such a doctor was too new and lacked sufficient medical experience, or that fellow was too old and behind the times. . . . If they encountered a medical dispute between a doctor and a patient's family, they were very happy to talk about the previous doctor's demerits with the family members." See Fan Shouyuan, "Zhe ye suan shi yichang susong" [It is also a medical lawsuit], *Yishi huikan* [Medical Practice Journal] 9, 1–2 (1937): 9–32, cited in Zhang Bin, "Qianxi minguo shiqi de yishi jiufen" [Brief analysis of medical disputes during the Republic of China], *Zhongguo yixue lunlixue* [Medical Ethics of China] 16, no. 6 (December 2003): 23.

14. Chun'anxian renmin weiyuanhui weishengke [Health bureau of Chun'an County People's Committee], "Yi zhengdun gonggu tigao zhiliang, qinjian ban weisheng shiye" [Strengthening and improving medical service through adjustment, doing health work frugally].

15. Zhou Yonggan, interview, November 6, 2009.

16. Xu Peichun, interview, November 19, 2009.

17. Potter and Potter, *China's Peasants*, 116–17; Huaiyin Li, *Village China under Socialism and Reform: A Micro History, 1948–2008* (Stanford, CA: Stanford University Press, 2009), 204.

18. Zhang Ahhua, interview, April 24, 2004.

19. Yan Shengyu, interview, May 27, 2007.

20. Niu Shuiying, interview, January 8, 2005.

21. However, conscious or unconscious competition for professional prestige was still noticeable during the 1970s among doctors in medical units at different levels. As Chen Zhicheng recalled, "At that time, we referred patients to higher-up hospitals. Doctors there always criticized patient families for the delayed referral: 'If patient had been sent here one or two hours later, he would have died!' Actually, they just want to show that their medical proficiency was better than ours and that without them, patients would definitely die." Chen Zhicheng, interview, October 9, 2010.

22. Unschuld, *Medical Ethics in Imperial China*, vii.

23. Farquhar, "Market Magic," 242.

24. Hu Zaohua, interview, March 25, 2004.

25. William Hinton, *Shenfan* (New York: Random House, 1983), 106–9; and Martin King Whyte and William L. Parish, *Urban Life in Contemporary China* (Chicago: University of Chicago Press, 1984), 18–19.

26. Potter and Potter, *China's Peasants*, 306–11. See also Philip C. C. Huang, *The Peasant Family and Rural Development in the Yangzi Delta, 1350–1988* (Stanford, CA: Stanford University Press, 1990), 288–304; and Gao, *Gao Village*, 30.

27. Potter and Potter, *China's Peasants*, 311.

28. Zhang, *Gaobie lixiang*, 428–30.

29. Chun'anxian weishengju geming weiyuanhui [Revolutionary committee of the Health Bureau of Chun'an County], "Guanyu zhaoshou yipi weisheng renyuan de baogao" [Report on recruiting a batch of medical personnel], October 27, 1971, CAA, vol. 36-1-46.

30. Jiang Jingting, interview, April 20, 2004; and Chen Zhicheng, interview, January 6, 2005.

31. Zhou Yonggan, interview, April 21, 2004.

32. Yuhangxian weishengju [Yuhang County Health Bureau], "Guanyu gongshe weishengyuan nei gongzuo de chijiaoyisheng de daiyu wenti" [Payment of barefoot doctors working in commune clinics], March 27, 1979, YHA, vol. 42-2-31.

33. Chen Zhicheng, interview, January 10, 2005; and Zhou Yonggan, interview, May 20, 2004.

34. Shen Xianbing, interview, January 10, 2005; and Xu Shuilin, interview, September 23, 2005.

35. Chen Zhicheng, interview, January 6, 2005; and Xu Shuilin, interview, September 23, 2005.

36. Zhang Ahhua, interview, May 24, 2004.

37. Jiandexian weishengju, "Nongcun weisheng gongzuo jiben qingkuang."

38. Henderson and Cohen found that the promotion system ceased during the Cultural Revolution. There was no upward mobility for medical professionals working in hospitals. In contrast, downward mobility and uncertainty were the main features. See Henderson and Cohen, *Chinese Hospital*, 86, 32–39.

39. Reinhard Spree, *Health and Social Class in Imperial Germany: A Social History of Mortality, Morbidity and Inequality* (New York: St. Martin's Place, 1988), 158.

40. Kleinman, *Patients and Healers in the Context of Culture*, 214.

41. Yuhangxian weishengju [Yuhang County Health Bureau], "Guanyu Shen Yutian feifa xingyi zaocheng yanzhong houguo de tongbao" [A notice on serious results caused by Shen Yutian's illegal medical practice], August 16, 1974, SDA.

42. Guowuyuan [The State Council], "Guanyu quanguo weisheng gongzuo huiyi de baogao" [Report on national health work meeting], August 5, 1975, HZA, vol. 132-4-128; and Li Baochang, "Wei wuchan jieji laogu zhanling nongcun weisheng zhendi jianchi douzheng" [Keep fighting to occupy the rural health front firmly for the proletariat], in *Chijiao yisheng xianjin shiji huibian: Chijiao yisheng zhuozhuang chengzhang* [Collection of model deeds of barefoot doctors: Barefoot doctors are growing up quickly] (Beijing: Renmin weisheng chubanshe, 1975), vol. 3, 115–16.

43. Yuhangxian weishengju [Yuhang County Health Bureau], "Xianwei fushuji Sun Xuchun tongzhi zai xian dierjie hezuo yiliao chijiaoyisheng dabiao dahui bimushi shang de jianghua" [Vice secretary of the committee of the Communist Party of China of Yuhang County Comrade Sun Xuchun's speech at the closing ceremony of the county cooperative medical service and barefoot doctor representative meeting], October 26, 1976, YHA, vol. 42-1-39.

44. Zhejiangsheng weishengju, Zhejiangsheng nongyeju [Zhejiang Provincial Health Bureau, Zhejiang Provincial Agricultural Bureau], "Zhejiangsheng nongcun hezuo yiliao banfa (shixing)" [Program for rural cooperative medical service in Zhejiang Province (temporary)], November 8, 1979, CAA, vol. 36-1-62.

45. Shen Guanrong, interview, January 11, 2005.

46. Luo Linyuan, interview, January 5, 2005.

47. He Weisheng, interview, March 23, 2004.

48. Liu, "Change and Continuity of Yi Medical Culture," 237–38.

49. Katherine Gould-Martin, "Hot Cold Clean Poison and Dirt: Chinese Folk Medical Categories," Social Science & Medicine 12 (January 1978): 41.

50. Yuhangxian weishengju, "Guanyu Shen Yutian feifa xingyi zaocheng yanzhong houguo de tongbao."

51. Ibid.

52. Jonathan Spence, "Commentary on Historical Perspectives and Ch'ing Medical Systems," in Medicine in Chinese Cultures: Comparative Studies of Health Care in Chinese and Other Societies, ed. Arthur Kleinman, Peter Kunstadter, E. Russell Alexander, and James L. Gale (Bethesda, MD: National Library of Health, 1975), 81; Sivin, Traditional Medicine in Contemporary China, 21.

53. Lei, "Fu zeren de yisheng yu you xinyang de bingren," 85.

54. Kleinman, Patients and Healers in the Context of Culture, 259–310.

55. Cunningham and Andrews, Western Medicine as Contested Knowledge, 11.

56. Ibid., 6.

57. Henderson and Cohen, Chinese Hospital, 112.

58. Chen, Medicine in Rural China, 81.

59. Hsun-yuan Yao, "The Second Year of the Rural Health Experiment in Ting Hsien, China," The Milkbank Memorial Fund Quarterly Bulletin 10, no. 1 (January 1932): 53–66.

60. F. P. Lisowski, "Emergence and Development of the Barefoot Doctor in China," in History of the Professionalisation of Medicine: Proceedings of the 3rd International Symposium on the Comparative History of Medicine—East and West, ed. Teizo Ogawa (Osaka: Taniguchi Foundation, 1987), 154.

61. Wen Yiqun, "Zhongguo chijiao yisheng chansheng he cunzai de shehui wenhua yuanyin fenxi" [Social-cultural analysis of the emergence of barefoot doctors in China], in Cong chijiao yisheng dao xiangcun yisheng [From barefoot doctors to village doctors], ed. Zhang Kaining (Kunming: Yunnan renmin chubanshe, 2002), 325.

62. Yang Nianqun further argues that when barefoot doctors were renamed village doctors and incorporated into the market economy in 1985, the bottom tier of the medical system lost the dual constraints of kinship affection and the political system. The medical care of villagers and barefoot doctors' epidemic prevention duties were seriously impaired. In some areas, the epidemic prevention mobilization network was no longer effectively organized. Yang, Zaizao "bingren," 380–94; and

"Fangyi xingwei yu kongjian zhengzhi" [Epidemic prevention and spatial politics], *Dushu* [Reading], 7 (2003): 25–33.

63. Liu Junyang, "Wo dangle banian chijiao yisheng" [I was a barefoot doctor for eight years], *HZRB*, December 8, 2003.

64. Ibid.

65. "Hezuo yiliao genshen yemao: Shandongsheng Changwei diqu de diaocha baogao" [Cooperative medical services are flourishing: Investigative report of the cooperative medical services in Changwei area, Shandong Province], in *Hezuo yiliao hao* [Cooperative medical services are excellent], ed. Wei Ge (Shanghai: Shanghai renmin chubanshe, 1974), 23; Chen, *Medicine in Rural China*, 78, 201.

66. Porter and Porter, *Patient's Progress*, 13; and Nancy Theriot, "Negotiating Illness: Doctors, Patients, and Families in the Nineteenth Century," *Journal of the History of Behavior Sciences* 37, no. 4 (October 2001): 351.

67. Stanley Joel Reiser, *Technological Medicine: The Changing World of Doctors and Patients* (New York: Cambridge University Press, 2009), 7–8.

68. Reiser, *Medicine and the Reign of Technology*, 36.

69. Liu, "Wo dangle banian chijiao yisheng."

70. Shang Guo, "Guoguo" [Guoguo], in *Qingchun fangchengshi: Wushi ge beijing nüzhiqing de zishu* [Youth formula: Accounts by 50 Beijing female educated youth], ed. Liu Zhonglu (Beijing: Beijing daxue chubanshe, 2000), 340.

71. Fuyangxian weishengju geming weiyuanhui [The revolutionary committee of the Fuyang County Health Bureau], "Guanyu wufu yian miding zaocheng zhongdu shigu de baogao" [Report on the accidental poisoning caused by mistaking ethylamine pyridine dosage], August 1, 1972, FYA, vol. 74-3-15.

72. Marilynn M. Rosenthal and Jay R. Greiner, "The Barefoot Doctor of China: From Political Creation to Professionalization," *Human Organization* 41, no. 4 (1982): 338–39; and Scheid, *Chinese Medicine in Contemporary China*, 96.

73. Chen Zhicheng, interview, November 6, 2009.

74. Maurice Meisner, *Mao's China and After: A History of the People's Republic* (New York: Free Press, 1999), 427–48.

75. Scheid, *Chinese Medicine in Contemporary China*, 81; and Henderson, "Issues in the Modernization of Medicine in China," 201.

76. Lin'anxian weishengzhi bianzhuan weiyuanhui, *Lin'anxian weishengzhi*, 146.

77. Fuyangxian weishengju, "Quansheng weisheng gongzuo huiyi wenjian."

78. Zhejiangsheng weishengju [Zhejiang Province Health Department], "Guanyu dui nongcun chijiaoyisheng kaohe fazheng de tongzhi" [Notice on holding barefoot doctor examinations and issuing certificates], October 6, 1979, FYA, vol. 74-3-36.

79. Chun'anxian weishengju [Chun'an County Health Bureau], "Guanyu jingxin xiangcun yisheng kaoshi kaohe fazheng de tongzhi" [Notice on holding village doctor examinations, assessment, and issuing certificates], December 1981, CAA, vol. 36-1-64.

80. Chun'anxian weishengju [Chun'an County Health Bureau], "Guanyu renzhen zuohao xiangcun yisheng kaoshi kaohe gongzuo juti yijian de tongzhi" [Notice on holding village doctor examinations seriously], November 15, 1982, CAA, vol. 30-2/4-232-5.

81. Fang Benpei, interview, January 14, 2006.

82. Chun'an xianzhi bianzhuan weiyuanhui, *Chun'an xianzhi*, 193.

83. "Chijiao yisheng de kunao" [Barefoot doctors' dilemmas], *RMRB*, August 10, 1980.

84. Yuhangxian weishengju [Yuhang County Health Bureau], "Qing yanjiu luoshi chijiao yisheng daiyu zhengce" [Please study and implement payment policies for barefoot doctors], December 1980, YHA, vol. 42-2-59.

85. Weishengbu [The Ministry of Health], "Guanyu heli jiejue chijiao yisheng buzhu wenti de baogao" [Report on properly solving subsidy problems for barefoot doctors], *Guowuyuan gongbao* [The State Council Bulletin], February 16, 1981.

86. Ren, *Hangzhou shizhi*, 9:17.

87. Gao, *Gao Village*, 171.

88. Wang, "Xuexi jizhi yu shiying nengli," 122.

89. In a recent study, Jane Duckett argued that the collapse of the cooperative medical service was not simply a consequence of economic decollectivization after 1978. It was more precisely the result of a 1981 reversal in Ministry of Health, which was due to elite leadership and ideological changes in late 1970s. See Jane Duckett, "Challenging the Economic Reform Paradigm: Policy and Politics in the Early 1980s Collapse of the Rural Cooperative Medical System," *China Quarterly* 205 (March 2011): 80–95.

90. Yan Shengyu, interview, November 23, 2009.

91. Ibid.

92. The barefoot doctor examinations were held starting in 1981, but actual progress varied within the seven counties under the jurisdiction of Hangzhou Prefecture.

93. Niu Shuiying, interview, January 11, 2005; and Yan Shengyu, interview, May 27, 2004.

94. Luo Zhengfu, interview, November 23, 2009. This process also occurred in other parts of China. In Xiangfen County, Shanxi Province, most of those who were classified as health aides stopped providing health care and became farmers because they could not compete with the better-educated barefoot doctors. See Jia, "Chinese Medicine in Post-Mao China," 47.

95. Henderson, "Issues in the Modernization of Medicine in China," 206; and Chen, *Medicine in Rural China*, 170.

96. Duckett, *The Chinese State's Retreat from Health*, 6–7; Kleinman and Watson, "SARS in Social and Historical Context," 1–16; Blumenthal and Hsiao, "Privatization and Its Contents," 1165–69; Liu, "China's Public Health-Care System," 532–38; Wang, "Zhongguo gonggong weisheng de weiji yu zhuanji," 52–88; Gu Xin and Fang Liming, "Ziyuanxing yu qiangzhixing zhijian, Zhongguo nongcun hezuo yiliao de zhidu qianruxing yu fazhan ke chixuxing" [Between being voluntary and compulsory: Chinese rural cooperative service's institutional embeddedness and sustainable development], *Shehuixue yanjiu* [Sociology Study Journal], 5 (2004): 1–18; Liu Yuanli, William C. L. Hsiao, Qing Li, Xingzhu Liu, and Minghui Ren, "Transformation of China's Rural Health Care Financing," *Social Science & Medicine* 41, no. 8 (October 1995): 1085; and Charlotte Cailliez, "The Collapse of the Rural Health System," *China Perspective* 18 (1998): 36–43.

97. Some scholars have made positive comments on the rural health situation after the rural reforms. Martin King White and Zhongxin Sun argue that "despite sharp reductions in medical insurance coverage, rising medical care costs and unequal access, China has made dramatic progress in improving the health of its population

since market reforms were launched." See Martin King White and Zhongxin Sun, "The Impact of China's Market Reforms on the Health of Chinese Citizens: Examining Two Puzzles," *China: An International Journal* 8, no. 1 (March 2010): 1–32; Judith Banister argues that the public health situation in China has improved dramatically since 1949, as well as since the beginning of the economic reforms. See Judith Banister, "Population, Public Health and Environment in China," *China Quarterly* 156 (December 1998): 1015. Huang Yanzhong claims that, contrary to widespread alarmist reports, China has not witnessed a measurable decline in the overall public health status. See Huang Yanzhong, "Bringing the Local State Back In: The Political Economy of Public Health in Rural China," *Journal of Contemporary China* 13, no. 39 (2004): 367–70. For similar comments, see Deborah Davis, "Chinese Social Welfare: Policies and Outcomes," in "The People's Republic of China after 40 Years," special issue, *China Quarterly* 119 (September 1989): 590; Gerald Bloom and Gu Xingyuan, "Introduction to Health Sector Reform in China," *IDS Bulletin* 28, no. 1 (1997): 1–11; Gail Henderson, "Trends in Health Services Utilisations in Eight Provinces, 1989–1993," *Social Science & Medicine* 47, no. 12 (1998): 1957–71; Kaufman, "SARS and China's Health-Care Response," 59; and Organization for Economic Cooperation and Development, *OECD Economic Survey China 2010*, 227.

98. Wang and Wang, *Zhongguo renkou: Zhejiang fence*, 345.

99. Chen, *Medicine in Rural China*, 169.

100. Yang, "Fangyi xingwei yu kongjian zhengzhi," 25–33.

101. For the development of medicine, health and epidemic prevention after 1978, see Chen, *Medicine in Rural China*, 142–73.

102. Yuhangxian weisheng fangyizhan, *Yuhangxian weisheng fangyizhi*, 105–10.

103. Yu Fuquan, interview, May 12, 2004.

104. Luo Zhengfu, interview, November 23, 2009.

105. Xu Shuilin, interview, November 5, 2009.

106. Zhu Shouhua, interview, January 5, 2005.

107. Khng, "Trends in the Utilization of Traditional Chinese Medicines," 123.

108. Fuyangshi weishengju [Fuyang City Health Bureau], ed., *Fuyangxian xingzhengcun weishengshi guanli ruogan guiding* [A few regulations concerning village clinic management] (Fuyang: Fuyangxian weishengju, 1990).

109. Chen Minzhang, "Chen Minzhang tongzhi zai yijiubawunian quanguo weishengtingjuzhang huiyi shang de zongjie jianghua" [Minister of Health Comrade Chen Minzhang's summary speech at the National Health Bureau Directors' Meeting in 1985], January 24, 1985, cited in Ma Hong, ed., *Zhongguo gaige quanshu: Yiliao weisheng tizhi gaigejuan* [China reform: Medical and health system reform] (Dalian: Dalian chubanshe, 1992), 137.

Chapter Seven

1. Unrelated to this topic, the third significant change in Chinese medicine is globalization. In his discussion of Chinese medicine and globalization, Scheid argued that "globalization [also] refers to the dispersion of Chinese medicine throughout the world, where it is now practiced in an increasing number of different settings."

He further pointed out that "after a century of struggle against domination by Western medicine of modernization and revolution, Chinese medicine now stands at the threshold of emergence as a truly global medicine." See Scheid, *Chinese Medicine in Contemporary China*, 268–69. Similarly, Mei Zhan also proposed the term "worlding" to refer to the translocal process of marketization and globalization of traditional Chinese medicine. See Mei Zhan, "A Doctor of the Highest Caliber Treats an Illness Before It Happens," *Medical Anthropology* 28, no. 2 (2009): 172; and *Other-Worldly: Making Chinese Medicine through Transnational Frames* (Durham, NC: Duke University Press. 2009). However, this does not mean that Chinese medicine has a dominant position outside China, where it is still an "alternative medicine."

2. Scheid, *Chinese Medicine in Contemporary China*, 128.

Bibliography

Primary Sources

Archives

Changyang County Archives, Hubei Province
Chuansha County Archives, Shanghai Municipality
Chun'an County Archives, Zhejiang Province
Fuyang City Archives, Zhejiang Province
Hangzhou Prefecture Archives, Zhejiang Province
Jiande City Archives, Zhejiang Province
Jiangsu Province Archives, Jiangsu Province
Lin'an City Archives, Zhejiang Province
Nanjing Prefecture Archives, Jiangsu Province
National Archives, London, UK
Pudong New District Archives, Shanghai Municipality
Rockefeller Archival Center, USA
Sandun Township Integrated Chinese and Western Medicine Hospital, Hangzhou City, Zhejiang Province
Shanghai Municipality Archives, Shanghai Municipality
Xiaoshan District Archives, Hangzhou City, Zhejiang Province
Yuhang District Archives, Hangzhou City, Zhejiang Province
Zhejiang Province Archives, Zhejiang Province

Gazetteers

Chun'an xianzhi bianzhuan weiyuanhui [Editorial board of Chun'an County Gazetteer], ed. *Chun'anxianzhi* [Chun'an County Gazetteer]. Shanghai: Hanyu dacidian chubanshe, 1990.

Chun'anxian jihua weiyuanhui [Chun'an County Planning Committee], ed. *Chun'anxian guomin jingji tongji ziliao, 1949–1978* [Statistical data of Chun'an County national economy, 1949–1978]. Chun'an: Chun'anxian jihua weiyuanhui, 1980.

Fan Zhangyou, ed. *Tonglu xianzhi* [Tonglu County Gazetteer]. Hangzhou: Zhejiang renmin chubanshe, 1991.

Fan Zushu, *Hangsu yifeng* [Hangzhou Custom]. Hangzhou: Liuyi shuju, 1928.

Fei Hei, ed. *Xiaoshan xianzhi* [Xiaoshan County Gazetteer]. Hangzhou: Zhejiang renmin chubanshe, 1987.

Fujiansheng weishengzhi bianzhuan weiyuanhui [Editorial board of Fujian Province Health Gazetteer], ed. *Fujiansheng weishengzhi* [Fujian Province Health Gazetteer]. Fuzhou: Fujiansheng weishengzhi bianzhuan weiyuanhui, 1989.

Hangzhou yiyao shangyezhi bianzhuan weiyuanhui [Editorial board of Hangzhou Pharmaceutical Commerce Gazetteer], ed. *Hangzhou yiyao shangyezhi* [Hangzhou Pharmaceutical Commerce Gazetteer]. Beijing: Zhongguo qingnian chubanshe, 1990.

Hangzhoushi weisheng fangyizhan [Hangzhou Prefecture Sanitation and Epidemic-Prevention Station], ed. *Yiqing ziliao huibian, 1950–1979* [Compiled data of epidemic disease prevention, 1950–1979]. Hangzhou: Hangzhoushi fangyizhan, 1982.

Hangzhoushi weishengju [Hangzhou Prefecture Health Bureau], ed. *Hangzhoushi weisheng gongzuo dashiji, 1949–2000* [Chronicles of health work in Hangzhou, 1949–2000]. Hangzhou: Hangzhoushi weishengju, 2002.

Hangzhoushi weishengju Hangzhoushi weishengzhi bianji weiyuanhui [Editorial board of Hangzhou Prefecture Health Gazetteer of Hangzhou Prefecture Health Bureau], ed. *Hangzhoushi weishengzhi* [Hangzhou Prefecture Health Gazetteer]. Hangzhou: Hangzhoushi weishengju, 2000.

Hubeisheng difangzhi bianzhuan weiyuanhui [Editorial board of Hubei Province Local Gazetteer], ed. *Hubei shengzhi: Weisheng* [Hubei Province Gazetteer: Health]. Vol. 2. Wuhan: Hubei renmin chubanshe, 2000.

Jiangsusheng difangzhi bianzhuan weiyuanhui [Editorial board of Jiangsu Province Local Gazetteer], ed. *Jiangsu shengzhi: Weishengzhi* [Jiangsu Province Gazetteer: Health]. Nanjing: Jiangsu guji chubanshe, 1999.

Jinyunxian yiyaozhi bianzhuan xiaozu [Editorial team of Jinyun CountyMedical and Pharmaceutical Gazetteer], ed. *Jinyunxian yiyaozhi* [Jinyun County Medical and Pharmaceutical Gazetteer]. Jinyun: Jinyunxian yinshuachang, 1990.

Lin'an xianzhi bianzhuan weiyuanhui [Editorial board of Lin'an County Gazetteer], ed. *Lin'an xianzhi* [Lin'an County Gazetteer]. Shanghai: Hanyu dacidian chubanshe, 1992.

Lin'anxian weishengzhi bianzhuan weiyuanhui [Editorial board of Lin'an County Health Gazetteer], ed. *Lin'anxian weishengzhi* [Lin'an County Health Gazetteer]. Lin'an: Lin'anxian weishengju, 1992.

Ren Zhentai, ed. *Hangzhou shizhi* [Hangzhou Prefecture Gazetteer].12 vols. Beijing: Zhonghua shuju, 1995–2001.

Shen Qingyang, ed. *Yuhangxian jiangcunxiang xueyi de tulangzhong* [Folk healers in Jiang Village Township, Yuhang County]. Jiang Village, 2009.

Shi Fu, ed. *Jinhua xianzhi* [Jinhua County Gazetteer]. Hangzhou: Zhejiang renmin chubanshe, 1992.

Sichuansheng yiyao weishengzhi bianzhuan weiyuanhui [Editorial board of Sichuan Province Pharmaceutical and Health Gazetteer], ed. *Sichuansheng yiyao weishengzhi* [Sichuan Province Pharmaceutical and Health Gazetteer]. Chengdu: Sichuan kexue jishu chubanshe, 1991.

Wang Kewu, Wang Lieting, and He Songtang, eds. *Zhejiang nüeji kongzhi* [Malaria control in Zhejiang Province]. Hangzhou: Zhejiangsheng weisheng fangyizhan, 1996.

Wang Qing, ed. *Yuhang shizhi* [Yuhang City Gazetteer]. Beijing: Zhonghuashuju, 2000.

Wang Wenzhi, ed. *Fuyang xianzhi* [Fuyang County Gazetteer]. Hangzhou: Zhejiang renmin chubanshe, 1993.

Wu Shichun, ed. *Qianhong cunzhi* [Qianhong Village Gazetteer]. Yiwu: Qianhong cunzhi bianzhuan weiyuanhui, 1996.

Xiaoshan weishengju [Xiaoshan County Health Bureau], ed. *Xiaoshan weishengzhi* [Xiaoshan County Health Gazetteer]. Hangzhou: Zhejiang daxue chubanshe, 1989.

Xiaoshanshi weisheng fangyizhan [Xiaoshan City Sanitation and Epidemic-Prevention Station], ed. *Xiaoshan weisheng fangyizhi* [Xiaoshan City Sanitation and Epidemic-Prevention Gazetteer]. Xiaoshan: Xiaoshanshi weisheng fangyizhan, 1996.

Xu Yuangen, ed. *Fuyangxian weishengzhi* [Fuyang County Health Gazetteer]. Beijing: Zhongguo yiyao keji chubanshe, 1991.

Yan Youxiang, ed. *Jiandexian yiyao weishengzhi* [Jiande County Pharmaceutical and Health Gazetteer]. Jiande: Jiandexian weishengju, 1985.

Yang Lixing and Shi Guanzhen, eds. *Xinchangxian weishengzhi* [Xinchang County Health Gazetteer]. Shanghai: Tongji daxue chubanshe, 1992, 161.

Ying Yiping, ed. *Wuyixian weishengzhi* [Wuyi County Health Gazetteer]. Wuyi: Wuyixian weishengju, 1992.

Yu Guangyan, ed. *Chun'anxian weishengzhi* [Chun'an County Health Gazetteer]. Chun'an: Chun'anxian renmin zhengfu jiguan yinshuachang, 1998.

Yuhangxian diming weiyuanhui [Yuhang County Geographic Name Committee], ed. *Yuhangxian dimingzhi* [Yuhang County Geographic Name Gazetteer]. Yuhang: Yuhangxian diming weiyuanhui, 1987.

Yuhangxian weisheng fangyizhan [Yuhang County Sanitation and Epidemic-Prevention Station], ed. *Yuhangxian weisheng fangyizhi* [Yuhang County Sanitation and Epidemic-Prevention Gazetteer]. Yuhang: Yuhangxian weisheng fangyizhan, 1990.

Yuhangxian weishengju weishengzhi bianzhuanzu [Editorial board of Yuhang County Health Gazetteer], ed. *Yuhangxian weishengzhi* [Yuhang County Health Gazetteer]. Yuhang: Yuhangxian weishengju, 1988.

Yunnansheng difangzhi bianzhuan weiyuanhui [Editorial board of Yunnan Province Local Gazetteer], ed. *Yunnan shengzhi: Weishengzhi* [Yunnan Province Gazetteer: Health Gazetteer]. Kunming: Yunnan renmin chubanshe, 2002.

Zhang Binhua, ed. *Chongfu zhenzhi* [Chongfu Township Gazetteer]. Shanghai: Shanghai shudian chubanshe, 1994.

Zhejiang fangzhi bianjibu [Editorial board of Zhejiang Province Gazetteer], ed. *Zhejiang wengge jishi* [Chronicles of the Cultural Revolution in Zhejiang]. Hangzhou: Zhejiang fangzhi bianjibu, 1989.

Zhejiangsheng tongjiju [Zhejiang Province Bureau of Statistics], ed. *Zhejiang tongji nianjian 1990* [Zhejiang Statistical Year Book 1990]. Hangzhou: Zhejiangsheng tongjiju, 1990.

———. *Zhejiang tongji nianjian1989* [Zhejiang Statistical Year Book 1989]. Hangzhou: Zhejiangsheng tongjiju, 1989.

———. *Zhejiang tongji nianjian1988* [Zhejiang Statistical Year Book 1988]. Hangzhou: Zhejiangsheng tongjiju, 1988.

———. *Zhejiang tongji nianjian1985* [Zhejiang Statistical Year Book 1985]. Hangzhou: Zhejiangsheng tongjiju, 1985.

———. *Zhejiang tongji nianjian1984* [Zhejiang Statistical Year Book 1984]. Hangzhou: Zhejiangsheng tongjiju, 1984.

Zhejiangsheng yiyaozhi bianzhuan weiyuanhui [Editorial board of Zhejiang Province Pharmaceutical Gazetteer], ed. *Zhejiangsheng yiyaozhi* [Zhejiang Province Pharmaceutical Gazetteer]. Beijing: Fangzhi chubanshe, 2003.

Zhengxie Hangzhoushi weiyuanhui wenshi ziliao gongzuo weiyuanhui [The cultural and historical data committee of Hangzhou Prefecture political consultative committee], ed. *Hangzhou wenshi ziliao* [Hangzhou Cultural and Historical Data]. 24 vols. Hangzhou: 1982–2000.

Zhongguo jiaoyu nianjian bianjibu [Editorial board of China Education Yearbook], ed. *Zhongguo jiaoyu nianjian 1949–1981* [China Education Year Book]. Beijing: Zhongguo dabaike quanshu chubanshe, 1984.

Zhongguo weisheng nianjian bianzhuan weiyuanhui [Editorial board of China health yearbook], ed. *Zhongguo weisheng nianjian 1990* [China Health Yearbook 1990]. Beijing: Renmin weisheng chubanshe, 1991.

———. *Zhongguo weisheng nianjian 1983* [China Health Yearbook 1983]. Beijing: Renmin weisheng chubanshe, 1983.

Zhongguo yiyao gongsi [China Pharmaceutical Company], ed. *Zhongguo yiyao shangye shigao* [The history of pharmaceutical commerce in China]. Shanghai: Shanghai shehui kexueyuan chubanshe, 1990.

Zhou Jinkui, ed. *Jiande xianzhi* [Jiande County Gazetteer]. Hangzhou: Zhejiang renmin chubanshe, 1986.

Zhou Lingen, ed. *Yuhang zhenzhi* [Yuhang Township Gazetteer]. Hangzhou: Zhejiang renmin chubanshe, 1990.

Zhou Ruhan, ed. *Yuhang xianzhi* [Yuhang County Gazetteer]. Hangzhou: Zhejiang renmin chubanshe, 1990.

Barefoot Doctors' Medical Textbooks

Chuanshaxian jiangzhen gongshe chijiao yisheng [Barefoot doctors of Jiangzhen Commune, Chuansha County], ed. *Chijiao yisheng changyong yaowu* [Common medicines prescribed by barefoot doctors]. Shanghai: Shanghai renmin chubanshe, 1975.

Guangdongsheng zhiwu yanjiusuo caiyao zhishi bianxiezu [Editorial team of knowledge for collecting herbal medicine, Guangdong Province Botanical Research Institute], ed. *Caiyao zhishi* [Knowledge of collecting herbal medicine]. Guangzhou: Guangdong renmin chubanshe, 1977.

Hangzhoushi disan renmin yiyuan ji hongyi peixunban jiaocai bianweihui [Hangzhou City No. 3 People's Hospital andEditorial board of red doctor training class textbooks], ed. *Gongnong yiliao weisheng shouce* [Worker and peasant health manual]. Hangzhou: Hangzhou Health Revolutionary Committee, 1969.

Hangzhoushi jihua shengyu bangongshi [Hangzhou Prefecture Family Planning Office], ed. *Renkou fei kongzhibuxing* [The population must be controlled]. Hangzhou: Hangzhoushi jihua shengyu bangongshi, 1978.

Hangzhoushi weisheng fangyizhan [Hangzhou Prefecture Sanitation and Epidemic-Prevention Station], ed. *Jiji yufang huxidao chuanranbing* [Actively preventing infectious respiratory diseases]. Hangzhou: Hangzhoushi weisheng fangyizhan geweihui, 1970.

Hangzhoushi weisheng fangyizhan geming weiyuanhui [Revolutionary Committee of Hangzhou Prefecture Sanitation and Epidemic-Prevention Station], ed. *Nongyao shiyong yu zhongdu fangzhi* [Pesticide usage and poisoning prevention]. Hangzhou: Hangzhoushi weisheng fangyizhan geweihui, 1971.

Hunan Province Revolutionary Health Committee, ed. *A Barefoot Doctor's Manual: A Guide to Traditional Chinese and Modern Medicine, Revised and Enlarged Edition.* Cloudburst Press, 1977.

Nanfang shisan shengshi "liangguang" "wugai" xuexiban ["Two controls and five reforms" class for thirteen provinces and municipalities in Southern China], ed. *Nanfang nongcun weisheng "liangguan" "wugai" ziliao huibian* [Compiled documents of "two controls and five reforms" in rural Southern China]. Beijing: Renmin weisheng chubanshe, 1975.

Shanghaishi Chuanshaxian Jiangzhen gongshe weishengyuan [Jiangzhen Commune Clinic of Chuansha County, Shanghai Municipality], ed. *Chijiao yisheng jiaocai: Gong nanfang diqu fuxun shiyong* [Barefoot doctor textbooks: For retraining in Southern China]. Beijing: Renmin weisheng chubanshe, 1974.

Shanghaishi diyi remin yiyuan erke [Pediatrics Department of Shanghai Municipal No. 1 People's Hospital], ed. *Ertong changyong yaowu* [Common medicines for children]. Shanghai: Shanghai kexue jishu chubanshe, 1966.

Shanghaishi zhongyi xueyuan, Zhejiangsheng zhongyi xueyuan, Zhejiangsheng zhongyi yanjiuyuan [Shanghai Chinese Medicine College, Zhejiang Chinese Medicine College, and Zhejiang Chinese Medicine Research Institute], ed. *Chijiao yisheng shouce* [Barefoot doctor's manual]. Shanghai: Shanghai kexue jishu chubanshe, 1969.

Sidel, Victor W., ed. *A Barefoot Doctor's Manual: Practical Chinese Medicine and Health.* New York: Gramercy, 1985.

Zhejiang xuexichongbing fangzhishi bianweihui [Editorial board of the History of schistosomiasis prevention and treatment in Zhejiang Province], ed. *Zhejiang xuexichongbing fangzhishi* [The history of schistosomiasis prevention and treatment in Zhejiang Province]. Shanghai: Shanghai kexue jishu chubanshe, 1992.

Zhejiangsheng geweihui shengchan zhihuizu weishengju [Health Bureau of the Production Directing Team of Zhejiang Province Revolutionary Committee], ed. *Zhejiang minjian changyong caoyao* [Common folk herbal medicines in Zhejiang Province]. 3 vols. Hangzhou: Zhejiang renmin chubanshe, 1970–72.

Zhejiangsheng weisheng xuanchuan xiezuozu [Zhejiang Province Health Propaganda Coordinating Team], ed. *Weisheng fangyi shouce* [Sanitation and epidemic-prevention manual]. Hangzhou: Zhejiangsheng weisheng xuanchuan xiezuozu, 1974.

Zhejiangsheng weishengting [Zhejiang Province Health Department], ed. *Nongcun weishengyuan keben* [Rural health worker's textbook]. Hangzhou: Zhejiang renmin chubanshe, 1966.

Zhejiangsheng weishengting [Zhejiang Provincial Health Department], *Zhejiangsheng xiangcun yisheng jiben yaowu mulu* [The basic catalogue of pharmaceuticals prescribed by village doctors in Zhejiang Province]. March 16, 2006.

Zheng Simin. *Jishengchongbing zhishi* [Knowledge of parasitic diseases]. Shanghai: Shanghai renmin chubanshe, 1973.

Collections of Documents

Chijiao yisheng xianjin shiji huibian [Collection of model deeds of barefoot doctors]. Beijing: Renmin weisheng chubanshe, 1974.

Chijiao yisheng xianjin shiji huibian: Chijiao yisheng zhuozhuang chengzhang [Collection of model deeds of barefoot doctors: Barefoot doctors are growing up quickly]. Vol. 3. Beijing: Renmin weisheng chubanshe, 1975.

Cihai (xiudinggao): yiyao weisheng fence [Unabridged comprehensive dictionary (revised edition): Medicine, pharmaceutical and health]. Shanghai: Shanghai cishu chubanshe, 1978.

Fuyangshi weishengju [Fuyang City Health Bureau], ed. *Fuyangxian xingzhengcun weishengshi guanli ruogan guiding* [A few regulations concerning village clinic management]. Fuyang: Fuyangxian weishengju, 1990.

Guowuyuan [The State Council]. *Guowuyuan gongbao* [State Council Gazetteer], 1957, 1958, 1981.

Jianshe weiyuanhui diaocha Zhejiang jingjisuo [Zhejiang Institute of Economics Survey of Construction Commission]. *Zhejiang lin'an nongcun diaocha* [Rural survey of Lin'an County, Zhejiang Province]. Hangzhou: Jianshe weiyuanhui diaocha Zhejiang jingjisuo, 1931.

Laodong renshibu laodong kexue yanjiusuo [Labor Research Institute of the Ministry of Labor and Personnel], ed. *Zhonghua renmin gongheguo laodong fagui xuanbian* [Collected labor laws and regulations of the People's Republic of China]. Beijing: Laodong renshi chubanshe, 1988.

Liu Zhonglu, ed. *Qingchun fangchengshi: Wushi ge Beijing nüzhiqing de zishu* [Youth formula: Stories told by 50 Beijing female educated youth]. Beijing: Beijing daxue chubanshe, 1995.

Mao Zedong. *Jianguo yilai Mao Zedong wengao* [Mao Zedong manuscript since the founding of the People's Republic of China]. Beijing: Zhongyang wenxian chubanshe, 1992.

Renmin ribao [The People's Daily]. "Renmin ribao quanwen shujuku guangpan, 1946–2008" [CD-ROM of Full Text Database of the *People's Daily*, 1946–2008].

Shanghai renmin chubanshe [Shanghai People's Press], ed. *Hezuo yiliao hao* [Cooperative medical services are excellent]. Shanghai: Shanghai renmin chubanshe, 1974.

Wei Ge, ed. *Hezuo yiliao hao* [Cooperative medical services are excellent]. Shanghai: Shanghai renmin chubanshe, 1974.

Zhang Zaitong and Xian Rijin, eds. *Minguo yiyao weisheng fagui xuanbian, 1912–1948* [Collection of medical and health regulations of the Republic of China, 1912–1948]. Jinan: Shangdong daxue chubanshe, 1990.

Zhejiangsheng weisheng fangyizhan [Zhejiang Province Sanitation and Epidemic-Prevention Station], ed. *Zhejiangsheng yiqing ziliao huibian, 1950–1979* [Compiled data of epidemic diseases in Zhejiang Province, 1950–1979]. Hangzhou: Zhejiangsheng weisheng fangyizhan, 1982.

———. *Zhejiangsheng yiqing ziliao huibian, 1980–1989* [Compiled data of epidemic diseases in Zhejiang Province, 1980–1989]. Hangzhou: Zhejiangsheng weisheng fangyizhan, 1994.

Zhonggong zhongyang wenxian yanjiushi [Literature Research Office of the Central Committee of the Chinese Communist Party], ed. *Jianguo yilai zhongyao wenxian xuanbian* [Collected important documents since the founding of the People's Republic of China]. Vol.3. Beijing: Zhongyang wenxian chubanshe, 1992.

Zhonghua renmin gongheguo weishengbu bangongting [General Office of the Ministry of Health of the People's Republic of China], ed. *Zhonghua renmin gongheguo weisheng fagui xuanbian, 1978–1980* [Collected legal documents of the People's Republic of China, 1978–1980]. Beijing: Falü chubanshe, 1982.

Zhongyang renmin zhengfu fazhi weiyuanhui [The Legal Affairs Committee of the Central Government], ed. *Zhongyang renmin zhengfu faling huibian (1949–1950)* [Collection of law documents of the central government, 1949–1950]. Beijing: Falü chubanshe, 1982.

Newspapers

Dongnan ribao [Southeastern Daily]
Fuyang ribao [Fuyang Daily]
Hangzhou ribao [Hangzhou Daily]
Jiankangbao [Health Care Newspaper]
Qianjiang wanbao [Qianjiang Evening News]
Renmin ribao [People's Daily]
Xinjingbao [The Beijing News]
Xinmin wanbao [Xinmin Evening News]
Zhejiang ribao [Zhejiang Daily]
Zhejiang weishengbao [Zhejiang Health Newspaper]

Magazines

Beijing zhongyi [Beijing Journal of Chinese Medicine]
Chijiao yisheng zazhi [Journal of Barefoot Doctors]
Current Scene: Development in Mainland China
Fujian zhongyiyao [Fujian Chinese Medicine Journal]
Gongnongbing huabao [Pictorial of Workers, Peasants, and Soldiers]
Guangji yikan [Guangji Hospital Medical Journal]
Guangxi chijiao yisheng [Guangxi Barefoot Doctor's Journal]
Guangxi weisheng [Journal of Guangxi Health]
Guowuyuan gongbao [The State Council Bulletin]

Hongqi [Red Flag]
Peking Review
Renmin baojian [People's Health Care]
Shanghai diyi yixueyuan xuebao [No.1 Shanghai Medical College Journal]
Xin yixue [New Medicine]
Xin zhongyiyao [New Chinese Medicine]
Yishi huikan [Medical Practice Journal]
Yiyao shijie [Medicine and Pharmaceutical World]
Zhejiang weisheng tongxun [Zhejiang Health Correspondence]
Zhejiang zhongyiyao zazhi [Zhejiang Chinese Medicine Journal]
Zhongguo chuantong yixue [Chinese Traditional Medicine]
Zhonghua yixue zazhi [China Medical Journal]

Films

Chunmiao. Directed by Xie Jin. Shanghai Film Factory, 1975.
Hongyu. Directed by Cui Wei. Beijing Film Factory, 1975.
Yanmin hupan. Directed by Gao Tianhong. Changchun Film Factory, 1975.

Secondary Sources

Anderson, Warwick. "Biomedicine in Chinese East Asia: From Semicolonial to Post-colonial?" In Leung and Furth, *Health and Hygiene in Chinese East Asia*, 273–78.
Andrews, Bridie. "The Making of Modern Chinese Medicine, 1895–1937." PhD diss., University of Cambridge, 1996.
Arnold, David. *Colonizing the Body: State Medicine and Epidemic Disease in Nineteenth-Century India.* Berkeley: University of California Press, 1993.
———, ed. *Imperial Medicine and Indigenous Societies.* Manchester: Manchester University Press, 1988.
Banister, Judith. *China's Changing Population.* Stanford, CA: Stanford University Press, 1987.
———. "Population, Public Health and Environment in China." *China Quarterly* 156 (December 1998): 986–1015.
Barnes, Linda L. *Needles, Herbs, Gods and Ghosts: China, Healing and the West to 1848.* Cambridge, MA: Harvard University Press, 2005.
Bastid, Marianne. "Economic Necessity and Political Ideals in Educational Reform during the Cultural Revolution." *China Quarterly* 42 (April–June 1970): 16–45.
Beijing yixueyuan yingyu jiaoyanshi hanying changyong yixue cihui bianxiezu [Editorial team of Chinese-English common medical vocabularies of the Beijing Medical College English teaching and research office], ed. *Hanying changyong yixue cihui* [Chinese-English common medical vocabularies]. Beijing: Renmin weisheng chubanshe, 1982.
Benedict, Carol. "Bubonic Plague in Nineteenth-Century China." *Modern China* 14, no. 2 (April 1988): 107–55.

————. "Policing the Sick: Plague and the Origins of State Medicine in Late Imperial China." *Late Imperial China* 14, no. 2 (December 1993): 60–77.

Bernstein, Thomas. *Up to the Mountains and Down to the Villages: The Transfer of Youth from Urban to Rural China.* New Haven, CT: Yale University Press, 1977.

Bibeau, Gilles. "From China to Africa: The Same Impossible Synthesis between Traditional and Western Medicines." *Social Science & Medicine* 21 (1985): 937–43.

Blendon, Robert J. "Can China's Health Care Be Transplanted without Chinese Economic Policies?" *New England Journal of Medicine* 300, no.26 (June 1979): 1453–58.

Bloom, Gerald, and Gu Xingyuan. "Introduction to Health Sector Reform in China." *IDS Bulletin* 28, no. 1 (1997): 1–11.

Blumenthal, David, and William Hsiao. "Privatization and Its Discontents—The Evolving Chinese Health Care System." *New England Journal of Medicine* 353, no. 11 (September 2005): 1165–69.

Bonavia, David. "The Fate of the 'New Born Things' of China's Cultural Revolution." *Pacific Affairs* 51, no.2 (Summer 1978): 177–94.

Borowy, Iris, ed. *Uneasy Encounters: The Politics of Medicine and Health in China 1900–1937.* New York: Peter Lang, 2009.

Bowers, John Z. *Western Medicine in a Chinese Palace: Peking Union Medical College, 1917–1951.* Philadelphia: Josiah Macy Jr. Foundation, 1972.

Bray, Francesca. "Chinese Medicine." In Bynum and Porter, *Companion Encyclopedia of the History of Medicine,* 728–54.

————. *Technology and Gender: Fabrics of Power in Late Imperial China.* Berkeley: University of California Press, 1997.

Brown, E. Richard. "Rockefeller Medicine in China: Professionalism and Imperialism." *China Notes* (Fall 1981): 174–81.

Burnham, John. *How the Idea of Profession Changed the Writing of Medical History.* London: Wellcome Institute for the History of Medicine, 1998.

Bynum, William. *Science and the Practice of Medicine in the Nineteenth Century.* Cambridge: Cambridge University Press, 1994.

Bynum, W. F., and Roy Porter, eds. *Companion Encyclopedia of the History of Medicine.* Vol. 2. London: Routledge, 1993.

Cai Jingfen. *Zhongguo yixue tongshi* [The general history of Chinese medicine]. Beijing: Renmin weisheng chubanshe, 2000.

Cailliez, Charlotte. "The Collapse of the Rural Health System." *China Perspective* 18 (1998): 36–43.

Cao Jinqing, Zhang Letian, and Chen Zhongya. *Dangdai zhebei xiangcun de shehui wenhun bianqian* [Social and cultural changes in contemporary Northern Zhejiang rural society]. Shanghai: Shanghai yuandong chubanshe, 2001.

Cass, Victoria B. "Female Healers in the Ming and the Lodge of Ritual and Ceremony." *Journal of the American Oriental Society* 106, no.1 (January-March 1986): 233–45.

Chan, Alan K. L., Gregory K. Clancey, and Hui-Chieh Loy, eds. *Historical Perspectives on East Asian Science, Technology and Medicine.* Singapore: Singapore University Press, 2001.

Chang Chia-che. "The Therapeutic Tug of War: The Imperial Physician-Patient Relationships in the Era of Dowager Cixi (1874–1908)." PhD diss., University of Pennsylvania, 1998.

Chang Chung-li. *The Income of the Chinese Gentry.* Seattle: University of Washington Press, 1962.

Chao, Yüan-ling. "The Ideal Physician in Late Imperial China: The Question of Sanshi 三世." *East Asian Science, Technology, and Medicine* 17 (2000): 66–93.

———. *Medicine and Society in Late Imperial China: A Study of Physicians in Suzhou, 1600–1850.* New York: Peter Lang, 2009.

Chen Bangxian. *Zhongguo yixueshi* [Chinese medical history]. Beijing: Shangwu yinshuguan, 1998.

Chen Cunren. *Wo de yiwu shengya* [My medical career]. Guilin: Guangxi shifan daxue chubanshe, 2007.

———. *Yinyuan shidai shenghuoshi* [The life history of the silver era]. Guilin: Guangxi shifan daxue chubanshe, 2007.

Chen Tejun and Mark Selden. "The Origins and Social Consequences of China's Hukou System." *China Quarterly* 139 (September 1994): 644–68.

Chen Zhongwu. "Medical Services in China." In *Modern Chinese Medicine.* Vol. 3 of *Chinese Health Care,* edited by Chen Haifeng and Zhu Chao, 644–68. Singapore: P. G. Publishing, 1984.

Chen, C. C. *Medicine in Rural China: A Personal Account.* Berkeley: University of California Press, 1989.

———. "Ting Hsien and the Public Health Movement in China." *Milbank Memorial Fund Quarterly* 15 (October 1937): 380–90.

Chen, Meei Shai. "The Great Reversal: Transformation of Health Care in the People's Republic of China." In *The Blackwell Companion to Medical Sociology,* edited by William C. Cockerham, 456–82. Oxford: Blackwell, 2001.

Chen, Pi-Chao. "The Chinese Model of Rural Health Service," in *Population and Health Policy in the People's Republic of China.* Occasional Monograph Series, No. 9. Washington: Interdisciplinary Communications Program, Smithsonian Institution, 1976.

Chen, Zhu. "Launch of the Health-Care Reform Plan in China." *Lancet* 373, no. 9672 (April 2009): 1322–24.

Cheung, Yuet-Wah. *Missionary Medicine in China: A Study of Two Canadian Protestant Missions in China before 1937.* Lanham, ND: University of America Press, 1988.

Cochran, Sherman. *Chinese Medicine Men: Consumer Culture in China and Southeast Asia.* Cambridge, MA: Harvard University Press, 2006.

Connor, Linda H. "Healing Powers in Contemporary China." In *Healing Powers and Modernity: Traditional Medicine, Shamanism, and Science in Asian Societies,* edited by Linda H. Connor and Geoffrey Samuel, 3–24. Westport, CT: Bergin & Garvey, 2000.

Croizier, Ralph. "Medicine and Modernization in China: An Historical Overview." In *Medicine in Chinese Culture: Comparative Studies of Health Care in Chinese and Other Societies,* edited by Arthur Kleinman, Peter Kunstadter, E. Russell Alexander, and James L. Gale, 21–35. Bethesda, MD: National Institutes of Health, 1975.

———. "Medicine, Modernization, and Cultural Crisis in China and India." *Comparative Studies in Society and History* 12 (July 1970): 275–91.

———. *Traditional Medicine in Modern China: Science, Nationalism, and the Tensions of Cultural Change.* Cambridge, MA: Harvard University Press, 1968.

Cullen, Christopher. "Patients and Healers in Late Imperial China: Evidence from the *Jinpingmei.*" *History of Science* 31, no. 2 (June 1993): 99–150.

———. "Yi'an (Case Statement): The Origins of a Genre of Chinese Medical Literature." In *Innovation in Chinese Medicine,* edited by Elisabeth Hsu, 297–323. Cambridge: Cambridge University Press, 2001.

Cunningham, Andrew, and Bridie Andrews. *Western Medicine as Contested Knowledge.* Manchester: Manchester University Press, 1997.

Davis, Deborah. "Chinese Social Welfare: Policies and Outcomes." In "The People's Republic of China after 40 Years." Special issue. *China Quarterly* 119 (September 1989): 577–97.

De Grunchè, Kingston. *Doctor Apricot of "Heaven Below": The Story of the Hangchow Medical Mission.* London: Marshall Brothers, 1911.

———. *Dr. D. Duncan of Hangchow, Known in China as Dr. Apricot of Heaven Below.* London: Marshall Morgan & Scott, Ltd., 1930.

Ding Hong, Wu Lijuan, Yuan Fang, Yang Shanfa, and Dong Wenjing. "Xiangcun yisheng kangshengsu yu jisu shiyong fenxi" [The analysis of antibiotics and hormones prescribed by village doctors]. *Yixue yu zhexue* [Medicine and Philosophy] 26, no. 10 (October 2005): 33–34.

Ding Xueliang. "Yingdui SARS weiji de sanzhong tizhi: Qiangzhi, fazhi, ruozhi" [Three systems responding toward SARS crisis: Mandatory, legal, and weak methods]. Accessed March 20, 2011. http://www.aisixiang.com/data/7243.html.

Dong, Hengjin, Lennart Bogg, Clas Rehnberg, and Vinod Diwan. "Drug Policy in China: Pharmaceuticals Distribution in Rural Areas." *Social Science & Medicine* 48, no. 6 (March 1999): 777–86.

Duckett, Jane. "Challenging the Economic Reform Paradigm: Policy and Politics in the Early 1980s Collapse of the Rural Cooperative Medical System." *China Quarterly* 205 (March 2011): 80–95.

———. *The Chinese State's Retreat from Health: Policy and the Politics of Retrenchment.* Abingdon, UK: Routledge, 2010.

Elling, Ray H. "Medical Systems as Changing Social Systems." *Social Science & Medicine,* 12 (April 1978): 107–15.

Elman, Benjamin. *A Cultural History of Modern Science in China.* Cambridge, MA: Harvard University Press, 2006.

———. *From Philosophy to Philology: Intellectual and Social Aspects of Change in Late Imperial China.* Los Angeles: UCLA Asian Pacific Monograph Series, 2001.

———. *On Their Own Terms: Science in China, 1550–1900.* Cambridge, MA: Harvard University Press, 2005.

Ernst, Waltraud. "Plural Medicine, Tradition and Modernity: Historical and Contemporary Perspective: Views from Below and Above." In *Plural Medicine, Tradition and Modernity, 1800–2000,* edited by Waltraud Ernst, 1–17. New York: Routledge, 2002.

Establet, Florence Bretelle. "Resistance and Receptivity: French Colonial Medicine in Southwest China, 1893–1930." *Modern China* 25, no. 2 (April 1999): 171–203.

Fan Rusen and Ji Tianshu. "Jindai beifang yaoping gongying tixi de jiangou" [The development of a pharmaceutical supply and marketing system in modern North China]. *Zhongguo lishi dili lunchong* [Collections of Essays on Chinese Historical Geography] 18, no. 2 (June 2003): 104–13.

Fang, Xiaoping. "Dedicated to a Medical Career in the 'Heaven Below': Duncan David Main's Correspondence, 1914–1926." Research Report, Rockefeller Archive Center (RAC), 2008.

———. "Sexual Misconduct and Punishment in Chinese Hospital in the 1960s and 1970s." *Nan nü: Men, Women, and Gender in China* 14, no. 2 (2012): 1–35

———. "From Union Clinics to Barefoot Doctors: Village Healers, Medical Pluralism, and State Medicine in Chinese Villages." *Journal of Modern Chinese History* 2, no. 2 (2008): 223–41.

———. "The Global Cholera Pandemic Reaches Chinese Villages: Population Mobility, Political Control, and Economic Incentives in Epidemic Prevention, 1962–1964." Modern Asian Studies, forthcoming.

———. "Western Medicine since 1949." In *Encyclopaedia of Modern China*, edited by David Pong, 579–80. New York: Charles Scribner's Sons, 2009.

———. "Zhongguo nongcun de chijiao yisheng yu hezuo yiliao zhidu: Zhejiangsheng Fuyangxian de gean yanjiu" [Barefoot doctors and cooperative medical services in rural China: A case study of Fuyang County, Zhejiang Province]. *Ershiyi shiji* [Twenty-First Century] 79 (October 2003): 87–98.

Farquhar, Judith. "Eating Chinese Medicine." *Cultural Anthropology* 9, no. 4 (November 1994): 471–97.

———. *Knowing Practice: The Clinical Encounter of Chinese Medicine*. Boulder, CO: Westview, 1994.

———. "Market Magic: Getting Rich and Getting Personal in Medicine after Mao." *American Ethnologist* 23, no. 2 (May 1996): 239–57.

———. "Problems of Knowledge in Contemporary China." *Social Science & Medicine* 24 (1987): 1013–21.

Feng Xueshan, Tang Shenglan, Gerald Bloom, Malcolm Segall, and Gu Xingyuan. "Cooperative Medical Schemes in Contemporary Rural China." *Social Science & Medicine* 41, no. 8 (October 1995): 1111–18.

Ferguson, Mary E. *China Medical Board and Peking Union Medical College*. New York: China Medical Board, 1970.

Field, Mark G. "Health and the Polity: Communist China and Soviet Russia." *Studies in Comparative Communism* 7, no. 4 (Winter 1974): 420–25.

Forster, Keith. *Rebellion and Factionalism in a Chinese Province: Zhejiang, 1966–1976*. Armonk, NY: M. E. Sharpe, 1990.

Fox, Daniel M. "Medical Institutions and the State." In Bynum and Porter, *Companion Encyclopedia of the History of Medicine*, 1210–18.

Freidson, Eliot. "How Dominant Are the Professions?" In Hafferty and McKinlay, *Changing Medical Profession: An International Perspective*, 54–68.

———. "The Profession of Medicine." In *The Sociology and Politics of Health: A Reader*, edited by Michael Purdy and David Banks, 130–34. New York: Routledge, 2001.

———. *Profession of Medicine: A Study of the Sociology of Applied Knowledge*. Chicago: University of Chicago Press, 1988.

———. "The Sociology of Medicine," *Current Sociology* 10, no. 11 (1962): 123–92.

Frenk, Julio, and Luis Duran-Arenas. "The Medical Profession and the State." In Hafferty and McKinlay, *Changing Medical Profession*, 124–37.

Friedman, Edward, Paul G. Pickowicz, and Mark Selden. *Revolution, Resistance, and Reform in Village China*. New Haven, CT: Yale University Press, 2005.

Furth, Charlotte. *A Flourishing Yin: Gender in China's Medical History, 960–1665*. Berkeley: University of California Press, 1999.

————. "Hygienic Modernity in Chinese East Asia." In Leung and Furth, *Health and Hygiene in Chinese East Asia*, 1–21.

Gao, Mobo C. F. *Gao Village: A Portrait of Rural Life in Modern China.* Honolulu: University of Hawai'i Press, 1999.

Gao, James Z. *The Communist Takeover of Hangzhou: The Transformation of City and Cadre, 1949–1954.* Honolulu: University of Hawai'i Press, 2004.

Gao Ming and Qian Haoping. "Beida nüboshihou yao kan weishengyuan" [A woman postdoctoral fellow of Peking University would like to cancel township clinics]. *Yiyao chanye zixun* [Medicine and Management Industry Information] 3, no. 7 (March 2006): 54–56.

Gardner, John, and Wilt Idema. "China's Educational Revolution." In *Authority, Participation and Cultural Changes in China*, edited by Stuart R. Schram, 257–90. Cambridge: Cambridge University Press, 1973.

Ge Zichang. "Zhongguo diyige nü chijiao yisheng de quzhe rensheng" [The intricate life of the first Chinese female barefoot doctor]. *Guizhou wenshi tiandi* [Guizhou Literature and History World] 2 (2001): 30–38.

Geiger, H. Jack. "Health Care in the People's Republic of China: Implications for the United States." In *Culture and Healing in Asian Societies: Anthropological, Psychiatric and Public Health Studies*, edited by Arthur Kleinman, Peter Kunstadter, E. Russell Alexander, and James L. Gate, 379–89. Boston: G. K. Hall, 1978.

Geyndt, De Willy. *From Barefoot Doctor to Village Doctor in Rural China.* The World Bank Technical Paper, Asia Technical Department Series. Washington, DC: The World Bank, 1992.

Gish, Oscar. "The Political Economy of Primary Care and 'Health by the People': An Historical Explanation." *Journal of Opinion* 9, no. 3 (Autumn 1979): 6–13.

Goldschmidt, Asaf. *The Evolution of Chinese Medicine: Song Dynasty, 960–1200.* Abingdon, UK: Routledge, 2008.

Goldstein, Joshua. "Scissors, Surveys, and Psycho-Prophylactics: Prenatal Health Care Campaigns and State Building in China, 1949–1954." *Journal of Historical Sociology* 11, no.2 (June 1998): 153–84.

Gong Youlong and Chao Limin. "Shanghaixian de chijiao yisheng" [Barefoot doctors in Shanghai County]. *Shanghai diyi yixueyuan xuebao* [No.1 Shanghai Medical College Journal] 1 (1982): 76–79.

Good, Charles M. *Ethno-Medical Systems in Africa: Patterns of Traditional Medicine in Rural and Urban Kenya.* New York: Guilford, 1987.

Goodkin, Karen Marcia. "In Mao's Shadow: Local Health System Praxis, Process, and Politics in Deng Xiaoping's China." PhD diss., University of Connecticut, 1998.

Gould-Martin, Katherine. "Hot Cold Clean Poison and Dirt: Chinese Folk Medical Categories." *Social Science & Medicine* 12 (January 1978): 39–46.

Granshaw, Lindsay, and Roy Porter, eds. *The Hospital in History.* London: Routledge, 1989.

Grant, Joanna. *A Chinese Physician: Wang Ji and the "Stone Mountain Medical Case Histories."* New York: Routledge-Curzon, 2003.

Gross, Miriam. "Chasing Snails: Anti-Schistosomiasis Campaigns in the People's Republic of China." PhD diss., University of California, San Diego, 2010.

Grypma, Sonya. *Healing Henan: Canadian Nurses at the North China Mission, 1888–1947.* Vancouver: UBC Press, 2008.

Gu Xin and Fang Liming. "Ziyuanxing yu qiangzhixing zhijian: Zhongguo nongcun hezuo yiliao de zhidu qianruxing yu fazhan ke chixuxing" [Between being voluntary and compulsory: Chinese rural cooperative service's institutional embeddedness and sustainable development]. *Shehuixue yanjiu* [Sociology Study Journal] 5 (2004): 1–18.

Hafferty, Frederic W., and John B. McKinlay. *The Changing Medical Profession: An International Perspective.* New York: Oxford University Press, 1993.

Hahn, Robert A., and Arthur Kleinman. "Biomedical Practice and Anthropological Theory: Frameworks and Directions." *Annual Review of Anthropology*, 12 (1983): 305–33.

Hai Wen, Wang Jian, Chen Qiulin, Zhao Zhong, and Hou Zhengang. "Nongcun weisheng fuwu tixi tantao" [Discussion on rural health service system]. China Center for Economic Research and China Academy of Healty Policy, Peking University, May 12, 2003.

Halstead, Scott B., and Yu Yong-xin. "Human Viral Vaccine in China." In *Science and Medicine in Twentieth-Century China: Research and Education*, edited by John Z. Bowers, J. William Hess, and Nathan Sivin, 141–54. Ann Arbor, MI: Center for Chinese Studies, University of Michigan, 1988.

Han, Dongping. "Impact of the Cultural Revolution on Rural Education and Economic Development." *Modern China* 27, no. 1 (January 2001): 59–90.

———. *The Unknown Cultural Revolution: Education Reforms and Their Impact on China's Rural Development.* New York: Garland, 2000.

Hanson, Marta. "Conceptual Blind Spots, Media Blindfolds: The Case of SARS and Traditional Chinese Medicine." In Leung and Furth, *Health and Hygiene in Chinese East Asia*, 228–54.

———. "Inventing a Tradition in Chinese Medicine: From Universal Canon to Local Medical Knowledge in South China, the Seventeenth to the Nineteenth Century." PhD diss., University of Pennsylvania, 1997.

———. "Merchants of Medicine: Huizhou Mercantile Consciousness, Morality, and Medical Patronage in Seventeenth-Century China." In *East Asian Science: Tradition and Beyond*, edited by KeizôHashimoto, Catherine Jami, and Lowell Skar, 207–14. Osaka: Kansai University Press, 1995.

Hardon, Anita P. "The Use of Modern Pharmaceuticals in a Filipino Village: Doctors' Prescription and Self Medication." *Social Science & Medicine* 25, no. 3 (1987): 277–92.

He Zhaoxiong. *Zhongguo yide shi* [The history of Chinese medical ethics]. Shanghai: Shanghai yike daxue chunbanshe, 1988.

Heller, Peter S. "The Strategy of Health-Sector Planning in Public Health in the People's Republic of China." In *Medicine and Health in China*, edited by M. Wegman and T. Lin. New York: Josiah Macy Jr. Foundation, 1973.

Henderson, Gail. "Issues in the Modernization of Medicine in China." In *Science and Technology in Post-Mao China*, edited by Denis Fred Simon and Merle Goldman, 199–221. Cambridge, MA: Harvard University Press, 1989.

———. "Physicians in China: Assessing the Impact of Ideology and Organization." In Hafferty and McKinlay, *Changing Medical Profession*, 184–96.

———. "Trends in Health Services Utilisations in Eight Provinces, 1989–1993." *Social Science & Medicine* 47, no. 12 (1998): 1957–71.

Henderson, Gail, and Myron Cohen. *The Chinese Hospital: A Socialist Work Unit.* New Haven, CT: Yale University Press, 1984.

Hershatter, Gail. "Birthing Stories: Rural Midwives in 1950s China." In *Dilemmas of Victory: The Early Years of the People's Republic of China,* edited by Jeremy Brown and Paul G. Pickowicz, 337–58. Cambridge, MA: Harvard University Press, 2007.

——. "The Gender of Memory: Rural Chinese Women and the 1950s." *Signs: Journal of Women in Culture and Society* 28, no. 1 (Fall 2002): 43–70.

Hillier, Sheilam, and J. A. Jewell. "Chinese Traditional Medicines and Modern Western Medicine: Integration and Separation in China." In Hillier and Jewell, *Health Care and Traditional Medicine in China,* 306–35.

Hillier, Sheilam and J. A. Jewell, eds. *Health Care and Traditional Medicine in China, 1800–1982.* London: Routledge & Kegan Paul, 1983.

Hinrichs, T. J. "New Geographies of Chinese Medicine." In *Osiris.* 2nd ser., vol. 13, *Beyond Joseph Needham: Science, Technology, and Medicine in East and Southeast Asia,* edited by Morris F. Low, 287–325. Chicago: University of Chicago Press, 1998.

Hinton, William. *Shenfan.* New York: Random House, 1983.

Horn, Joshua S. *Away with All Pests: An English Surgeon in People's China, 1954–1969.* New York: Hamlyn, 1969.

Hsia, Tao-tai. "Law on Public Health." In *Medicine and Public Heath in the People's Republic of China,* edited by Joseph R. Quinn, 109–35. Bethesda, MD: National Institutes of Health, 1972.

Hsu, Elisabeth. "The Medicine from China Has Rapid Effects: Chinese Medicine Patients in Tanzania." *Anthropology & Medicine* 9, no. 3 (2002): 291–313.

——. "The Reception of Western Medicine in China: Examples from Yunnan" In *Science and Empires, Boston Studies in the Philosophy of Science,* edited by Patrick Petitjean, Catherine Jami, and Anne Marie Moulin, 89–101. Vol. 136. Dordrecht: Kluwer, 1992.

——. *The Transmission of Chinese Medicine.* Cambridge: Cambridge University Press, 1999.

Hu Shiming and Eli Saifman. *Toward a New World Outlook: A Documentary History of Education in the People's Republic of China.* New York: AMS Press, 1976.

Huang, Phillip C. C. *The Peasant Family and Rural Development in the Yangzi Delta, 1350–1988.* Stanford, CA: Stanford University Press, 1990.

——. "Rural Class Struggle in the Chinese Revolution: Representational and Objective Realities from the Land Reform to the Cultural Revolution." *Modern China* 21, no. 1 (January 1995): 105–43.

Huang Shumin. "Transforming China's Collective Health Care System: A Village Study." *Social Science & Medicine* 27, no. 9 (1988): 879–89.

Huang Shuze and Lin Shixiao, eds. *Dangdai zhongguo de weisheng shiye* [Health Development in Contemporary China]. Vols. 1 and 2. Beijing: Zhongguo shehui kexue chubanshe, 1986.

Huang Yanzhong. "Bringing the Local State Back In: The Political Economy of Public Health in Rural China." *Journal of Contemporary China* 13, no. 39 (May 2004): 367–90.

Hyde, Sandra Teresa. *Eating Spring Rice: The Cultural Politics of AIDS in Southwest China.* Berkeley: University of California Press, 2007.

Jackson, Sukhan, Adrian C. Sleigh, Li Peng, and Liu Xi-li. "Health Finance in Rural Henan: Low Premium Insurance Compared to the Out-of-Pocket System." *China Quarterly* 181 (2005): 137–57.

Jewson, N. D. "The Disappearance of the Sick-Man from Medical Cosmology." *Sociology* 10, no. 2 (1976): 225–44.

Jia, Huanguang. "Chinese Medicine in Post-Mao China: Standardization and the Context of Modern Science." PhD diss., University of North Carolina–Chapel Hill, 1997.

Jiang Zhushan. "Wanming Jiangnan Qi Biaojia jiazu de richang shenghuoshi: Yi yibing guanxi weili de tantao" [The daily life of the Qi Biaojia family in late Ming Jiangnan: A focus on doctor-patient relations]. *Dushi wenhua yanjiu* [Urban Culture Studies] 1 (2006): 181–212.

Jin Wenguan. "Tantan xiangcun funu de weisheng wenti" [On the issue of rural women's health]. *Chusheng yuekan* [The Sound of the Hoe Monthly] 1, no. 7 (1935): 10–13.

Jing Jun. *Dingxian shiyan: Shequ yixue yu huabei nongcun* [Ding County experiment: Community medicine and rural North China]. Beijing: Department of Sociology, Tsinghua University, 2004.

Kaptchuk, Ted J., Peter Goldman, David A Stone, and William B Stason. "Do Medical Devices Have Enhanced Placebo Effects?" *Journal of Clinical Epidemiology* 53, no.8 (2000): 786–92.

Karchmer, Eric I. "Chinese Medicine in Action: On the Postcoloniality of Medical Practice in China." *Medical Anthropology* 29, no. 3 (2010): 226–52.

Kaufman, Joan. "SARS and China's Health-Care Response: Better to be Both Red and Expert!" In *SARS in China: Prelude to Pandemic?* edited byArthur Kleinman and James L. Watson. Stanford, CA: Stanford University Press, 2006.

Khng, Christopher Houng Chin. "Trends in the Utilization of Traditional Chinese Medicines in Rural China: A Case Study of Yuhang County, Zhejiang Province." Master's Thesis, University of Guelph, 2001.

Kleinman, Arthur. "Lessons from a Clinical Approach to Medical Anthropological Research." *Medical Anthropology Newsletter* 8, no.4 (August 1977): 11–15.

———. *Patients and Healers in the Context of Culture: An Exploration of the Borderland between Anthropology, Medicine, and Psychiatry.* Berkeley: University of California Press, 1980.

Kleinman, Arthur, and James L. Watson. "SARS in Social and Historical Context." In *SARS in China: Prelude to Pandemic?* Edited by Arthur Kleinman and James L. Watson, 1–16. Stanford, CA: Stanford University Press, 2006.

Klotzbucher, Sascha, Peter Lässig, Qin Jiangmei, and Susanne Weigelin-Schwiedrzik. "What's New in the 'New Rural Co-Operative Medical System'? An Assessment in One Kazak County of the Xinjiang Uyghur Autonomous Region," *China Quarterly* 201 (March 2010): 38–57.

Kwok, Pui-Lan. *Chinese Women and Christianity, 1860–1927.* Atlanta: Scholars Press, 1992.

Lampton, David. "Economics, Politics, and the Determinants of Policy Outcomes in China: Post-Cultural Revolutionary Health Policy." *Australia and New Zealand Journal of Sociology* 12, no.1 (1976): 43–49.

——. *Health, Conflict, and the Chinese Political System*, Michigan Papers in Chinese Studies, No. 1. Ann Arbor, MI: Center for Chinese Studies, University of Michigan, 1974.

——. "Health Policy during the Great Leap Forward." *China Quarterly* 60 (December 1974): 668–98.

——. "Performance and the Chinese Political System: A Preliminary Assessment of Education and Health Policies." *China Quarterly* 75 (September 1978): 509–39.

——. *The Politics of Medicine in China: The Policy Process*, 1949–1977. Boulder, CO: Westview, 1977.

——. "Public Health and Politics in China's Past Two Decades." *Health Services Report* 87, no. 10 (December 1972): 895–904.

Landy, David. *Culture, Disease, and Healing: Studies in Medical Anthropology*. New York: Macmillan, 1977.

——. "Role Adaptation: Traditional Curers under the Impact of Western Medicine." *American Ethnologist* 1, no. 1 (February 1974): 103–27.

Langwick, Stacy. "From Non-Aligned Medicines to Market-Based Herbals: China's Relationship to the Shifting Politics of Traditional Medicine in Tanzania." *Medical Anthropology* 29, no. 3 (2010): 15–43.

Lee, Liming. "The Current State of Public Health in China." *Annual Review of Public Health* 25 (2004): 327–29.

Lee Sung. "WHO and the Developing World: The Contest for Ideology." In *Western Medicine as Contested Knowledge*, edited by Andrew Cunningham and Bridie Andrews, 24–45. Manchester: Manchester University Press, 1997.

Lei Jin. "From Mainstream to Marginal? Trends in the Use of Chinese Medicine in China from 1991 to 2004." *Social Science & Medicine* 71, no. 6 (September 2010): 1063–67.

Lei, Sean Hsiang-lin. "Fu zeren de yisheng yu you xinyang de bingren: Zhongxiyi lunzheng yu yibing guanxi zai minguo shiqi de zhuanbian" [Accountable doctor and loyal patient: The transformation of doctor-patient relationships in the Republican period]. *Xinshixue* [New History] 14, no. 1 (March 2003): 45–96.

——. "When Chinese Medicine Encountered the State: 1910–1949." PhD diss., University of Chicago, 1999.

——. "When Chinese Medicine Encountered the State, 1928–1937." Accessed June 30, 2009. http://www.ihp.sinica.edu.tw/~medicine/active/years/hl.PDF.

Leslie, Charles. *Asian Medical Systems: A Comparative Study*. Berkeley: University of California Press, 1976.

Leslie, Charles, and Allan Young, eds. *Path to Asian Medical Knowledge*. Berkeley: University of California Press, 1992.

Leung, Angela Ki Che. "Dignity of the Nation, Gender Equality, or Charity for All? Options for the First Modern Chinese Women Doctors." In *The Dignity of Nations: Equality, Competition, and Honor in East Asian Nationalism*, edited by Sechin Y. S. Chien and John Fitzgerald, 71–92. Hong Kong: Hong Kong University Press, 2006.

——. "Medical Instruction and Popularization in Ming-Qing China." *Late Imperial China* 24 (June 2003): 130–52.

———. "Medical Learning from the Song to the Ming." In *The Song-Yuan-Ming Transition in Chinese History*, edited by Paul Jakov Smith and Richard Von Glahn, 374–400. Cambridge, MA: Harvard University Asia Center, 2003.

———. *Medicine for Women in Imperial China*. Leidon: Brill, 2006.

———. "Mingdai shehui zhong de yiyao" [Medicines and pharmaceuticals in Ming society]. *Faguo hanxue* [French Sinology] 6 (2002): 345–61.

———. "Organized Medicine in Ming-Qing China: State and Private Medical Institutions in the Lower Yangzi Region." *Late Imperial China* 8, no. 1 (1987): 134–66.

———. "Women Practicing Medicine in Pre-Modern China." In *Chinese Women in the Imperial Past: New Perspectives*, edited by H. Zurndorfer, 101–34. Leiden: Brill Academic, 1999.

———. "Yiliaoshi yu zhongguo xiandaixing wenti" [The medical history and modernity]. *Zhongguo shehui lishi pinglun* [China Social History Review] 8 (2007): 1–18.

Leung, Angela Ki Che, and Charlotte Furth, eds. *Health and Hygiene in Chinese East Asia: Policies and Publics in the Long Twentieth Century*. Durham, NC: Duke University Press, 2010.

Lewis, Milton J., and Kerrie L. MacPherson, *Public Health in Asia and the Practice: Historical and Comparative Perspectives*. London: Routledge, 2008.

Lewis, Thomas. *The Youngest Science: Notes of a Medicine-Watcher*. New York: Viking Press, 1983.

Li Decheng. "Chijiao yisheng yanjiu shuping" [Comments on studies of barefoot doctors]. *Zhongguo weisheng chuji baojian* [Chinese Primary Health Care] 21, no. 1 (January 2007): 6–8.

Li, Huaiyin. *Village China under Socialism and Reform: A Micro History, 1948–2008*. Stanford, CA: Stanford University Press, 2009.

LiJinghan. *Dingxian shehui gaikuang diaocha* [Social survey of Ding County]. Shanghai: Shanghai shudian, 1992.

———. *Zhongguo nongcun wenti* [China's Rural issues]. Changsha: Shangwu yishuguan, 1939.

Li Jingwei and Stella Quah. *The Triumph of Practicality: Tradition and Modernity in Health Care Utilization in Selected Asian Counters*. Singapore: Social Issues in Southeast Asia, Institute of Southeast Asia, 1989.

Li Peiliang and Xu Huiying. "Yiliao weishengwang" [Medical and health network]. In *Renmin gongshe yu nongcun fazhan: Taishanxian doushan gongshe de jingyan* [People's commune and rural development: Experiences of Doushan Commune, Taishan County], edited by Li Peiliang and Liu Zhaojia, 59–95. Hong Kong: Chinese University of Hong Kong Press, 1981.

Li Ting'an. *Zhongguo xiangcun weisheng wenti* [Chinese rural health issue]. Shanghai: Shangwu yinshuguan, 1935.

Li Yushang, "The Elimination of Schistosomiasis in Jiaxing and Haining Counties, 1948–1958." In Leung and Furth, *Health and Hygiene in Chinese East Asia*, 204–27.

Lin Qianliang. "Zhejiang jiefangqian de zhongyi jiaoyu" [Chinese medical education in Zhejiang before liberation]. *Zhejiang wenshi ziliao* [Zhejiang Historical Data] 16 (June 1980): 143–53.

Lisowski, F. P. "Emergence and Development of the Barefoot Doctor in China." In *History of the Professionalisation of Medicine: Proceedings of the 3rd International Symposium on the Comparative History of Medicine—East and West*, edited by Teizo Ogawa,129–65. Osaka: Taniguchi Foundation, 1987.

Litsios, Socrates. "The Long and Difficult Road to Alma-Ata: A Personal Reflection." *International Journal of Health Services* 32, no. 4 (2002): 709–32.

Liu Jingzhen and Li Bozhong. "Duotai, biyun, yu jueyu—Song, Yuan, Ming, Qing shiqi jiangzhe diqu de jueyu fangfa jiqi yunyong yu chuanbo" [Abortion, contraception, and sterilization: Sterilization methods and their application in Jiangsu and Zhejiang areas in the Song-Yuan-Ming-Qing periods]. *Zhongguo xueshu* [China Scholarship] 1 (2000): 71–99.

Liu Luya. "Jiuzhongguo de zhiyao gongye" [The pharmaceutical industry in old China]. *Lishi dang'an* [Historical Archives] 2 (1995): 105–12.

Liu Xiaoxing. "Change and Continuity of Yi Medical Culture in Southwest China." PhD diss., University of Illinois at Urbana-Champaign, 1995.

Liu Yuanli. "China's Public Health-Care System: Facing the Challenges." *Bulletin of the World Health Organization* 82, no. 7 (July 2004): 532–38.

———. "China's Public Health-Care System: Facing the Challenges." *Bulletin of the World Health Organization* 82, no. 7 (July 2004): 532–38.

Liu Yuanli, William C. L. Hsiao, Qing Li, Xingzhu Liu, and Minghui Ren. "Transformation of China's Rural Health Care Financing." *Social Science & Medicine* 41, no. 8 (October 1995): 1085–93.

Liu Zhongyi. *Cong chijiao yisheng dao meiguo dafu: Yige meiguo yixue zhuanjia de bansheng zishu* [From barefoot doctor to American doctor: An autobiography of half the life of an American medical professor]. Shanghai: Shanghai renmin chubanshe, 1994.

Lo, Vivienne. "But Is it [History of] Medicine? Twenty Years in the History of the Healing Arts of China." *Social History of Medicine* 22, no. 2 (August 2009): 283–303.

Lora-Wainwright, Anna. "Using Local Resources: Barefoot Doctors and Bone Manipulation in Rural Langzhong, Sichuan Province, PRC." *Asian Medicine: Tradition and Modernity* 1, no. 2 (2005): 470–89.

Lu Gwei-djen and Joseph Needham. *Celestial Lancets: A History and Rationale of Acupuncture and Moxa.* New York: Cambridge University Press, 1980.

Lu Qianlu. "Minjian de jibing yu yiyao" [Folk diseases and pharmaceutical]. *Zhejiang minzhong jiaoyu* [Mass Education in Zhejiang] 1 (1947):17–18.

Lucas, AnElissa. "Changing Medical Models in China: Organizational Options or Obstacles?" *China Quarterly* 83 (September 1980): 461–89.

———. *Chinese Medical Modernization: Comparative Policy Continuities, 1930s–1980s.* New York: Praeger, 1982.

Ma Boying. *Zhongwai yixue wenhua jiaoliushi* [The history of intercultural medicine communication between China and foreign countries]. Shanghai: Wenhui chubanshe, 1993.

Ma Boying, Gao Xi, and Hong Zhongli. *Zhongguo yixue wenhuashi* [Chinese cultural history of medicine]. Shanghai: Shanghai renmin chubanshe, 1994.

Ma Hong, ed. *Zhongguo gaige quanshu: Yiliao weisheng tizhi gaigejuan* [China reform: Medical and health system reform]. Dalian: Dalian chubanshe, 1992.

MacPherson, Kerrie L. *A Wilderness of Marshes: The Origins of Public Health in Shanghai, 1843–1893.* Hong Kong: Oxford University Press, 1987.

Mann, Felix. "Chinese Traditional Medicine: A Practitioner's View." *China Quarterly* 23 (July–September 1965): 28–36.

McElroy, Ann, and Patricia K. Townsend. *Medical Anthropology in Ecological Perspective.* Boulder, CO: Westview, 1985.

Meisner, Maurice. *Mao's China: A History of the People's Republic.* New York: Free Press, 1977.

———. *Mao's China and After: A History of the People's Republic.* New York: Free Press, 1999.

Miao Yubing. "Jiefangqian Hangzhoushi de difang weisheng yiliao" [Local health and medicine in Hangzhou before liberation]. In *Hangzhou wenshi zilliao* [Hangzhou Cultural and Historical Data], vol. 6, edited by Zhengxie Hangzhoushi weiyuanhui wenshi ziliao gongzuo weiyuanhui [The Cultural and Historical Data Committee of Hangzhou Prefecture Political Consultative Committee], 75–81. Hangzhou: Zhengxie Hangzhoushi weiyuanhui wenshi ziliao gongzuo weiyuanhui, 1988.

Minden, Karen. *Bamboo Stone: The Evolution of A Chinese Medical Elite.* Toronto: University of Toronto Press, 1994.

"Missing the Barefoot Doctors." *Economist* 385, no. 8550 (October 13, 2007): 27–30.

Needham, Joseph, and Lu Gwei-Djen. "China and the Origins of Qualifying Examinations in Medicine." In *Clerks and Craftsmen in China and the West: Lectures and Addresses on the History of Science and Technology,* edited by Joseph Needham, 379–95. Cambridge: Cambridge University Press, 1970.

Oksenberg, Michel. "The Chinese Policy Process and the Public Health Issue: An Arena Approach." *Studies in Comparative Communism* 7, no. 4 (Winter 1974): 375–408.

Organization for Economic Cooperation and Development. *OECD Economic Survey China 2010.* Vol. 2010/6. Paris: OECD Publications, February 2010.

Parmelee, Donna, Gail Henderson, and Myron Cohen. "Medicine under Socialism: Some Observations on Yugoslavia and China." *Social Sciences & Medicine* 16, no. 15 (1982): 1389–96.

Pepper, Suzanne. *Radicalism and Education Reform in 20th Century China: The Search for an Ideal Development Model.* New York: Cambridge University Press, 1996.

Peterson, Glen. *The Power of Words: Literacy and Revolution in South China, 1949–95.* Vancouver: UBC Press, 1997.

Peterson, M. Jeanne. *Medical Profession in Mid-Victorian London.* Berkeley: University of California Press, 1978.

Porter, Dorothy, and Roy Porter. *Patient's Progress: Doctors and Doctoring in Eighteenth-Century England.* Oxford: Polity in Association with Basil Blackwell, 1989.

Porter, Roy. "The Patient in England, C1660–C1800." In *Medicine in Society: Historical Essays,* edited by Andrew Wear, 91–118. Cambridge: Cambridge University Press, 1992.

———. "The Patient's View: Doing Medical History from Below." *Theory and Society* 14, no. 2 (March 1985): 175–98.

Potter, Sulamith Heins, and Jack M. Potter. *China's Peasants: The Anthropology of a Revolution.* Cambridge: Cambridge University Press, 1990.

Press, Irwin. "Problems in the Definition and Classification of Medical Systems." *Social Science & Medicine* 14 B, no. 1 (February 1980): 45–57.

Qi Moujia, ed. *Dangdai zhongguo de yiyao shiye* [Pharmaceuticals in contemporary China]. Beijing: Zhongguo shehui kexue chubanshe, 1988.

Qian Xinzhong. *Zhongguo weisheng shiye fazhan yu juece* [Health development and decision-making in China]. Beijing: Zhongguo yiyao keji chubanshe, 1992.

Qiao Qiming. *Zhongguo nongcun shehui jingjixue* [Social Economics of Rural China]. Shanghai: Shanghai shudian, 1992.

Qiu Shiting, ed. "1929 nian fandui feizhi zhongyi zhongyao de douzheng" [The struggle against the abolishment of Chinese medicine doctors and Chinese pharmaceuticals in 1929]. In *Hangzhou wenshi ziliao* [Hangzhou Cultural and Historical Data], vol.7, edited by Zhengxie Hangzhoushi weiyuanhui wenshi ziliao gongzuo weiyuanhui [The cultural and historical data committee of Hangzhou Prefecture political consultative committee], 67–85. Hangzhou: Zhengxie Hangzhoushi weiyuanhui wenshi ziliao gongzuo weiyuanhui, 1986.

Quah, Stella. "Health and Culture." In *The Blackwell Companion to Medical Sociology*, edited by William C. Cockerham, 23–42. Oxford: Blackwell, 2001.

Quah, Stella R., and Li Jingwei. "Marriage of Convenience: Traditional and Modern Medicine in the People's Republic of China." In *The Triumph of Practicality: Tradition and Modernity in Health Care Utilization in Selected Asian Counters*, edited by Stella R. Quah, 19–42. Singapore: Social Issues in Southeast Asia, Institute of Southeast Asia, 1989.

Reiser, Stanley Joel. *Technological Medicine: The Changing World of Doctors and Patients.* Cambridge: Cambridge University Press, 2009.

———. *Medicine and the Reign of Technology.* Cambridge: Cambridge University Press, 1978.

Renshaw, Michelle. *Accommodating the Chinese: The American Hospital in China, 1880–1920.* New York: Routledge, 2005.

Rice, Edward Earl. *Mao's Way.* Berkeley: University of California Press, 1972.

Ritzer, George, and David Walczak. "Rationalization and the Deprofessionalization of Physicians." *Social Forces* 67, no. 1 (September 1988): 1–22.

Robinson, Jean C. "Decentralization, Money, and Power: The Case of People-Run Schools in China." *Comparative Education Review* 30, no1 (February 1986): 73–88.

Rogaski, Ruth. *Hygienic Modernity: Meanings of Health and Disease in Treaty-Port China.* Berkeley: University of California Press, 2004.

———. "Nature, Annihilation, and Modernity: China's Korean War Germ-Warfare Experience Reconsidered." *Journal of Asian Studies*, 61, no. 2 (May 2002): 381–415.

Rosenberg, Charles. *The Care of Strangers: the Rise of America's Hospital System.* New York: Basic Books, 1987.

Rosenthal, Marilynn M., and Jay R. Greiner. "The Barefoot Doctor of China: From Political Creation to Professionalization." *Human Organization* 41, no. 4 (1982): 330–41.

Scheid, Volker. *Chinese Medicine in Contemporary China: Plurality and Synthesis.* Durham, NC: Duke University Press, 2002.

———. *Currents of Tradition in Chinese Medicine, 1626–2006*. Seattle, WA: Eastland, 2007.

———. "Kexue and guanxixue: Plurality, Tradition and Modernity in Contemporary Chinese Medicine." In *Plural Medicine, Tradition and Modernity, 1800–2000*, edited by Ernst Waltraud, 130–52. New York: Routledge, 2002.

———. "Shaping Chinese Medicine: Two Cases from Contemporary China." In *Innovation in Chinese Medicine*, edited by Elisabeth Hsu, 370–404. Cambridge: Cambridge University Press, 2001.

Schneider, Joseph, and Wang Laihua. *Giving Care, Writing Self: A "New Ethnography."* New York: Peter Lang, 2000.

Schwartz, Jonathan, R. Gregory Evans, and Sarah Greenberg. "Evolution of Health Provision in Pre-SARS China: The Changing Nature of Disease Prevention." *China Review* 7, no. 1 (Spring 2007): 81–104.

Shao Jing, "Hospitalizing Traditional Chinese Medicine: Identity, Knowledge and Reification." PhD diss., University of Chicago, 1999.

Shorter, Edward. "The History of the Doctor-Patient Relationship." In Bynum and Roy, *Companion Encyclopedia of the History of Medicine*, 783–800.

Sidel, Ruth. *Women and Child Care in China: A Firsthand Report*. New York: Penguin Books, 1976.

Sidel, Victor W. "The Barefoot Doctors of the People's Republic of China." *New England Journal of Medicine* 286, no.24 (1972): 1292–1300.

Sidel, Victor W., and Ruth Sidel. *Serve the People: Observations on Medicine in the People's Republic of China*. Boston: Beacon Press, 1973.

Sigerist, Henry E. *Civilization and Disease*. Chicago: University of Chicago Press, 1970.

———. *A History of Medicine*. Vol. 2, *Early Greek, Hindu, and Persian Medicine*. New York: Oxford University Press, 1961.

———. On the Sociology of Medicine. New York: MD Publications, 1960.

———. "The Social History of Medicine," paper presented to the California Academy of Medicine in San Francisco, March 11, 1940. In *Henry E. Sigerist on the History of Medicine*, edited by Felix Marti-Ibanez, 25–33. New York: MD Publications, 1960.

Sivin, Nathan. *Medicine, Philosophy and Religion in Ancient China: Researches and Reflections*. Brookfield, VT: Variorum, 1995.

———. "Editor's Introduction." In *Science and Civilisation in China*. Vol. 6, *Biology and Biological Technology, Part VI: Medicine*, 1–37. Cambridge: Cambridge University Press, 2000.

———. "The History of Chinese Medicine: Now and Anon." *Positions* 6, no. 3 (Winter 1998): 731–62.

———. "Science and Medicine in Chinese History." In *Heritage of China: Contemporary Perspectives on Chinese Civilization*, edited by Paul S. Ropp, 164–96. Berkeley: University of California Press, 1990.

———. "Text and Experience in Classical Chinese Medicine." In *Knowledge and the Scholarly Medical Traditions*, edited by Don Bates, 177–204. Cambridge: Cambridge University Press, 1995.

———. *Traditional Medicine in Contemporary China: A Partial Translation of Revised Outline of Chinese Medicine*. Ann Arbor, MI: Center for Chinese Studies, University of Michigan, 1987.

Skinner, William. "Marketing and Social Structure in Rural China," Part I. In *Peasant Society: A Reader*, edited by Jack M. Potter, May N. Diaz, and George M. Foster, 63–98. Boston: Little, Brown, 1967.

Spence, Jonathan. "Commentary on Historical Perspectives and Ch'ing Medical Systems." In *Medicine in Chinese Cultures: Comparative Studies of Health Care in Chinese and Other Societies*, edited by Arthur Kleinman, Peter Kunstadter, E. Russell Alexander, and James L. Gale, 77–84. Bethesda, MD: National Institutions of Health, 1975.

Spree, Reinhard. *Health and Social Class in Imperial Germany: A Social History of Mortality, Morbidity and Inequality*. New York: St. Martin's Place, 1988.

Stoner, Bradley P. "Understanding Medical Systems: Traditional, Modern, and Syncretic Health Care Alternatives in Medically Pluralistic Societies." *Medial Anthropology Quarterly* 17, no. 2 (1986): 44–48.

Summers, William C. "Congruence in Chinese and Western Medicine from 1830–1911: Smallpox, Plague and Cholera." *Yale Journal of Biology and Medicine* 67 (1994): 23–32.

Sun, Xiaoyun, Sukhan Jackson, Gordon A. Carmichael, and Adrian C. Sleigh. "Prescribing Behaviour of Village Doctors under China's New Cooperative Medical Scheme." *Social Science & Medicine* 68, no. 10 (May 2009): 1775–79.

Szto, Peter Paul. "The Accommodation of Insanity in Canton, China, 1857–1935." PhD diss., University of Pennsylvania, 2002.

Taylor, Kim. *Chinese Medicine in Early Communist China, 1945–1963*. London: Routledge Curzon, 2005.

———. "Divergent Interests and Cultivated Misunderstanding: The Influence of the West on Modern Chinese Medicine," *Social History of Medicine* 17, no. 1 (2004): 93–111.

Theriot, Nancy. "Negotiating Illness: Doctors, Patients, and Families in the Nineteenth Century." *Journal of the History of Behavior Sciences* 37, no. 4 (October 2001): 349–68.

Thornton, Patricia M. "Crisis and Governance: SARS and the Resilience of the Chinese Body Politic." *China Journal* 61 (January 2009): 23–48.

Tomes, Nancy. "Oral History in the History of Medicine." *Journal of American History* 78, no. 2 (September 1991): 44–48.

Turner, Bryan. *The Body and Society: Explorations in Social Theory*. London: Sage, 1996.

Unger, Jonathan. "Cultural Revolution Conflict in the Villages." *China Quarterly* 153 (March 1998): 82–106.

Unschuld, Paul. "Epistemological Issues and Changing Legitimization: Traditional Chinese Medicine in the Twentieth Century." In *Paths to Asian Medical Knowledge*, edited by Charles Leslie and Allan Young, 44–61. Berkeley: University of California Press, 1992.

———. "Medical History in Chinese Studies: A Personal Perspective on Achievements, Approaches, Expectations." In *Xingbie yu yiliao* [Gender and medical history], edited by Huang Kewu, 127–64. Taibei: Academia Sinica, 2002.

———. *Medical Ethics in Imperial China: A Study in Historical Anthropology*. Berkeley: University of California Press, 1979.

———. *Medicine in China: A History of Ideas*. Berkeley: University of California Press, 1985.

————. *Medicine in China: Historical Artifacts and Images*. Munich: Prestel Verlag, 2000.

————. *What is Medicine? Western and Eastern Approaches to Healing*. Berkeley: University of California Press, 2009.

Wang, Fei-ling. *Organizing through Division and Exclusion: China's Hukou System*. Stanford, CA: Stanford University Press, 2005.

Wang Hongman. *Daguo weisheng zhinan: Zhongguo nongcun yiliao weisheng xianzhuang yu zhidu gaige tantao* [The dilemma of a big country: Present situations of rural health in China and discussion on system reform]. Beijing: Beijing University Press, 2004.

Wang, Jun. "A Life History of Ren Yingqiu: Historical Problems, Mythology, Continuity and Difference in Chinese Medical Modernity." PhD diss., University of North Carolina–Chapel Hill, 2003.

Wang, Liping. "Paradise for Sale: Urban Space and Tourism in the Social Transformation of Hangzhou, 1589–1937." PhD diss., University of California, San Diego, 1997.

Wang Shaoguang. "Xuexi jizhi yu shiying nengli: Zhongguo nongcun hezuo yiliao tizhi bianqian de qishi" [Learning and adapting: The case of rural health-care financing in China]. *Zhongguo shehui kexue* [Social Sciences in China] 6 (2008): 111–33.

————. "Zhongguo gonggong weisheng de weiji yu zhuanji" [China's public health: Crisis and opportunity]. *Bijiao* [Comparative Studies] 7 (2003): 52–88.

Wang Sijun and Wang Ruizi, eds. *Zhongguo renkou: Zhejiang fence* [China population: Zhejiang]. Beijing: Zhongguo caizheng jingji chubanshe, 1988.

Warren, Kenneth S. "'Farewell to the Plague Spirit': Chairman Mao's Crusade against Schistosomiasis." In *Science and Medicine in Twentieth-Century China: Research and Education*, edited by John Z. Bowers, J. William Hess, and Nathan Sivin, 123–40. Ann Arbor, MI: Center for Chinese Studies, University of Michigan, 1988.

Wei Dongpeng. "Transmission and Natural Regulations of Infection with Ascaris Lumbricoides in Rural Community in China." *Journal of Parasitology* 84, no. 2 (April 1998): 252–58.

Wen Yiqun. "Zhongguo chijiao yisheng chansheng he cunzai de shehui wenhua yuanyin fenxi" [The social-cultural analysis of the emergence of barefoot doctors in China]. In *Cong chijiao yisheng dao xiangcun yisheng* [From barefoot doctors to village doctors], edited by Zhang Kaining, 313–34. Kunming: Yunnan renmin chubanshe, 2002.

White, Martin King, and Zhongxin Sun. "The Impact of China's Market Reforms on the Health of Chinese Citizens: Examining Two Puzzles." *China: An International Journal* 8, no. 1 (March 2010): 1–32.

White, Sydney D. "Deciphering 'Integrated Chinese and Western Medicine' in the Rural Lijiang Basin: State Policy and Local Practice(s) in Socialist China." *Social Science & Medicine* 49, no. 10 (1999): 1333–47.

————. "From Barefoot Doctor to Village Doctor in Tiger Springs Village: A Case Study of Rural Health Care Transformations in Socialist China." *Human Organization* 57, no. 4 (Winter 1998): 480–90.

————. "Medicines and Modernities in Socialist China: Medical Pluralism, the State, and Naxi Identities in the Lijiang Basin." In *Healing Powers and Modernity: Traditional Medicine, Shamanism, and Science in Asian Societies*, edited by Linda H. Connor and Geoffrey Samuel, 171–96. Westport, CT: Bergin & Garvey, 2000.

Whyte, Martin King, and William L. Parish. *Urban Life in Contemporary China*. Chicago: University of Chicago Press, 1984.

Wilenski, Peter. *The Delivery of Health Services in the People's Republic of China*. Ottawa: International Development Research Centre, 1976.

Wong, K. C., and Wu Lien-Teh. *History of Chinese Medicine: Being a Chronicle of Medical Happenings in China from Ancient Times to the Present Period*. 2nd ed. Shanghai: National Quarantine Service, 1936.

World Bank. *Financing Health Care: Issues and Options for China*. Washington, DC: The World Bank, 1997.

———. *China: Long-Term Issues and Options in the Health Transition*. Washington, DC: The World Bank, 1992.

World Health Organization. *Primary Health Care: The Chinese Experience: Report of an Inter-Regional Seminar*. Geneva: World Health Organization, 1983.

———. *The Promotion and Development of Traditional Medicine: Report*. Geneva: World Health Organization, 1978.

———. *The Use of Essential Drugs: Report of a WHO Expert Committee*. Technical Report Series, 685. Geneva: World Health Organization, 1983.

World Health Organization and the United Nations Children's Fund. "Primary Health Care: A Joint Report by the Director-General of the World Health Organization and the Executive Director of the United Nations Children's Fund." International Conference on Primary Health Care, Alma-Ata, USSR, September 1978.

Worsley, Peter. "Non-Western Medical Systems." *Annual Review of Anthropology* 11, no. 1 (1982): 315–48.

Wu Fengsi. "Double Mobilization: Transnational Advocacy Network for China's Environment and Public Health." PhD diss., University of Maryland, 2005.

Wu Lien-Teh, *Plague Fighter: The Autobiography of a Modern Chinese Physician*. Cambridge, UK: W. Heffer & Sons, 1959.

———. "A Hundred Years of Modern Medicine in China." *Chinese Medical Journal* 50, no. 2 (February 1936): 152–54.

Wu, Yi-li. "The Bamboo Grove Monastery and Popular Gynecology in Qing China." *Late Imperial China* 21, no. 1 (June 2000): 41–76.

———. "Transmitted Secrets: The Doctors of Low Yangzi Region in Popular Gynecology in Late Imperial China." PhD diss., Yale University, 1998.

———. *Reproducing Women: Medicine, Metaphor, and Childbirth in Late Imperial China*. Berkeley: University of California Press, 2010.

Wu Yiyi. "A Medical Line of Many Masters: A Prosopographical Study of Liu Wansu and His Disciples from Jin to the Early Ming." *Chinese Science* 11 (1993–94): 36–65.

Xu Liangying and Fan Dainian. *Science and Socialist Construction in China*. Translated by C. Hsu. Armonk, NY: M. E. Sharpe, 1980.

Xu Tong. "Combing Traditional Chinese Medicine and Modern Western Medicine." In *The Role of Traditional Chinese Medicine in primary Health Care in China*, edited by O. Akerele, G. Stott, and Lu Weibo, 34–36. Manila: World Health Organization, 1985.

Xu Xiaoqun. "National Essence vs. Science: Chinese Native Physicians' Fight for Legitimacy, 1912–1937." *Modern Asian Studies* 31, no. 4 (October 1997): 847–77.

―――. *Chinese Professionals and the Republican State: The Rise of Professional Associations in Shanghai, 1912–1937*. New York: Cambridge University Press, 2001.

Xu Xifan. "Fangzhizhu xuexichongbing" [Preventing schistosomiasis]. *Dongnan ribao* [Southeastern Daily], December 12, 1948.

Xue, Yong. "'Treasure Night Soil as If It Were Gold': Economic and Ecological Links between Urban and Rural Areas in Late Imperial Jiangnan." *Late Imperial China* 26, no. 1 (June 2005): 41–71.

Yan Xinzhe. *Nongcun shehuixue gaiyao* [General survey of rural sociology]. Shanghai: Shanghai shudian, 1992.

Yan Yunxiang. *Flow of Gifts: Reciprocity and Social Networks in a Chinese Village*. Stanford, CA: Stanford University Press, 1996.

―――. "Rural Youth and Youth Culture in North China." *Culture, Medicine, and Psychiatry* 23, no. 1 (March 1999): 75–97.

Yang, Mayfair Mei-Hui. *Gifts, Favors, and Banquets: The Art of Social Relationships in China*. Ithaca, NY: Cornell University Press, 1994.

Yang Nianqun. "Disease Prevention, Social Mobilization and Spatial Politics: The Anti-Germ Warfare Incident of 1952 and the Patriotic Health Campaign." *Chinese Historical Review* 11, no. 2 (Fall 2004): 155–82.

―――. "Fangyi xingwei yu kongjian zhengzhi" [Epidemic prevention and spatial politics]. *Dushu* [Reading] 7 (2003): 25–33.

―――. "The Memory of Barefoot Doctor System." In *Governance of Life in Chinese Moral Experience: The Quest for an Adequate Life*, edited by Everett Zhang, Arthur Kleinman, and Tu Weiming, 131–45. London: Routledge, 2011.

―――. *Zaizao "bingren": Zhongxiyi chongtuxia de zhengzhi kongjian, 1832–1985* [Remaking "patients": Spatial politics in the conflicts between Chinese and Western medicine, 1832–1985]. Beijing: Zhongguo renmin daxue chubanshe, 2006.

Yang Xiao. *The Making of a Peasant Doctor*. Beijing: Foreign Language Press, 1976.

Yao, Hsun-yuan. "The Second Year of the Rural Health Experiment in Ting Hsien, China." *The Milkbank Memorial Fund Quarterly Bulletin* 10, no. 1 (January 1932): 53–66.

Ye Xiaoqing. "Regulating the Medical Profession in China: Health Policies of the Nationalist Government." In *Historical Perspectives on East Asian Science, Technology and Medicine*, edited by Alan K. L. Chan, Gregory K. Clancey, and Hui-Chieh Loy, 198–213. Singapore: Singapore University Press, World Scientific, 2001.

Yip Ka-Che. "Health and Nationalist Reconstruction: Rural Health in Nationalist China, 1928–1937." *Modern Asian Studies* 26, no. 2 (May 1992): 395–415.

―――. *Health and National Reconstruction in Nationalist China: The Development of Modern Health Services, 1928–1937*. Ann Arbor, MI: Association for Asian Studies, 1995.

Yu Hui. "Zhongguo zhengfu yaoye guanzhi zhidu xingcheng zhangai de fenxi" [The analysis of obstacles formed by Chinese government pharmaceutical management institutions]. *Guanli shijie* [Management World], Part I, 5 (1997): 126–35; Part II, 6 (1997): 87–95.

Yu Xinzhong. *Qingdai jiangnan de wenyi he shehui* [The plague and society in Jiangnan area in the Qing Dynasty]. Beijing: zhongguo renmin daxue chubanshe, 2003.

Zaccarini, M. Cristina. "Modern Medicine in Twentieth-Century Jiangxi, Anhui, Fujian and Sichuan: Competition, Negotiation and Cooperation." *Social History of Medicine* 23, no. 2 (2010): 338–55.

Zhan, Mei. "A Doctor of the Highest Caliber Treats an Illness Before It Happens." *Medical Anthropology* 28, no. 2 (2009): 166–88.

———. *Other-Worldly: Making Chinese Medicine through Transnational Frames*. Durham, NC: Duke University Press. 2009.

Zhang Bin. "Qianxi minguo shiqi de yishi jiufen" [Brief analysis of medical disputes during the Republic of China]. *Zhongguo yixue lunlixue* [Medical Ethics of China] 16, no. 6 (December 2003): 22–24.

Zhang Daqing. *Zhongguo jindai jibing shehuishi (1912–1937)* [A social history of diseases in modern China, 1912–1937]. Jinan: Shangdong jiaoyu chubanshe, 2006.

Zhang Daqing and Paul Unschuld. "China's BarefootDoctor: Past, Present, and Future." *Lancet* 372, no. 9653 (November 29, 2008): 1865–67.

Zhang Kaining. *Cong chijiao yisheng dao xiangcun yisheng* [From barefoot doctors to village doctors]. Kunming: Yunnan renmin chubanshe, 2002.

Zhang Letian. *Gaobie lixiang: renmin gongshe zhidu yanjiu* [Farewell to ideals: A study of the people's commune system]. Shanghai: Dongfang chuban zhongxin, 1998.

Zhang Xiaobo and Ravi Kanbur. "Spatial Inequality in Education and Health Care in China." *China Economic Review* 6, no. 2 (2005): 189–204.

Zhang Yuhuan and K. Rose. *Who Can Ride the Dragon?: An Exploration of the Cultural Roots of Traditional Chinese Medicine*. Brookline, MA: Paradigm, 1999.

Zhang Zikuang, "Guanyu woguo nongcun hezuo yiliao baojian zhidu de huiguxing yanjiu" [Retrospective research on rural cooperative medical services]. *Zhongguo nongcun weisheng shiye guanli* [China Rural Health Administration Journal] 14, no. 6 (1994): 4–9.

Zhao Hongjun. "Chinese versus Western Medicine: A History of Their Relations in theTwentieth Century." *Chinese Science* 10 (1991): 21–37.

Zheng Zihua. *Leyuan xiongfeng* [Glorious wind of Leyuan]. Hong Kong: Tianma tushu youxian gongsi, 2003.

Zhou Shouqi, Gu Xingyuan, and Zhu Aorong. "Zhongguo nongcun jiankang baozhang zhidu de yanjiu jinzhan" [Research progress on China rural health-care institutions]. *Zhongguo nongcun weisheng shiye guanli* [China Rural Health Management] 14, no. 9 (1994): 7–12.

Zhu Chao. *Xin zhongguo yixue jiaoyushi* [The history of medical education in new China]. Beijing: Beijing yike daxue, Zhongguo xiehe yike daxue lianhe chubanshe, 1990.

Zhu Deming, "Jindai Hangzhou zhongyaodian gouchen" [The history of Chinese medicine shops in modern Hangzhou], *Zhonghua yishi zazhi* [Chinese Journal of Medical History] 36, no. 4 (October 2006): 243–45.

———. *Zhejiang yiyaoshi* [The history of medicine and pharmaceuticals in Zhejiang]. Beijing: Renmin junyi chubanshe, 1999.

Zhu Ling. "Zhengfu yu nongcun jiben yiliao baojian baozhang zhidu xuanze" [The government and options for alternative medical and health systems in rural areas]. *Zhongguo shehui kexue* [Social Sciences in China] 4 (2000): 89–99.

Zhu, Naisu, Zhihua Ling, Jie Shen, J. M. Lane, and Shanlin Hu. "Factors Associated with the Decline of the Cooperative Medical Systems and Barefoot Doctors in Rural China." *Bulletin of the World Health Organization* 67 (1989): 431–41.

Zhu Yong. "Jibing zai geming zhong de mingyun" [The destiny of diseases in revolution]. *Shuwu* [The Study] 6 (2006): 70–76.

Index

abortion, 45, 143, 145, 161

accounting, 24, 34, 70, 78–79, 111

accreditation. *See* regulation and registration

acknowledgments (*daxie*) of gratitude, 151

acupuncture: barefoot doctors, 56, 167; commune clinics, 56, 134; Cultural Revolution, 95–97; healing styles, 99–103, 105, 109; heat stroke, 23, 26, 34, 36, 57, 73; legitimization, 181, 204n8, 206n25; new techniques (*xinzhen liaofa*), 59

administrative changes, 179

administrative villages, 168, 187

agricultural collectivization. *See* collectivization

agricultural cooperatives, 25, 127

agricultural household identity. *See* rural household registration status

agricultural labor: barefoot doctors, 48, 152–53, 155, 159; health workers' participation in, 27, 31, 151, 161; women's participation in, 72

agricultural production, 25, 27, 68, 127, 238n85

"Ah Bao, Mr." (*Ah Bao xiansheng*). *See* Chen Hongting

anatomy, 59

ancestral halls, 22

Anhui Province: Chinese medical knowledge, 42; cooperative medical service, 216n80; Jiuhua Mountain, 44; map, xiv; pharmaceuticals, 106; rural economic reforms, 167

antibiotics, 78–79, 101–5, 108, 120–21, 123, 164, 181, 189–91, 231n67, 239n121, 240n125

antisepsis, 167

appendicitis, 46, 137, 140, 231n67

apprenticeship. *See* medical apprenticeship

artificial respiration, 167

ascariasis, 69, 193

aspirin, 94

assistant medical practitioners (*zhiye zhuli yishi*), 179–80, 183

association members, 29

awards, 62–63, 157

bad elements, 47

Bamboo Temple (*zhulinsi*), Xiaoshan County, Zhejiang, 22

bannong banyi. See "half-peasant, half-doctors"

barefoot doctors (*chijiao yisheng*): age, 31, 49–51, 63; authority, 166, 171, 175–76; career and social mobility, 30–31, 157–60, 171, 175, 177, 246n38; case records, 164; characteristics, 47–54; commune clinics and, 32, 48, 57, 61, 65, 98–99, 142–46, 148–50, 158–60, 165–66, 182; disintegration of program (1980s), 152, 166–72, 175, 181, 247n62; "doctors wearing shoes," 152–53; dual role, 139–45, 147; educational background, 43–44, 47–49, 53–54, 60, 98, 175; emergence (1968), 47, 152, 154, 162–63, 177, 181, 211–12n115; gender, 51–53, 85; group identity, 151–76, 183; healing styles, 95–104, 109–13, 123; hospitalization, 125; infectious diseases, 70; knowledge structure, 62–63, 66; legitimacy, 171; medical encounters, 136–37;

healing styles, 102, 106, 108; infectious diseases, 82–84; map, xiv; medical community, 126, 134; medical knowledge, 43–45, 63–65; pharmaceuticals, 73–76, 79–80, 85, 87, 92, 120, 122; postsocialist era, 180; private medical practitioners, 36; sending-down policy, 38–40; social epidemiology, 67–72; state investment in health infrastructure, 29; township clinics, 148; village doctors, 167; Western medicine shops, 73–74

healers: classification of, 208n56; diagnosis, 151; differentiation and reorganization, 25–26, 41; marginalization of competitors, 161–62, 175, 183, 245n13; socialist villages, 37. *See also* barefoot doctors; doctors; folk healers; itinerant doctors; medical practitioners; physicians; religious healers; supernatural healers; village healers

healing styles, 94–124, 222n25, 235n46; revolutionary discourse and daily practice, 95–101

health care workers. *See* barefoot doctors; health workers

health infrastructure, state investment in, 29, 131

health service stations, 179–83

health workers (*weishengyuan*): agricultural labor, 151; barefoot doctors and, 139, 145, 159, 163, 175; educational background, 54; epidemic prevention, 140; gender, 52; "half-peasant, half-doctors," 30–31, 41, 47, 54, 139, 149; pharmaceuticals, 105; selection, 27, 44, 48–49; state supervision, 28; training, 25, 30, 55–56, 139, 149

health-care contracts, 25

heat stroke, 21–22, 57, 73, 77, 118

heat-stroke acupuncturists, 23, 26, 34, 36, 57, 73

herbal medicine. *See* Chinese herbal medicine

herbalists, 21, 36

hierarchical medical system, 41, 125, 132, 137–39, 182–83. *See also* three-tier medical system; two-tier state medical system

home-based medical encounters, 21, 125–27, 129, 131, 134–36, 139, 149–50, 182, 185–86

hongbao. See Red Storm

Hongyu (film, 1975), 96–98, 234n9

hookworm, 28, 68, 70

hospitals: childbirth, 169, 171; clinics and, 149; emergence, 209n88; family accompanying patients (*see* family); healing styles, 102, 122, 124, 182; medical community and coordination, 129–32; medical publications, 59; medical training, 44–45, 55–56; missionary (*see* Christian missionaries); pharmaceuticals, 74–75, 120; power relationships, 162; promotion system, 246n38; quality of services, 166; referral to, 134–36, 139–40, 143, 148, 150; sectional medical service, 242n39; sending down policy, 38–40; townships, 122, 175, 180; treatment in, 125–27. *See also* county hospitals; minihospitals; Western hospitals

house calls. *See* home-based medical encounters

household registration system (*hujizhi*), 29, 153, 179

household responsibility system, 119, 168, 215n65

Hua Guofeng, 147

hygiene. *See* sanitation and hygiene

identity. *See* barefoot doctors

ideological principles: barefoot doctors, 31–32, 177; Cultural Revolution, 37; medical systems, 182, 184; Nationalist, 40; pharmaceuticals, 92–93. *See also* politics; revolutionary discourse; rural economic reforms

imperial China, 4, 8, 10, 13, 15–16, 20, 22, 42–43, 49, 100, 185, 210n103

income. *See* business; finance

infant mortality, 51–52

CPSIA information can be obtained at www.ICGtesting.com
Printed in the USA
LVOW10s2319060815

448998LV00001B/13/P